Operationalizing Trauma-Informed Care Through Systemic Support, Ethical Accountability, and Intersectional Awareness

Sara Morgan Pickett
https://orcid.org/0009-0002-2858-8320
Western Kentucky University, USA

IGI Global
Scientific Publishing
Publishing Tomorrow's Research Today

Vice President of Editorial	Melissa Wagner
Director of Acquisitions	Mikaela Felty
Director of Book Development	Jocelynn Hessler
Production Manager	Mike Brehm
Cover Design	Jose Rosado

Published in the United States of America by
IGI Global Scientific Publishing
701 East Chocolate Avenue
Hershey, PA, 17033, USA
Tel: 717-533-8845 | Fax: 717-533-7115
Website: https://www.igi-global.com E-mail: cust@igi-global.com

Library of Congress Cataloging-in-Publication Data

Names: Pickett, Sara Morgan, 1983- editor
Title: Operationalizing trauma-informed care through systemic support, ethical accountability, and intersectional awareness / edited by Sara Morgan Pickett.
Description: Hershey PA : IGI Global Scientific Publishing, 2027. | Includes bibliographical references and index. | Summary: "This book explores trauma-informed care as both a clinical framework and a social justice imperative. It examines how sustainable trauma-informed systems are implemented and evaluated, and how providers can challenge harmful structures while upholding equitable, accountable care"-- Provided by publisher.
Identifiers: LCCN 2026009774 (print) | LCCN 2026009775 (ebook) | ISBN 9798337385976 hardcover | ISBN 9798337385983 paperback | ISBN 9798337385990 ebook
Subjects: LCSH: Psychic trauma--Patients--Care | Mental health services--United States
Classification: LCC RC552.T7 .O64 2026 (print) | LCC RC552.T7 (ebook) | DDC 616.85/21--dc23/eng/20260521
LC record available at https://lccn.loc.gov/2026009774
LC ebook record available at https://lccn.loc.gov/2026009775

British Cataloguing in Publication Data
A Cataloguing in Publication record for this book is available from the British Library.

Table of Contents

Detailed Table of Contents

Trauma-informed care frameworks have emerged as essential approaches in health, social services, and educational settings, emphasizing the recognition, understanding, and response to the widespread impact of trauma on individuals. The foundations of TIC are rooted in research on adverse childhood experiences (ACEs), psychological trauma, and the neurobiological, social, and emotional consequences of traumatic events. Central principles include safety, trustworthiness, empowerment, collaboration, and cultural sensitivity, which guide organizations and practitioners in creating supportive environments that prevent re-traumatization and promote healing. TIC frameworks have evolved from individual-focused interventions to systemic approaches, integrating trauma awareness into policies, organizational cultures, and community practices. This evolution reflects an increasing understanding of the complex interplay between trauma, social determinants of health, and structural inequities. Contemporary TIC models emphasize interdisciplinary collaboration, evidence-based interventions.

Vulnerable populations—people with historically marginalized backgrounds—face an increased risk of employment exploitation, housing instability, poverty and financial precarity. This chapter aims to provide a deeper understanding of the historical context that reinforces and perpetuates trauma for vulnerable people, discuss multicultural considerations mental health professionals should take into consideration, and offer trauma-informed care approaches that empower individuals and promote healing.

The Pew Research Center (2018) recorded that 8 out of 10 individuals endorse a religious and/or a spiritual identity. Religious/ spiritual abuse is defined as the "mistreatment of an individual through mental or physical means by weakening, undermining, distorting, or decreasing their spiritual integrity." R/S abuse can result in various forms of trauma that distort one's image of God or a higher power and spiritual identity. Purity culture at its core posits that an individual's moral worth, particularly for women, is inextricably tied to their sexual "purity"—defined as a total absence of sexual thought, desire, or action outside of heterosexual marriage. The act of spiritual bullying can be observed in the extreme form of conversion practice. Ongoing and repetitive traumatic events of any kind can lead to long-term psychological and physiological consequences in addition to a potential spiritual crisis. Clinicians, health care providers, and spiritual caregivers can offer effective trauma-informed care

Trauma-informed care has matured around acute events but remains under-theorized for the chronic relational deprivation accumulating in long-term family systems, where adults perform functional roles for decades while their emotional identity becomes progressively unseen.This chapter argues such under-recognition constitutes cumulative relational trauma. It introduces the Dual-Track Emotional System, which distinguishes a functional responsibility system from a personal emotional system and traces how dominance of the first attenuates the second. A heuristic illustration from the literature shows how role engulfment, identity attenuation, and relational deprivation converge in one individual over time. The chapter centers both the role-strained adult and the unseen primary partner, who carries their own betrayal trauma.The framework is operationalized through an assessment protocol, clinical heuristics, organizational implementation suggestions, and reflective-practice guidance. Ethical accountability and intersectional awareness frame the application, with attention to misuse risks.

This chapter examines storytelling in trauma contexts as a political practice shaped by power, history, and social location rather than an inherently therapeutic act. Challenging dominant assumptions that healing requires disclosure, it shows how compelled or premature storytelling can reproduce harm, particularly for marginalized survivors. Drawing on trauma studies, decolonial theory, and epistemic justice, the chapter introduces narrative sovereignty as an ethical framework that affirms survivors' rights to author, withhold, revise, or reclaim their stories on their own terms, including through silence, art, ritual, or collective action. It distinguishes between internal trauma integration and external narration, emphasizing consent, autonomy, and harm reduction as core principles of ethical story work. Beyond individual therapy, the chapter centers collective storytelling practices such as art activism, zines, and community archives- as sites of resistance and healing that situate trauma within structural and historical contexts.

This chapter examines community-based and collective healing approaches within trauma-informed care frameworks, focusing on evaluation methodologies and measurement strategies for systemic implementation. Drawing from intersectional perspectives and evidence-based research, the chapter explores how collective trauma responses—including historical, racial, and community-level adversities—require healing models that extend beyond individual clinical interventions. The discussion integrates cultural considerations, community-driven practices, and systems-level accountability measures. Through critical analysis of existing evaluation frameworks, the chapter proposes comprehensive assessment tools that capture both process and outcome measures across multiple ecological levels.

This chapter argues that trauma recovery is inseparable from the systems that shape survivors' lives. Through the lenses of advocacy, policy, and activism, it demonstrates how trauma-informed care must extend beyond individual intervention to address the structural conditions that produce and perpetuate harm. Advocacy offers concrete, immediate support as survivors navigate housing, healthcare, employment, and legal systems. Policy establishes the broader conditions under which safety, stability, and access become possible. Activism mobilizes collective power to challenge inequities, shift narratives, and demand systemic change. Integrating these lenses reveals trauma recovery as both an individual and collective process, requiring coordinated efforts across practitioners, organizations, and communities. The chapter concludes with a call to stewardship, inviting readers to recognize their spheres of influence and to participate in creating conditions where justice, dignity, and healing can take root. Trauma-informed care becomes not only a practice, but a shared responsibility.

This chapter explores the critical transition from individual trauma-informed clinical practice to the development of trauma-informed systems. While trauma-informed care is widely endorsed, the author argues that meaningful change requires institutional accountability and structural transformation across counseling, healthcare, and human service sectors. The chapter examines the organizational readiness and cultural foundations necessary to support trauma-informed values, emphasizing leadership commitment, workforce sustainability, and the mitigation of secondary traumatic stress. An intersectional lens examines how systems can actively prevent retraumatization for marginalized populations, particularly women and gender-diverse individuals. By distinguishing between program, organization, and system-level implementation, this chapter provides a practical roadmap for embedding safety and equity into policy. The author proposes specific evaluation strategies to move institutions beyond symbolic language toward measurable, sustainable, and transformative standards of care.

This chapter reframes professional ethics through an intersectional, trauma-informed lens, emphasizing that "neutral" approaches often overlook how trauma, oppression, and structural inequities shape client experiences and ethical decision-making. The chapter invites readers to map power across interpersonal, organizational, policy, and historical levels, inviting practitioners to engage in reflexivity through positionality tools and to navigate common tensions. The chapter offers practical guidance on confidentiality, safety-forward documentation, technology security, culturally responsive collaboration, and disability justice.

Culturally responsive contemplative practices offer transformative pathways of healing for women navigating trauma within contexts of systemic oppression. Grounded in intersectionality and trauma-informed care, these approaches extend beyond symptom reduction to restore dignity, cultural identity, and collective agency. This chapter examines how contemplative practices, when rooted in cultural reclamation and relational accountability, disrupt reductionist wellness models and resist epistemic hierarchies. While emerging neuroscience suggests meaningful shifts in attention and regulation, healing must also be understood through lived experience, community knowledge, and justice-centered sustainability. Ultimately, culturally responsive contemplative practice is advanced not merely as a clinical intervention but as an epistemological shift that reorients counseling, education, and research toward equity, relational care, and collective flourishing.

Preface

INTRODUCTION

Trauma-informed care has emerged as one of the most influential frameworks for understanding and responding to the pervasive impact of trauma across clinical, educational, organizational, and community settings. Yet as the concept has gained widespread recognition, important questions remain regarding its implementation, ethical foundations, and capacity to address the broader social, cultural, and structural conditions that contribute to trauma and shape pathways to healing. This volume, *Operationalizing Trauma-Informed Care Through Systemic Support, Ethical Accountability, and Intersectional Awareness*, was developed in response to those questions and the growing need for approaches that move beyond theory into meaningful, equitable practice.

The chapters collected in this book reflect a shared commitment to understanding trauma-informed care not only as a clinical framework but also as a social justice imperative. While trauma-informed principles have traditionally focused on creating safety, trust, empowerment, and collaboration within therapeutic relationships, the contributors to this volume demonstrate that these principles must also extend to the systems, institutions, and policies that influence the lives of individuals and communities. Trauma does not occur in isolation, nor can healing be fully understood apart from the social contexts in which people live. Therefore, effective trauma-informed care requires attention to systemic advocacy, ethical responsibility, cultural responsiveness, and intersectional awareness.

A central goal of this book is to bridge the gap between conceptual discussions of trauma-informed care and the practical realities of implementation. Existing scholarship often focuses either on clinical treatment techniques or on broad theoretical principles without offering sufficient guidance for translating those principles into sustainable practice. The contributors address this challenge by examining how trauma-informed approaches can be operationalized across diverse settings, including counseling, education, supervision, community-based interventions, organizational leadership, policy development, and institutional reform. Through research-informed analysis, applied examples, and practitioner perspectives, the chapters provide valuable insights into both the opportunities and complexities involved in creating trauma-informed systems.

Another distinguishing feature of this volume is its emphasis on feminist and intersectional perspectives. Trauma experiences and recovery processes are profoundly shaped by factors such as race, ethnicity, gender identity, sexual orientation, socioeconomic status, disability, culture, and other dimensions of identity. Traditional frameworks have often overlooked these realities, resulting in approaches that may unintentionally reinforce inequities or fail to address the lived experiences of marginalized populations. The contributors challenge universalized assumptions and highlight the importance of recognizing power, privilege, representation, and oppression as central considerations in ethical trauma-informed practice. In doing so, they advance a vision of care that is more inclusive, culturally responsive, and socially accountable.

The book also explores the evolving future of trauma-informed work. As communities continue to confront complex challenges—including social inequality, systemic violence, displacement, discrimination, and collective trauma—there is an increasing need for approaches that prioritize community-centered healing, interdisciplinary collaboration, and sustainable systems of support. The chapters encourage readers to consider how trauma-informed care can serve not only as a framework for individual recovery but also as a catalyst for organizational transformation, policy change, and collective well-being.

This volume is intended for an interdisciplinary audience of scholars, practitioners, educators, supervisors, policymakers, and students engaged in trauma-related work. It will be particularly valuable to counselor educators, mental health professionals, social workers, psychologists, marriage and family therapists, community advocates, and graduate students seeking to deepen their understanding of trauma-informed practice through a justice-oriented and intersectional lens. We hope readers will find both practical guidance and critical reflection within these pages, enabling them to strengthen their work and contribute to more equitable systems of care.

As editor, I am deeply grateful to the chapter authors whose expertise, scholarship, and dedication made this volume possible. Their contributions represent diverse perspectives and experiences, yet collectively they underscore a common message: trauma-informed care must be grounded not only in compassion and competence but also in accountability, equity, and a commitment to systemic change. It is my hope that this book will inspire continued dialogue, innovation, and action toward creating environments where individuals and communities can heal, thrive, and be fully supported.

I invite readers to engage critically with the ideas presented throughout this volume and to consider how trauma-informed principles can be translated into meaningful action within their own professional and community contexts. Through collective effort and ongoing reflection, we can continue advancing a vision of trauma-informed care that is ethical, inclusive, sustainable, and responsive to the realities of an increasingly interconnected world.

ORGANIZATION OF THE BOOK

The opening chapter establishes the conceptual and historical foundations of trauma-informed care (TIC), tracing its emergence from research on adverse childhood experiences, psychological trauma, and the long-term neurobiological, emotional, and social impacts of traumatic experiences. The chapter examines the evolution of trauma-informed frameworks from individual-level interventions to comprehensive systemic approaches that influence organizational culture, policy development, and community practice. By highlighting principles such as safety, trustworthiness, empowerment, collaboration, and cultural responsiveness, the chapter provides readers with an essential foundation for understanding the contemporary landscape of trauma-informed care and its growing role in addressing structural inequities and social determinants of health.

Chapter 2 expands the discussion by examining the relationship between economic trauma and structural violence. The chapter explores how poverty, employment exploitation, housing instability, and financial insecurity disproportionately affect individuals and communities that have historically experienced marginalization. By situating trauma within broader historical and social contexts, the chapter demonstrates how systemic inequalities perpetuate cycles of adversity and psychological harm. Particular attention is given to multicultural considerations and trauma-informed approaches that empower individuals while addressing the structural conditions that contribute to ongoing trauma exposure.

Chapter 3 addresses the often-overlooked topic of religious and spiritual harm within trauma-informed practice. Recognizing the central role that spirituality and religious identity play in the lives of many individuals, the chapter examines how spiritual abuse, purity culture, coercive religious practices, and conversion efforts can result in profound psychological, emotional, and spiritual trauma. The discussion highlights the long-term consequences of these experiences and emphasizes the importance of trauma-informed responses that support spiritual healing, identity reconstruction, and holistic well-being. The chapter offers valuable guidance for clinicians, healthcare providers, and spiritual caregivers working with individuals affected by religious and spiritual trauma.

Chapter 4 introduces a novel framework for understanding cumulative relational trauma arising from long-term role engulfment within family systems and intimate relationships. Moving beyond traditional conceptualizations of trauma that focus primarily on acute events, the chapter explores how chronic emotional invisibility, relational deprivation, and identity attenuation can accumulate over time. Through the Dual-Track Emotional System framework, readers are provided with practical tools for assessment, intervention, organizational implementation, and reflective practice. The chapter further emphasizes ethical accountability and intersectional awareness in applying trauma-informed approaches to complex relational dynamics.

Chapter 5 examines the trauma experienced by disabled and neurodivergent students within psychology training programs and clinical education settings. Using a trauma-informed and social justice framework, the chapter reveals how ableist program structures, discriminatory practices, exclusionary expectations, and institutional betrayal contribute to psychological harm among trainees. Through illustrative case studies, readers gain insight into the pervasive nature of disability-related oppression in educational and professional environments. The chapter concludes with actionable recommendations for creating more equitable, accessible, and accountable systems while maintaining professional rigor and ethical standards.

Chapter 6 advances the conversation by proposing a resilience-integrated approach to trauma treatment. Challenging traditional models that focus primarily on symptom reduction after traumatic exposure has ended, the chapter argues for the systematic development of resilience as a core component of trauma care. The PEACE Resilience Model is presented as a structured framework that incorporates resilience-building strategies across all phases of treatment, including stabilization, processing, and reintegration. The chapter offers practitioners an evidence-informed roadmap for fostering adaptive capacity, long-term psychological stability, and sustainable recovery among individuals facing ongoing or cumulative trauma.

Chapter 7 explores the complex relationship between trauma, storytelling, and power. The chapter challenges dominant assumptions that disclosure is inherently therapeutic and instead examines storytelling as a political and ethical practice shaped by social context, historical conditions, and power relations. Through the concept of narrative sovereignty, readers are encouraged to recognize survivors' rights to determine how, when, and whether their stories are shared. The chapter further highlights collective forms of storytelling, including art activism, community archives, and other forms of cultural expression, as powerful mechanisms for resistance, meaning-making, and healing.

Chapter 8 shifts attention to community-based and collective healing models within trauma-informed systems. Recognizing that many forms of trauma are experienced collectively through historical, racial, cultural, and community-level adversity, the chapter explores approaches that extend beyond individual clinical interventions. Particular emphasis is placed on evaluating and measuring the effectiveness of trauma-informed system implementation through comprehensive assessment frameworks that capture both process and outcome indicators across multiple ecological levels. The chapter contributes important insights into accountability, cultural responsiveness, and evidence-based evaluation within community-centered trauma work.

Chapter 9 broadens the scope of trauma recovery by examining the critical roles of advocacy, policy, and activism. The chapter demonstrates that healing cannot be fully understood apart from the social systems that shape access to resources, opportunities, and safety. By integrating individual support with collective action, the discussion illustrates how advocacy can address immediate needs, policy can establish conditions for stability and recovery, and activism can challenge the structural inequities that perpetuate harm. The chapter ultimately presents trauma-informed care as both a professional responsibility and a collective social endeavor.

Chapter 10 examines the practical realities of building and sustaining trauma-informed systems. The chapter argues that meaningful trauma-informed transformation requires more than individual clinical competence; it demands organizational commitment, leadership engagement, workforce support, and structural accountability. Through an intersectional lens, the discussion explores how institutions can reduce retraumatization, address inequities, and embed trauma-informed values into policies and procedures. Readers are provided with implementation strategies and evaluation tools designed to help organizations move from symbolic commitment to measurable and sustainable systems change.

Chapter 11 focuses on the ethical dimensions of trauma-informed practice through an intersectional framework. Challenging assumptions of neutrality in professional ethics, the chapter examines how power, oppression, identity, and structural inequities influence ethical decision-making and client experiences. Readers are introduced to practical tools for reflexivity, positionality assessment, confidentiality management, culturally responsive collaboration, disability justice, and technology-related ethical considerations. The chapter provides concrete guidance for navigating ethical complexities while maintaining accountability to diverse populations and contexts.

The concluding chapter looks toward future directions in trauma-informed care, feminism, and intersectionality. The chapter explores culturally responsive contemplative practices as transformative approaches to healing for individuals navigating trauma within systems of oppression. By integrating trauma-informed principles, intersectional analysis, cultural knowledge, and emerging research, the discussion advances a vision of healing that extends beyond symptom management to include dignity, empowerment, relational accountability, and collective flourishing. As a forward-looking conclusion to the volume, the chapter challenges readers to reimagine trauma-informed practice, education, and research through a justice-centered lens that promotes equity, sustainability, and meaningful social change.

CONCLUSION

As this volume demonstrates, trauma-informed care is far more than a set of clinical techniques or organizational best practices. At its core, it is a commitment to understanding the profound ways trauma shapes individuals, relationships, communities, and institutions, while simultaneously recognizing the responsibility to address the conditions that contribute to harm. The chapters in this book collectively illustrate that effective trauma-informed practice requires an integrated approach—one that combines clinical competence with systemic awareness, ethical accountability, cultural responsiveness, and a dedication to social justice.

Throughout these contributions, a common theme emerges: healing cannot be separated from context. Trauma is experienced within social, political, economic, cultural, and relational systems, and therefore recovery must be supported by environments that foster safety, dignity, equity, and empowerment. Whether examining structural violence, spiritual harm, disability justice, narrative sovereignty, collective healing, organizational transformation, or advocacy and policy reform, the authors challenge readers to expand their understanding of what trauma-informed care can and should encompass.

This volume also highlights the importance of intersectionality as a guiding framework for both scholarship and practice. By attending to the ways identity, power, privilege, and oppression influence trauma experiences and recovery processes, contributors offer a more nuanced and inclusive vision of care. Such perspectives are essential if trauma-informed systems are to remain responsive to the diverse realities of the individuals and communities they serve.

The future of trauma-informed care depends not only on continued research and innovation but also on the willingness of practitioners, educators, leaders, and policymakers to critically examine existing systems and advocate for meaningful change. Building trauma-informed organizations and communities requires ongoing reflection, collaboration, and accountability. It demands that we move beyond awareness toward action and beyond individual intervention toward collective responsibility.

As editor, I hope this book serves as both a scholarly resource and a catalyst for dialogue, reflection, and transformation. The insights presented throughout these chapters encourage us to envision trauma-informed care as an evolving and dynamic field, and that it continually adapts to emerging knowledge while remaining grounded in compassion, justice, and human dignity. It is my sincere hope that readers will leave this volume with a deeper understanding of trauma-informed practice and renewed commitment to fostering systems, relationships, and communities where healing, equity, and collective flourishing can thrive.

Ultimately, operationalizing trauma-informed care is not a destination but an ongoing process of learning, listening, and accountability. By embracing intersectional awareness, ethical responsibility, and systemic support, we can move closer to creating a world in which individuals and communities are not only protected from harm but are empowered to heal, grow, and flourish.

Sara Morgan Pickett
Western Kentucky University, USA

Acknowledgment

This volume would not have been possible without the dedication, expertise, and generosity of the chapter authors who contributed their scholarship, lived experiences, and professional wisdom to this project. I am deeply grateful to each contributor for engaging in this important work and for helping to advance conversations surrounding trauma-informed care, ethical accountability, systemic support, and intersectional awareness.

I would like to extend special thanks to Anne Schueler and Cambria Pickett, whose support, encouragement, and assistance throughout this project were invaluable. Your willingness to contribute your time, energy, and thoughtful perspectives helped make this volume possible.

I am also deeply grateful to Carly Stacy, Heidi Johnson, Kayla Ford, Bridgett Blakeman, Shane Self, Teli Hall, Kate Hess-Pace, and Dr. Andrew Wood. Whether through collaboration, friendship, scholarship, or ongoing support, your influence is reflected throughout this work.

I would also like to thank the reviewers whose thoughtful feedback strengthened this volume and helped ensure its scholarly rigor. Their expertise and careful consideration enhanced the quality of this text and challenged contributors to refine and strengthen their work.

Finally, I wish to express my deepest gratitude to my partner, whose unwavering support, patience, encouragement, and belief in me made this book possible. Throughout the many hours of writing, editing, and coordinating this project, you provided a constant source of strength and stability. Your willingness to celebrate successes, navigate challenges, and support this work behind the scenes has meant more than words can adequately express.

It is my sincere hope that this volume contributes to the ongoing advancement of trauma-informed and socially responsive practices across helping professions and encourages readers to continue fostering systems that promote healing, dignity, and equity for all.

Chapter 1
Foundations and Evolution of Trauma-Informed Care Frameworks

Sanjeev Kumar
http://orcid.org/0000-0002-7375-7341
Lovely Professional University, India

Pardeep Kumar
http://orcid.org/0000-0003-0308-7634
Lovely Professional University, India

ABSTRACT

Trauma-informed care frameworks have emerged as essential approaches in health, social services, and educational settings, emphasizing the recognition, understanding, and response to the widespread impact of trauma on individuals. The foundations of TIC are rooted in research on adverse childhood experiences (ACEs), psychological trauma, and the neurobiological, social, and emotional consequences of traumatic events. Central principles include safety, trustworthiness, empowerment, collaboration, and cultural sensitivity, which guide organizations and practitioners in creating supportive environments that prevent re-traumatization and promote healing. TIC frameworks have evolved from individual-focused interventions to systemic approaches, integrating trauma awareness into policies, organizational cultures, and community practices. This evolution reflects an increasing understanding of the complex interplay between trauma, social determinants of health, and structural inequities. Contemporary TIC models emphasize interdisciplinary collaboration, evidence-based interventions.

DOI: 10.4018/979-8-3373-8597-6.ch001

INTRODUCTION

The concept of Trauma-Informed Care (TIC) is a high-impact and transformative model in health, social services, and education spheres. It has developed and evolved to represent the altered conceptualization of the immense influence a trauma could have on the life of a specific person which can influence his or her emotional, psychological, physical and social functionality. Trauma is not confined to extreme or isolated qualities but the spectrum of experiences constituting it is very wide and it includes such experiences as abuse, neglect, being exposed to violence, chronic stress and structural inequity like discrimination and poverty. The realization that such experience may be long lastingly permanent has brought about the paradigm shift in service provision through the disapproval of models of service provision which are anchored on deficit and focusing on the models that underlie understanding, support and healing (Varghese & Emerson, 2022). TIC primarily revolves around the fact that traumatic experiences are commonplace and normal yet they have far-reaching health and well-being lifetime impacts. The History of Trauma-Informed Care is directly related to the study of Adverse Childhood Experiences (ACEs) which has proven to be a research breakthrough which has shown that early-life trauma is correlated with future health outcomes at a very high rate. Some of the experiences that are classified under the category of ACEs include the emotional, physical and sexual abuse, dysfunction in the household, substance or mental illness of one of the parents and parental exposure of domestic abuse. The study findings have indicated that people who have been exposed to ACEs group is extremely vulnerable to mental disorders, chronic illnesses, substance use, and poor social and work performance (Mahood et al., 2024). It is necessary to mention that the cumulative risk principle, with which the impact of trauma is not only that but, in most cases, compounded with time, was emphasized in the research of ACEs. This information has given TIC a strong empirical foundation, which implies that the interventions ought to take into account the long and short-term consequences of the trauma.

In addition to ACEs model, neurobiological studies have also come to play prominently in research on trauma with the view to offer information about the impacts of traumatic experiences on the brain and the body. It has been demonstrated that chronic stress and trauma adjust the neural pathways, regulation of stress response and influence memory, attention and change emotional processing. Some of the neurobiological mechanisms of the long-term effects of the trauma include the dysfunction of the hypothalamic-pituitary-adrenal (HPA) axis, the change in the activity of the brain parts (amygdala and hippocampus), and the modifications in the systems of neurotransmitters. Resting on such results, one may mention the significance of the approaches, which do not consider the behavior only but consider the physiological and cognitive effects of the trauma. TIC offers a holistic approach to understanding and remedy of human trauma by applying neurobiological, psychological and social approaches to the issue. TIC is based on paradigm shift. Instead of telling you what is wrong about you. practitioners have been proposed to inquire of you what has happened to you. It is through this reframing that empathy is developed, blame and pressures are reduced, practitioners are pushed to perceive behaviors and responses as adaptive, based on past experiences (Louw, 2024). It also focuses on the need to identify the signs and symptoms of such trauma that might very well be emotional dysregulation, hypervigilance, withdrawal, or inability to build a trusting relationship. TIC is used to aid the strength-based approach, recognition of the resilience in the individuals and their developmental abilities and offer delicate, aware and responsive care to the requirements of the individuals.

Safety, trustworthiness, collaboration, empowerment, and cultural sensitivity are the primary principles of Trauma-Informed Care that the implementation of TIC in any given setting is based on. Safety is not only about the physical safety, but also about establishing a space, which a person feels in their heart, and feels supported in it. Reliability and openness would be realized through effective communication, practices and expected interactions. The value of cooperation and support of peers is focused on the value of the collective decision-making process and the understanding of the fact that the recovery process is present most of the time in the relations and community contexts. Empowerment entails the development of independence and freedom of choices that render individuals assume the dominion of their lives and choices (Bargeman et al., 2022). The relevance, respectfulness, and fairness of the interventions are considered because cultural, historical, and gender factor are used to establish the fact that trauma is not evenly applied in social, cultural, and historical environments. All these are guided towards prevention of re-traumatization and good and humanized curing. The TIC models were first used at the level of individuals, which emphasized the trauma-informed work with the clients and patients. This area has extended overtime to include systemic and organizational approach. It is also available that organizations are institutionalizing trauma awareness in the policies, procedures and workplace cultures to an effort of ensuring that there is a trauma-sensitive workplace at all times. This involves educating its staff, educating on trauma-informed leadership, revising the protocol as an effort of preventing other triggers that contribute to re-traumatization, and feedback systems to ensure that things are able and will continue to improve (Holmes et al., 2023). Through incorporation of TIC concept in the organization and community architectural framework, the practitioners have come to understand that trauma is not a personal experience, but a communication problem, which has been revealed to structural inequity, discrimination, and unfavorable social determinants of health.

The initiation of TIC to systemic implication is associated with the appearance of the consciousness of the complex interaction of personal trauma with social determinants of health and community and society. One of them is that an oppressed, poor, or violence-stricken community in history can be traumatized intergenerationally i.e. the legacies of the past trauma still tend to trail the current generations. The trauma-informed systems put into consideration these larger environments and attempt to elicit latent assumptions that give rise to patterns of trauma exposure and recidivism of damage. This form of systemicness makes TIC even more relevant and effective to make sure that the interventions are personal, socially and culturally informed. Irrespective of the perceived advantages and the increasing popularity of TIC models, there are some difficulties to the implementation. Availability of resources can be a barrier to the full-scaled training programs and organizational redesign, and the workforce preparedness and capability is rather diverse in terms of industries. The question of standardized methods and individual care is a burden too because the organization must make sure that it remains loyal to the TIC principles and initiate interventions that would address the needs of its residents (Guevara et al., 2021). In addition, the outcomes and efficiency of TIC is an emerging subject and further studies are required to provide best practices and evidence-based practices. The TIC frameworks will not only be trauma responsive, but will develop resilience and well-being. TIC will lead to development of coping skills among individuals, restored trust and enhanced social bonds due to the provision of empowering and predictable environments. This, in its turn, leads to superior service outcomes, improved care utilization, and quality of life. TIC values endorse the notion of recovery as something that takes place repeatedly and continuously and not as an intervention among the organizations and practitioners, where the gist of a long-term support system and relational based approaches. Other than the effects of Trauma-informed care on people, the practice affects the organizational performance, service delivery, and the community well-being (Tebes et al., 2019). It has been noted that businesses who have implemented the TIC principles have enjoyed higher levels of employee satisfaction levels, less burnout, and more interdisciplinary group collaboration. Equity and inclusiveness are attained with the inclusion of trauma awareness in the policies and practices, responsiveness of particular services to a broad group of people and sensitivity of historical, cultural, and systemic contexts that influence how individuals perceive it. Finally, TIC is a paradigm shift, in which the human dignity, comprehension and healing are centralized and may serve as a prototype of the reference of the prolific effects of traumas on different levels. In a nutshell, Trauma-Informed Care is holistic and comprehensive approach to perception and reaction towards trauma. Consequently, the psychology, neurobiology, and social determinants of health, TIC is focusing on empathy, empowerment, and culturally relevant interventions due to the empirical research study which has been done on

ACEs (Champine et al., 2019). It is an indicator that it can comprehend the intricacy of the trauma-social and structural interactions better because it has been capable of formulating individual to systemic and organizational applications. TIC is not only assisting in creating the circumstances of safety, trust, collaboration, as well as empowerment, which facilitates individual healing to ensure that organizations and communities become more equitable, responsive, and efficient. TIC models provide an effective basis of health, social, and educational enhancement and well-being as a whole in a highly broad population given the fact that the field of knowledge in trauma is still being developed (Lynch et al., 2025).

FOUNDATIONS OF TRAUMA-INFORMED CARE

The theory of Trauma-Informed Care (TIC) is based on the reasonable expertise of multifaceted consequences of trauma on the individuals of the lifespan. The pinnacle of this finding is the contribution of Adverse Childhood Experiences (ACEs) who has offered concrete reasoning of the outcomes of childhood traumatizing events over a long period. ACEs can involve adverse childhood events, such as physical, emotional, or sexual abuse, neglect, dysfunction in a family combined with parental psychiatric disorder, substance abuse, or domestic violence. It is proved repeatedly that people who are exposed to ACE(s) more than one are exposed to a huge risk of a variety of negative outcomes, such as physical illnesses, mental disorders, drug use and low social and professional achievements. The model of ACEs is very keen on the cumulative aspect of the trauma where multiple or repeated exposure causes the probability of resulting in more adverse effects. It should be noted that the ACEs study reveals the significance of preventive and supportive interventions which can be adopted to control both short-term and long-term effects in an effort to offer a science behind TIC concepts. In addition to ACEs, the psychological and neurobiological impact of trauma ought to be familiar in order that a competitive TIC model would be implemented. Trauma is not a simple psychic process, it influences the brain formation, the mental functioning and feelings (Berring et al., 2024). The chronic stress and traumatic events may impede the maturation of the nervous system to modify the operation of the hypothalamic-pituitary-adrenal (HPA) axis to be able to regulate the state of the body in response to the stress. The transformations can result in the development of the stress susceptibility, emotional regulation problems, and susceptibility to anxiety, depression, and another mental dysfunction. The neuroimaging has depicted that structural and functional alterations in the major portions of the brain including amygdala, hippocampus and prefrontal cortex of threat detection, memory consolidation, and executive functions are present (Erickson & Harvey, 2023). There are also changes in autonomic nervous system that may occur in case of trauma and this may result in hyperarousal, hypervigilance or dissociation response to the situations that appear dangerous. TIC models offer a comprehensive approach of treating the interdependence of the trauma through a combination of neurobiological knowledge, psychological and social knowledge. Social and emotional impacts of the trauma also require practices that are informed by trauma. The traumatized persons cannot develop and sustain relationships, perform in the society and regulate their emotions. Part of the manifestations of the trauma can be social withdrawal, mistrust and authority or reactive behaviours that can be misinterpreted to mean defiance or noncompliance. The common emotional responses include shame, guilt, fear, and anger and can be complicated by stigma or lack of social knowledge about trauma. Furthermore, such structural influences as poverty, discrimination, and violence in the community are more likely to facilitate the trauma and increase the degree of stress and services to deal with. The significance of TIC is the fact that these social and emotional aspects are to be recognized as only in such circumstances, the need to develop safe, predictable and enabling environments where individuals may learn to be resilient and adopt adaptive coping mechanisms (Chafouleas et al., 2016). The TIC ideas bring out the fact that trauma is not a singular event but an experience with spill over effects in the other life spheres. Together with the intersectionality of ACEs, the neurobiological mechanisms, and the social-emotional factors, the practitioners and organizations will now be able to react to them in a more informed, compassionate and effective manner. The TIC frameworks are designed to detect such effects in due time as well as prevent and act on not only the individual but also the systemic aspects. The principles of TIC are based on the knowledge, which underlies their practices oriented to the concept of safety, trust, empowerment, collaboration, and cultural sensitivity. To conclude, one can mention that Trauma-Informed Care has three mutually dependent pillars, including awareness of negative childhood experiences, knowledge of the psychological and neurobiological effects of trauma, and awareness of its social and emotional effects. These pillars form the evidence-based foundation of the implementation of the TIC principles to the various settings, which include both clinical and educational setting and social service and community systems. Some of the lessons within this context refer to the minimization of the long-term consequences of the trauma, prevention of re-traumatization, and assisting the individuals to lead a complete life and become resilient. These are the key pillars, which are still under development and implementation of effective, compassionate, and equitable trauma-informed practice as the field advances.

CORE PRINCIPLES OF TRAUMA-INFORMED CARE

Trauma-Informed Care (TIC) practice, policy, and community practice have an edifice of essential principles that determine practice. These ideas are the pillars of the development of the setting that recognizes the omnipresence of consequences of trauma, the focus on the well-being, and the formation of the resilience. The essence of TIC is that traumatized people need a safe, conducive and enabling environment where they feel safe in accessing services and relationships without the fear of being re-traumatized. These concepts are connected and complementary to each other in the sense that they determine the relationship of the practitioner and the individual, the organization and their program organization and the community and the trauma victim. This is due to the fact that trauma-informed practice is based on safety. It goes as far as to imply the emotional and psychological protection as compared to physical protection. The trauma victims also become hypervigilant and thus they tend to believe that there is a threat where none exists. Another thing that needs to be taken into consideration to provide a safe environment is not only the physical location but also people communication. This comprises of routines, expectations and respectful communication (Cochran, 2019). The services will be consumed more likely at the time when people will be safe and able to reveal their needs and initiate the process of healing. The concept of safety also means a chance to identify the possible antecedents and reduce the conditions that could trigger traumatic reactions and make the environment as friendly as possible and not by accident potentially harmful. Safety is also accompanied by trustworthiness and transparency that is the secret of significant relations between people and service providers. The trauma may affect the trusting capacity of the subject especially those in positions of authority since there was the experience of being betrayed, neglected and abused in the past. Credibility is achieved through well-established, consistent and honest communication, establishing the right boundaries as well as being able to fulfill promises. This openness in its activities will facilitate the uncertainty and anxiety levels and establish a sense of reliability and predictability in its activities, expectations and decision making. The companies that hold the idea of the importance of trustworthiness are responsible and truthful and it sends a message to the people that their experience is not neglected but is appreciated. The use of trauma-informed practices is based on empowerment and choice that is agency of people managing themselves and their recovery (Elliott et al., 2005). The deprivation of the control or autonomy is possibly the part of the trauma and when a person has no chance to make a proper choice, it is very important to get an opportunity and re-establish one of the impressions of personal efficiency. Empowerment is the complement of the virtues of persons, choice and participation in the decision-making and decision-making. Choosing process does not only involve the choices of individuals in terms of treatment or services but also providing a chance to express preferences, choice goals and contributing to creation of new environment around people. One of the core requirements of resiliency and healed is developing a sense of control and confidence and being empowered and choose. The role of relationships in the process of recovery is manifested in collaboration and peer support. The trauma will alienate people and destroy the faith in interpersonal relationships. The collaborative methods are directed at decision making and collaboration between the practitioners, clients and community. Peer support - the association of the person with other individuals who have gone through it, receives confirmation, sympathy and hope. The teamwork cultures promote the exchange of knowledge, resources, respecting each other, and solving problems together. The principle of collaboration is also applied in the interdisciplinary teamwork in the organizational context, which implies ensuring that various perspectives and experiences are combined to deliver an all-inclusive and balanced care. The cultural, historical and gender sensitivity has the consciousness of the fact that, there is disparity in the experience of trauma in a social, cultural and historical situation. Reaction to trauma is prescribed by cultural norms and community histories, systemic oppression and gendered experiences. These are the dimensions to be determined in an attempt to offer equitable and effective care (Bargeman et al., 2021).

The consideration of race, ethnicity, socioeconomic status, sexual orientation, gender identity, and culture should also be offered culturally sensitive practices based on trauma. This competency requires practitioners to be self-reflective, practice cultural humility and purposeful learning and knowledge of the lived experience of the people with whom they offer care. It also involves identification of the larger structural and historical forces like colonization, discrimination and social marginalization, which add traumas and affect availability and provision of resources. These are the fundamental principles that constitute a formula of trauma-informed practice. They will help practitioners to establish predictable, attentive, and satisfying environments that will meet the needs of trauma victims (Peternelj-Taylor, 2018). TIC instills resilience, healing, and minimization of re-traumatization chances through focus on safety, trust, empowerment, collaboration, and cultural sensitivity. In addition, these principles are not fixed but they need to be implemented dynamically and adjusted to individual, organizational and community particular needs. All these principles integrated into practice, policy and culture may be seen as the shift towards the proactive rather than the reactive strategies with the priorities on the prevention, well-being and the holistic care. Fortunately, the general concepts of Trauma-Informed Care both offer a philosophy and change strategy to modify the manner of services delivery. They are a group of prisms upon which organizations, practitioners and communities can analyze what they are doing, what they can do better and make sure that the interaction is done based on the principle of respect, empathy and understanding (Berliner & Kolko, 2016). These values in the center of all care provision will help establish the environment where people will feel safe, valued, and empowered, and this will eventually lead to the recovery, resilience, and well-being. Core Principles of Trauma-Informed Care are shown in Table 1.

Table 1. Core principles of trauma-informed care

Principle	Description	Key Focus / Implementation
Safety	Creating physical, emotional, and psychological security for individuals	Predictable routines, clear expectations, minimizing triggers, supportive environment
Trustworthiness and Transparency	Building reliable and honest relationships to foster confidence	Clear communication, consistent actions, accountability, predictable decision-making
Empowerment and Choice	Supporting individual agency and promoting autonomy	Strengths-based approach, informed decision-making, goal-setting, options for participation
Collaboration and Peer Support	Encouraging partnership and shared decision-making	Interdisciplinary teamwork, peer connections, mutual respect, resource-sharing
Cultural, Historical, and Gender Sensitivity	Recognizing diversity and systemic influences on trauma experiences	Cultural humility, equity-focused practices, acknowledgment of historical and social context

EVOLUTION OF TRAUMA-INFORMED CARE FRAMEWORKS

The concept of Trauma-Informed Care (TIC) has been radically changing throughout the last several decades and converting the initial approaches that are individual-oriented into the generalized approaches that include organizations, systems, and communities. The specified trend is an indicator of greater consciousness on the ubiquity of trauma, the multidimensional nature of the interaction between individual and structural determinants, and the importance of the comprehensive approach to allow recovery and resilience. The most valuable contribution of TIC to the existing models is its historical development since it shows how the emphasis on the practices has grown to meet the trauma on different levels. First, the interventions that are individual-oriented were the basis of the trauma-informed practices to a great extent. These programs focused on direct therapeutic care of individuals who were traumatized with the perspective of treating them of symptoms and promoting coping without taking into consideration, personal recovery (Wilson et al., 2013). Several forms of evidence-based therapy that included cognitive-behavioral therapy (CBT), eye movement desensitization and reprocessing (EMDR), and trauma-focused psychotherapy were enforced by clinicians and counselors to assist their respective clients process their traumatic experiences to minimize emotional distress. The individual-based techniques were specifically applied to clinical practice that offered systematic ways of determining the existence of the presence of the trauma, information concerning the effects of trauma and personal recovery. Yet, though such interventions would provide people with the tremendous support, they might not always be helpful in terms of response to the environmental, organizational, or systemic factors that might still be involved in the presence and persistence of trauma or respondent to the recovery process. The trauma knowledge grew and the TIC models started to broaden their care to include systemic and organizational care models as opposed to the individual care they were initially made up of. Companies had also learnt that conditions under which the individuals are served can either be therapeutic or traumatizing without necessarily being so. Systemic approaches entail such an act of incorporating trauma consciousness into the organizational culture, the organizational policies as well as the organizational procedures (Goldstein et al., 2024). This involves introducing the staff training to make them more trauma literate, establishing the strategies of trauma-sensitive leadership, and introduction of organizational policies and procedures that are supportive of safety, trust, and collaboration. Systemic TIC also considers the wellbeing of work forces since it is known that a well-supported and trained work force is in the better position to offer quality and caring care. Trying to react to the trauma rather than being reactive, TIC may further move to the preventive level of intervention to help provide an improved overall service delivery and decrease the threat of re-traumatization. As far as the tenets of trauma-informed practices have been translated into more comprehensive policies, cultures and the practice within the community, the establishment of TIC has been as well. This systems integration means there is the realization that trauma is not a personal issue but a societal issue, which is unequal economically, has social determinants of health and is historically oppressed (Hartinger-Saunders et al., 2019). The Community-Based TIC deals with the integration of trauma awareness in community health programs, education, social services networks and community programs. One can develop policies that will minimize the exposure to trauma, expand the supply of the supportive resources, and weaken the other factors that contribute to the cumulative trauma like poverty, discrimination, and violence in the community. Culture and community practices have added TIC as well with an objective of collective resilience, peer support systems and mobilization of the effort of various sectors and the trauma response is also inclusive, comprehensive, and sustainable. The modern TIC models are preoccupied with the significance of the interdisciplinary teamwork, evidence-based practice, and cultural responsiveness (Downey & Greco, 2023).

The interdisciplinary approaches presuppose the involvement of specialists in the sphere of mental health, the area of social work, healthcare, education, and the community agencies to cover the complexity of the trauma. The evidence-based interventions undergo constant monitoring and modifications to make sure that the interventions can be effective in many populations as well as settings. Culturally responsive TIC acknowledges and accepts the fact that individuals respond to trauma differently based on cultural, historic, social influences and attempts to offer an equitable, inclusive, and respectful intervention to individuals, depending on personal identities and communal backgrounds. The characteristics of TIC development are also the presence of reactive approaches that transform into proactive and preventative ones (Wilson-Ching & Berger, 2024). TIC frameworks will help in preventing the expression of the trauma and its consequences by detecting traces of a trauma early and creating favorable conditions and address systemic issues to preclude these effects into the chronic consequences on the psyche or social life. This proactive nature takes into account the fact that principles of trauma-informed care are not restricted to the sphere of treatment only, but these must be incorporated into everyday routine of the practice, the policy and the organizational structure. Although this enormous progress has been made, the phenomenon of TIC development does not fare much. Community and system-wide interventions are resource-consuming in terms of training and coordination of the sector. The practices based on trauma require normalization and flexibility to treat the needs of individuals and the context of need by organizations. Moreover, continuous assessment and investigations are also required to determine results, determine the best practices and models to be improved and responsive to new learning regarding trauma and resilience. It can be mentioned that the development of the Trauma-Informed Care models is marked by the change of the previously practiced therapeutic interventions towards the systemic, organizational and community-wide practice (Kearns et al., 2026). The tendency is an indication of a more comprehensive knowledge of the complexity of the trauma, the need to focus on both individual and structural levels, the need to impose TIC principles on various levels of the society. In its formulation, TIC offers a more comprehensive, effective and sustainable means of servicing trauma victims and organizations and communities in the trauma affected areas to ensure healing, resilience and wellbeing in the varying environments.

ACEs, Neurobiology, and Social determinants in Trauma-Informed Care:

CEs are events that may have happened in childhood that have been potentially traumatized, including abuse, neglect, and dysfunction in the house. Studies indicate that the high ACE scores have a very close relationship with the development of mental health disorders, chronic diseases, and behavioral difficulties in the future. Knowledge about ACEs within the context of TIC enables the practitioners to understand that there is a high likelihood of having a lot of behaviors that are not misbehaviors, but merely coping reactions to a previous trauma. This turns the subject of inquiry into What is wrong with you? into What happened to you? Neurobiology is a discipline that describes the impact of trauma on the development and functioning of the brain. Stress in early developmental years may lead to an imbalance in the stress response system, especially of the amygdala, hippocampus and prefrontal cortex. This may cause increased fear reactions, emotional regulation and poor decision making. Through TIC frameworks, this knowledge is promoted and helps individuals to reconnect neural pathways and resilience through strategies that result in the creation of safety, predictability, and emotional regulation. Another factor in the exposure and recovery of the trauma is access to education, housing, and healthcare (social determinants of health). The individuals with the disadvantaged backgrounds are more likely to experience repeated traumas and inability to seek the support services. TIC models incorporate an understanding of such forces in the system to realize equitable, culturally aware, and accessible care. This is because ACEs, neurobiology and social determinants provide an integrated view of trauma research. These aspects also allow the Trauma-Informed Care frameworks to cease being concerned with the control of the symptoms but, instead, are directed at the healing of the human being as a whole being, establishing an environment in which recovery, empowerment, and well-being are enhanced.

CONTEMPORARY MODELS AND PRACTICES

The existing models of Trauma-Informed Care (TIC) are based on the principles and develop the paradigms to offer the evidence based, holistic and contextual specific approach to the issues of tackling the trauma. The contemporary TIC practice is interdisciplinary, is founded on the strict introduction of the evidence-based interventions, and non-discriminating methods of working, which address the needs of various groups of people. These models acknowledge that trauma is multifactorial and demands integrated approaches at the nexus of various systems, professional domains, and community settings in order to make a difference. Today interdisciplinary cooperation has become one of the TIC principles. Trauma has varied impacts on all spheres in life of an individual that may be physical, psychological, social life, performance in school or work. The collaboration of the team of professionals in different fields (mental health, medicine, social work, education, and community services) is required to achieve such complex needs. The multi-purposive, coordinated and holistic care encouraged by collaborative practices, entails the delivery of more comprehensive evaluations and treatment (Templeman & Robinson, 2011). An example is a child with certain trauma which can be helped by the combined efforts of a school counselor, pediatrician, social worker, and a family therapist who would be able to discuss different yet similar things about his or her experience. The interdisciplinary teamwork facilitates the consistency in the application of the trauma-informed principles throughout the points of contacts as well, which improves the continuity and effectiveness of the treatment. The other peculiarity of contemporary TIC models is evidence-based interventions. Studies have proved the effectiveness of trauma-focused cognitive behavioral therapy (TF-CBT), eye movement desensitization, and reprocessing (EMDR), somatic experiencing and other psychotherapy modes to respond to the requirements of the trauma symptoms. The evidence-based practices are based on scientific research articles and clinical results that provide interventions that are efficient, safe, and sensitive to individual preferences (Zembylas, 2014). The existing TIC models focus on measuring the effectiveness of the intervention and regular review of the results as well to enhance and refine the practice as well. Evidence-based strategies bring trauma-informed strategies more credible and reliable and offer the practitioner and the organization theoretically informed tools and practical ones, as well. The TIC models of the contemporary world imply the inclusion strategies with various populations. Different cultural, social, historical and economic environments have diverse experiences of trauma and one ought to be sensitive to this in a bid to provide effective care. The practices that will address the racial, ethnic, gender, sexual orientation, disability, and socio-economic status barriers will be inclusive TIC practices thus interventions will be accessible, equitable and culture functional. It neither simply refers to the change of clinical practices, but also the integration of culturally relevant models, community involvement in the decision-making and the significance of the systemic and historical trauma in the formation of the personal experience. Another concept is inclusivity that is also applied to the organizational policies and implies that the elements of diversity, equity, and inclusivity are embodied through the training of personnel, service provision, and community outreach. The current TIC models are supposed to serve every person equally, but with inclusiveness (primarily, people who are representatives of historically discriminated or disadvantaged groups). These preventative and aggressive measures are combined with such fundamental components and are aimed in current TIC. It is becoming implemented in cases where organizations and communities are getting trauma-informed instead of being done in cases where the situation is acute, or where crisis situations occur. The proactive stance would include the encouragement of the resilience, the formation of the positive networks, and the supply of the setting that will minimize the levels of exposure to the trauma to the minimum. Schools, health agencies and community organizations are integrating the TIC principles in their curriculum, training of staff, school policies and day to day operations as well as ensuring the knowledge of the trauma is a system culture and not a onetime program. Even technology and innovation even start to emerge in the existing TIC. More access to care, interdisciplinary contacts and personal care plans can be provided with the help of digital platforms, telehealth, and data-driven monitoring tools. Through these innovations the practitioners can follow the progress, to offer virtual assistance and access those populations, which might not be in position to access the traditional services (Kauffman et al., 2017).

Technology does not substitute the human based care, but it may be a complementary feature to increase access, effectiveness, and interaction. Even though the modern TIC models are improved, there is still a problem of implementation and sustainability. The organizational environment demands preserving the balance between standardization of the evidence-based practice and the flexibility to implement the flexibility in order to meet the needs of individuals and the community. Devotion to TIC tenets is a fact that should possess adequate resources, training and leadership provisions. It involves an ongoing revision, search and modification of it to allow that the current models can be effective, relevant and open on the fast-changing social and healthcare environment. In general, the modern paradigms and the methods of Trauma-Informed Care are focused on the teamwork in different disciplines, the evidence-based intervention introduction, and the integration of various population types. These approaches are a manifestation of a multidisciplinary view of trauma that introduces multimodal aspects, science, and cultural sensitivity to effective care. The modern models address the interests of the victims of the trauma by incorporating the concepts of TIC in the organizational cultures, work in the community, and collaboration between the professionals to provide a contributing role in creating the environment that facilitates the healing of the trauma victims, their resilience, and balanced support. Contemporary Models and Practices of Trauma-Informed Care are shown in table 2

Table 2. Contemporary models and practices of trauma-informed care; source

Component	Description	Key Focus / Implementation
Interdisciplinary Collaboration	Coordinated efforts among professionals from multiple disciplines to address the complex effects of trauma	Involves mental health, medical, social work, education, and community services; promotes holistic, consistent care across settings
Evidence-Based Interventions	Use of interventions validated by research to effectively address trauma symptoms	Trauma-focused CBT, EMDR, somatic experiencing; ongoing monitoring and adaptation based on outcomes
Inclusive Strategies for Diverse Populations	Ensuring interventions are culturally responsive, equitable, and accessible	Adapts practices for race, ethnicity, gender, disability, socioeconomic status; addresses systemic and historical trauma; engages communities in decision-making
Proactive and Preventive Approaches	Integrating TIC principles into routine practices to reduce trauma exposure and promote resilience	Embedding trauma-informed policies in schools, healthcare, and community programs; staff training and supportive environments
Technology and Innovation	Leveraging digital tools to enhance accessibility and coordination of care	Telehealth services, digital platforms for monitoring progress, data-driven communication among interdisciplinary teams

IMPLEMENTATION CHALLENGES

Though the concept of Trauma-Informed Care (TIC) models has demonstrated that the concept has many positive implications when it comes to serving individuals that experienced a traumatic experience, the implementation of the ideas into the spectrum of organizational, system, and community-related concerns is critical. These issues must be conversant in order to be in position to devise ways of enhancing adoption, sustainability and effectiveness. The allocation of resources and funding, the capability development and employee training, and the same practises on care delivery based on uniformity of care delivery versus the individual care delivery based care are some of the areas that are very critical. Resource and funding constraints are some of the obstacles that have been significantly used to stop implementation of the TIC. Trauma-informed programs offered by big-box can be expensive in terms of staff-training, organizational planning and redesigning, and the development of supporting policies and programs. Most organizations have limited financial and human resources, and more so those who practice in the social or healthcare fields that are not well-funded, and it is difficult to implement the TIC principles to their full potential. Limited resources can also determine access to expert interventions, tools, or technology that can be applied to encourage practices that are trauma-informed. Instead, organizations might be not in the state of being loyal to TIC frameworks unless the latter is adequately funded and will lead to inequality in application and performance. Planning is that solution to any resource concerns, lobbying as well as capitalization on resources that are available in the community through maximizing it. Workforce training and competency development is another cumbersome issue. Good TIC assumes the presence of knowledgeable personnel regarding the topic on trauma and its effects and trauma-related remedies. However, not all professionals receive professional training in their training or working lives and even the existing professionals might require the latest training to be qualified. The training interventions must not target to provide them with the theoretical knowledge only but provide them with the practical measures that can be implemented to address TIC principles to various settings and to various populations. Better still, the well-being of the staff members should be considered just like exposure of the staff members to the traumas that victims can cause, which may lead to the occurrence of secondary or vicarious traumas, burn out, and compassion fatigue. The organizations are therefore asked to invest in the skill building and the support systems, which are sustaining the personnel to remain afloat so that the workforce can be able to deliver trauma-based care at a sustainable effective rate. The third obstacle in the TIC implementation is that it is needed to find the balance between the standard practice and the personal care. Unified protocols and policies can help to guarantee homogeneity, accountability and selection of the evidence-based principles and, in certain cases, even conflict with the need of tailoring interventions to the unique requirements, culture and lived experience. Any population trauma is not similar and the response should be fluid enough to accommodate the various need, interests and situations. Organizations need to protest against the matter of maintaining a balance between a more routine approach to methodology, in respect of trauma-sensitivity, and freedom, safety, and empowerment. This balance could not be attained without good leadership, where someone ought to have the sense of direction on how an individual must flexibly utilize the principles and the exercise of incessant evaluation and response. These are not matters that simply can affect the application of TIC but rather larger systemic and societal imaginations of such a matter. Structural inequity can ignite trauma-informed actions and the cultural prejudices and inability to provide supportive resources in the undermine of these actions in areas of under-serving or marginalized populations. These are not all the contextual factors that organizations should take into consideration and check the equity-based strategies when planning, training and delivering services. It is necessary to work with the community stakeholders, policymakers and interdisciplinary teams to cover and make TIC programs more efficient to address systemic barriers. Irrespective of these issues, science, and practice point to the fact that these problems can be mitigated with the assistance of strategic planning, leadership commitment, and the constant appraisal. The companies, which consider the values of trauma-informed care, invest in the staff, use resources adequately, and those, who can change and be culturally adaptive, are in a better position to achieve the successful and sustainable TIC implementation. That is why the process of identifying and responding to the implementation issues should be introduced to introduce theoretical concepts of TIC into real and concrete outcomes that would help achieve resilience, healing, and well-being. In general, there is a great deal of concern related to the introduction of the Trauma-Informed Care models, including the absence of resources, training of working staff, the need to strike the balance between the standardization and non-standardized care. Any solution to such problems should be willed where resources are competent enough, developing constructive organizational cultures, and on liberal and inclusive paradigms. With the proactive strategy towards the above obstacles, organizations and communities shall be able to maximize their potential in providing efficient, sustainable and fair services in a trauma-informed manner and that will work in those who have already been traumatized.

IMPACT AND SIGNIFICANCE

The implications of TIC frameworks on individuals, institutions and societies are massive in terms of their resilience, service delivery and overall wellbeing. Introducing the knowledge of the trauma in the policies, practices, and relationship, TIC preconditions the provisions that support the recovery and introduce the positive long-term change. The fact that the effect and significance of these structures have been lost, informs the reader why they have become a key approach to health, social services and even in the educational institutions. The TIC impacts resilience in one of the most significant ways. The emotional regulation, social functioning, and adaptive coping disorientation caused by trauma may be handled by TIC principles and practices that may create the context within which the establishment of a feeling of safety, control, and self-efficacy may be re-established. TIC helps individuals to build adaptive coping mechanisms in coping with stress, experience processing and decision-making and managing difficulty through supportive relationships building empowerment and skill development. The safety, trust and collaboration will be likely to bring consistency and predictability needed to recover a person after previous trauma and this element makes him or her stronger in the end analysis. This emphasis on resilience highlights the ability to grow and recover as opposed to emphasizing the insufficiency or the pathology, which is the defining attribute of the strengths-based approach, which is the dominating characteristic of trauma-informed practice.

Trauma-Informed Care is an additional change that comes in handy in enhancing the service outcome within various types of facilities. The principles of TIC can be used to improve the level of engagement, satisfaction, and effectiveness of interventions in the healthcare, educational, and social service setting. The people will feel improved to fully engage in the services where they will feel heard, respected and empowered and the outcomes will be better since they will be more compliant to the treatment plan and less challenging behaviorally and, therefore, will reach the ultimate outcome. TIC in the case of organizations can result in an organization that is more integrated, stable and responsive in delivering care and this would close the gap between care and probability of re-traumatization. It is also concluded that the informed strategies relying on traumas can lead to decreased hospitalization, crisis services reduction, and improved educational and social functioning that imply the overall effect of TIC principles implementation in the various spheres. Well-being, holistically, is also the other important definition of TIC frameworks. Trauma does not affect mental health, but it has physical health, social relations, and the quality of life in general. TIC considers these areas to be related and proposes interventions grounded in the entire person and not limited symptoms. TIC reaches the people with a sense of agency and empowers them once more and allows them to develop significant relationships and follow their own agendas by providing people with enabling and supportive conditions. The holistic approaches take into consideration the social determinants of health, culture situation and systemic factors as well that the interventions provided are just, inclusive and sensitive to the larger determinants that influence the life of the individual. This consideration of the overall health will further expand the scope of TIC beyond the relief of symptoms in the short term and long-term recovery, level of life satisfaction (subjective) and social integration.

TIC also has an association with the worth of results within organizations and communities. The organizations which have embraced the implementation of the concept of trauma-informed practices were reported to have an improved degree of satisfaction among their staff members, a lower rate of burnout as well as a higher degree of transparency among the multidisciplinary teams. Such policies and practices based on trauma will play a significant role in establishing healthier and more supportive workplace cultures so that the personnel could effectively address the needs of their clientele and safeguard their welfare. At the community level, TIC could impact the health programs within the population, the education system and the social service programs and create the environment that minimizes the exposure to the traumatic condition, encourages recovery and social cohesion. Using TIC principles as the multiple layers embedded in the society will assist the communities to have better resources to transcend structural inequities, and also to accommodate the effects of the traumas and develop resiliency as a unit. That is, the influence and the perception of Trauma-Informed Care are numerous-dimensional and extensive. TIC frameworks are based on a holistic method of working with people who have already experienced trauma and they are more resilient, which improves the services outcomes and the well-being of people. They begin the focus to the proactive interventions and strengths-based models in which attention is paid to both the entire person and the surrounding. Moreover, TIC is just, inclusive and culturally responsive as a result, services provided are responsive to the needs of varied categories of people besides being responsive to systemic factors that lead to trauma. The application of the TIC principles is thus not the move in the personal care but the transition to the organizational culture and practice which is the communal one. Finally, one should also speak about Trauma-Informed Care because it is changing the perception of human behavior, service provision, and systemic responsibility. The overall and advanced outcomes of trauma in its identification, general and culturally competent services are inculcated in systems, which TIC creates recovery, resilience and wellbeing. It lacks a single level of impact; it possesses the organizational and community one, which can provide a comprehensive solution to the issue of the trauma treatment and creation of the positive results in the long-run.

PROGNOSIS OF TRAUMA-INFORMED CARE

Trauma-Informed Care (TIC) is already present on the market as an already developed model of helping a person who has experienced a traumatic event, and it still requires evolution in order to face new opportunities and challenges. Future of TIC is concerned with equity expansion, access expansion, research and innovation and continuation of change both internally and externally in the community. The following guidelines should most likely render trauma-informed practices within diverse settings more successful, comprehensive, and sustainable. The second stage of TIC is serious matter to augment equity and access. In spite of the increase of such access and quality disparities of trauma-informed services, accessibility of such services among marginalized populations, including racial and ethnic minorities, people with disabilities, LGBTQ+ communities, and the economically disadvantaged is still present. The identified steps that are to be undertaken will consist of shattering the obstacles of care, overcoming systemic inequities, and changing the trauma-informed practices into the more culturally responsive and accessible ones to everyone. It involves formulation of policies which would encourage inclusion, formulation of interventions founded on lived experience of the different populations, and the necessity to train practitioners to appreciate and address the needs of the historically underserved populations. As a way of making sure that TIC doctrines are beneficial to as many people as possible, it is necessary to widen equity and access as a way of ensuring that the trauma has been eradicated and social justice acquired.

The other future trend of TIC that is important to utilize is the use of research and innovation. The on-going studies regarding the neurobiological, psychological and social impact of the trauma is still working on the development of the best practices and perfecting the interventions. Evidence-based practices, data-driven approaches, and technological solutions will become a component of the TIC models of the future in an attempt to improve the assessment, treatment, and monitoring. New technologies like telehealth, online mental health workplace, and tools with the help of artificial intelligence can be used to make it more accessible, personal, and monitor the results in a more efficient way. In this case, the emerging area knowledge (i.e. the effects of community trauma, intergenerational trauma and systemic oppression) will be applied to create more specific and effective trauma-informed interventions. Incorporating the practical into the scientific knowledge, TIC could be receptive to the dynamic demands and could contribute as much as possible. Another important thing is to ensure that there is change in the mechanisms within the organization and the community but one must remember that the changes in the TIC practices should not be short-lived but rather need to be part of the organizational culture, policies and practices within the institutions. To achieve the organizational sustainability, the leaders are required to be committed, provide adequate resources, in-service training, and the periodic review of the trauma-informed practices. The community-level change, which promotes the healing and resiliency environments, and coordinates the work of the sectors, which involve healthcare, education, social services, and the local government, is one of the approaches that support the coordination of the work of the aforementioned sectors. TIC should also be applied in the organizational and community systems as the accountability mechanisms, the feedback and adjustment to the changing needs. Sustainability will also make sure that the principles of the trauma-informed will be upheld in the long-term so that the organizations and communities will effectively address the current and upcoming issues concerning trauma.

Prevention and early intervention are also given importance in the future of the TIC. The prevention strategies are based on the early identification of the exposure to traumas, interventions aiming to help before the appearance of the symptoms that can be extremely difficult to manage, and the resiliency of families, schools, and communities. Through the change in the models of trauma reacting and proactive action, the TIC can be used to reduce the long-term effects of the trauma and enhance the results in various spheres of life such as mental and physical well-being, social performance, and academic achievements. The TIC in the prevention segment considers the concepts of equity, inclusivity, and empowerment as the systemic factors are also likely to result in the persons being predisposed to trauma and to address these problems is needed to result in a significant change. Last but not least is the TIC of the future that places emphasis on collaboration and multidisciplinary approach. These issues such as poverty, violence among the community, and systemic oppression are both complex to the society and would involve interdisciplinary action and mobilization of experience in many spheres. The collaborative practices will be utilized so that the continuity of care should be ensured and the overall impact must be augmented so that the principles of trauma-informed practice are shared between the services and the contexts. Community involvement and the use of lived experience individuals in designing and evaluating trauma-sensitive programs also provide an extra assurance of the relevance, cultural responsiveness, and efficiency of interventions. Overall, the future perspectives of Trauma-Informed Care include the growth of equity and access, research use and innovations, as well as organizational and community sustainability of the change. It will be the following generation of the trauma-informed frameworks to ameliorate the healing outcomes, resilience, and well-being of the distinct populations who face systemic imbalances, and as the fresh knowledge and technology get assimilated and resulting in the merging of the TIC principles into the long-term systemic and community systems. The guidelines prove the willingness to adhere to the approach of continuous improvement, inclusion, and proactive that is based on the multifaceted and complex nature of trauma in the modern society.

CONCLUSION

The models of trauma-sensitive care have had a considerable impact on how companies and professionals perceive and respond to trauma. TIC is aimed at safety, trust, empowerment, collaboration, and cultural sensitivity based on the research on negative childhood experiences and the multifaceted effect of trauma. The history of the individual interventions and the shift towards the systemic one have revealed the importance of the introduction of the traumatic awareness into the policy and the organizational culture as well as the practices within the community. Even though the economic challenges of scarce resources and training of the staff remain relevant, the adoption of trauma-informed principles facilitate well-being, enhance the outcomes of the offered service, and contribute to the overall welfare. The frameworks help organizations to affix within systems and integrate in order to make environments more fair, supportive, and efficient to traumatized people.

REFERENCES

Bargeman, M., Abelson, J., Mulvale, G., Niec, A., Theuer, A., & Moll, S. (2022). Understanding the Conceptualization and Operationalization of Trauma-Informed Care Within and Across Systems: A Critical Interpretive Synthesis. *The Milbank Quarterly*, *100*(3), 785–853. DOI: 10.1111/1468-0009.12579

Bargeman, M., Smith, S., & Wekerle, C. (2021). Trauma-informed care as a rights-based "standard of care": A critical review. *Child Abuse & Neglect*, *119*, 104762. DOI: 10.1016/j.chiabu.2020.104762

Berliner, L., & Kolko, D. J. (2016). Trauma Informed Care: A Commentary and Critique. *Child Maltreatment*, *21*(2), 168–172. DOI: 10.1177/1077559516643785

Berring, L. L., Holm, T., Hansen, J. P., Delcomyn, C. L., Søndergaard, R., & Hvidhjelm, J. (2024). Implementing Trauma-Informed Care—Settings, Definitions, Interventions, Measures, and Implementation across Settings: A Scoping Review. *Healthcare (Basel)*, *12*(9), 908. DOI: 10.3390/healthcare12090908

Chafouleas, S. M., Johnson, A. H., Overstreet, S., & Santos, N. M. (2016). Toward a Blueprint for Trauma-Informed Service Delivery in Schools. *School Mental Health*, *8*(1), 144–162. DOI: 10.1007/s12310-015-9166-8

Champine, R. B., Lang, J. M., Nelson, A. M., Hanson, R. F., & Tebes, J. K. (2019). Systems Measures of a Trauma-Informed Approach: A Systematic Review. *American Journal of Community Psychology*, *64*(3–4), 418–437. DOI: 10.1002/ajcp.12388

Cochran, C. B. (2019). Infusing the Principles of Trauma-Informed Care Into Emergency Nursing: A Comprehensive Approach to Change Practice. *Journal of Forensic Nursing*, *15*(4), 206–213. DOI: 10.1097/JFN.0000000000000267

Downey, J., & Greco, J. (2023). Trauma sensitive schools: A comprehensive guide for the assessment planning and implementation of trauma informed frameworks. *Children and Youth Services Review*, *149*, 106930. DOI: 10.1016/j.childyouth.2023.106930

Elliott, D. E., Bjelajac, P., Fallot, R. D., Markoff, L. S., & Reed, B. G. (2005). Trauma-informed or trauma-denied: Principles and implementation of trauma-informed services for women. *Journal of Community Psychology*, *33*(4), 461–477. DOI: 10.1002/jcop.20063

Erickson, M., & Harvey, T. (2023). A Framework for a Structured Approach for Formulating a Trauma-Informed Environment. *Journal of Education*, *203*(3), 666–677. DOI: 10.1177/00220574211046811

Goldstein, E., Chokshi, B., Melendez-Torres, G., Rios, A., Jelley, M., & Lewis-O'Connor, A. (2024). Effectiveness of Trauma-Informed Care Implementation in Health Care Settings: Systematic Review of Reviews and Realist Synthesis. *The Permanente Journal*, *28*(1), 135–150. DOI: 10.7812/TPP/23.127

Guevara, A. M. M., Johnson, S. L., Elam, K., Rivas, T., Berendzen, H., & Gal-Szabo, D. E. (2021). What Does it Mean to be Trauma-Informed? A Multi-System Perspective from Practitioners Serving the Community. *Journal of Child and Family Studies*, *30*(11), 2860–2876. DOI: 10.1007/s10826-021-02094-z

Hartinger-Saunders, R. M., Jones, A. S., & Rittner, B. (2019). Improving Access to Trauma-Informed Adoption Services: Applying a Developmental Trauma Framework. *Journal of Child & Adolescent Trauma*, *12*(1), 119–130. DOI: 10.1007/s40653-016-0104-1

Holmes, M. R., King, J. A., Miller, E. K., King-White, D. L., Korsch-Williams, A. E., Johnson, E. M., Oliver, T. S., & Conard, I. T. (2023). Innovations in Trauma-Informed Care: Building the Nation's First System of Trauma-Informed Recreation Centers. *Behavioral Sciences (Basel, Switzerland)*, *13*(5), 394. DOI: 10.3390/bs13050394

Kauffman, J. M., Hallahan, D. P., & Pullen, P. C. (Eds.). (2017). *Handbook of Special Education* (2nd ed.). Routledge., DOI: 10.4324/9781315517698

Kearns, J., Davidson, G., Shannon, C., & Mulholland, C. (2026). How trauma-informed are we? A comparative framework analysis of early intervention service guidelines for psychosis and trauma-informed principles. *Psychosis*, •••, 1–19. DOI: 10.1080/17522439.2025.2603435

Louw, B. (2024). *Neonatal Opioid Withdrawal Syndrome: Speech-Language Pathologists and Interprofessional Care* (1st ed.). Routledge., DOI: 10.4324/9781003397267

Lynch, J. M., Stange, K. C., Dowrick, C., Getz, L., Meredith, P. J., Van Driel, M. L., Harris, M. G., Tillack, K., & Tapp, C. (2025). The sense of safety theoretical framework: A trauma-informed and healing-oriented approach for whole person care. *Frontiers in Psychology*, *15*, 1441493. DOI: 10.3389/fpsyg.2024.1441493

Mahood, E., Shahid, M., Gavin, N., Rahmann, A., Tadakamadla, S. K., & Kroon, J. (2024). Theories, Models, Frameworks, Guidelines, and Recommendations for Trauma-Informed Oral Healthcare Services: A Scoping Review. *Trauma, Violence & Abuse*, *25*(2), 869–884. DOI: 10.1177/15248380231165699

Peternelj-Taylor, C. (2018). Trauma-Informed Care: Responding to the Call for Action. *Journal of Forensic Nursing*, *14*(4), 185–186. DOI: 10.1097/JFN.0000000000000224

Tebes, J. K., Champine, R. B., Matlin, S. L., & Strambler, M. J. (2019). Population Health and Trauma-Informed Practice: Implications for Programs, Systems, and Policies. *American Journal of Community Psychology*, *64*(3–4), 494–508. DOI: 10.1002/ajcp.12382

Templeman, K., & Robinson, A. (2011). Integrative medicine models in contemporary primary health care. *Complementary Therapies in Medicine*, *19*(2), 84–92. DOI: 10.1016/j.ctim.2011.02.003

Varghese, L., & Emerson, A. (2022). Trauma-informed care in the primary care setting: An evolutionary analysis. *Journal of the American Association of Nurse Practitioners*, *34*(3), 465–473. DOI: 10.1097/JXX.0000000000000663

Wilson, C., Pence, D. M., & Conradi, L. (2013). Trauma-Informed Care. In C. Wilson, D. M. Pence, & L. Conradi, *Encyclopedia of Social Work*. NASW Press and Oxford University Press. DOI: 10.1093/acrefore/9780199975839.013.1063

Wilson-Ching, M., & Berger, E. (2024). Relationship building strategies within trauma informed frameworks in educational settings: A systematic literature review. *Current Psychology (New Brunswick, N.J.)*, *43*(4), 3464–3485. DOI: 10.1007/s12144-023-04590-5

Zembylas, T. (Ed.). (2014). *Artistic Practices* (0 ed.). Routledge., DOI: 10.4324/9781315863092

Chapter 2
Economic Trauma and Structural Violence

Albrina Burger
http://orcid.org/0009-0009-8804-5142
James Madison University, USA

ABSTRACT

Vulnerable populations—people with historically marginalized backgrounds—face an increased risk of employment exploitation, housing instability, poverty and financial precarity. This chapter aims to provide a deeper understanding of the historical context that reinforces and perpetuates trauma for vulnerable people, discuss multicultural considerations mental health professionals should take into consideration, and offer trauma-informed care approaches that empower individuals and promote healing.

INTRODUCTION

The American Dream is generally defined by one's financial status and achievements. Despite the perceived opportunities afforded to those living in America, many people are experiencing economic strains that are reinforced by flawed systemic infrastructures. Vulnerable populations marginalized by race, gender, age, culture, citizenship, ableism, language and sexual orientation are more likely to be afflicted by economic crises that reinforce unfeasible living wages, harsh workplace conditions, and unsafe or unstable housing status (Chun et al., 2023). Consequently, those negatively impacted by labor exploitation, housing insecurity, poverty, and financial precarity will not only suffer from these harsh trepidations, but they will

DOI: 10.4018/979-8-3373-8597-6.ch002

also experience severe mental health, traumatic and violent implications at the hands of perpetual instability (Baker, 2025).

Professional mental health workers—namely counselors, therapists and/or clinicians—are ethically bound to support clients with their diverse and overwhelming needs that derive from their economic insecurities (Duffey & Haberstroh, 2020). Furthermore, counselors should use an approach that is culturally empathetic and competent towards clients with a history of repeated traumatic experiences. This chapter calls for trauma-informed care that examines the different forms of economic trauma, acknowledges and identifies the unique barriers associated with economic trauma, and recognizes economic justice as a fundamental source of healing.

VULNERABLE POPULATIONS

The U.S. has a long-standing tradition of practices of oppressing groups of people who are not part of the superior White, heteronormative male species. Anyone considered exclusive of this group is devalued in different ways, and categorized as vulnerable. Vulnerable populations can be defined as people minoritized based on their gender, race, ethnicity, sexual identity, socioeconomic status and physical and/or intellectual impairment (Lewis et al., 2022). Vulnerable populations face a higher risk of illnesses, which are consequently attributed to lack of access to healthcare, economic instability, and poor living conditions (Ernstmeyer & Christman, 2022).

Lack of healthcare is often paralleled with lack of medical insurance (Zieff et al., 2020). The United States Census Bureau reported 310 million people, or 92%, living in America had health insurance for either part or the entire year in 2024, with 66.1% having private coverage (Bunch & Ketema, 2025). While insurance is designed to provide affordable health coverage for medical expenses and needs, 36% of Americans forwent getting insurance because of the cost, and 43% of Americans are not compliant with their prescriptions due to lack of affordability (Sparks et al., 2026). These statistics are even more alarming for sexually minoritized groups, such as LGBTQ+ populations who could benefit from medication that reduces the risk of contracting sexually transmitted viruses, diseases and infections.

The challenges surrounding affordable medical insurance impacts people of all backgrounds; people with compromised health conditions are at a higher risk. In consideration of populates who are considered inferior—based on age race, gender, sexual, cultural and/or ethnic identity—are more susceptible to mistreatment and lack of adequate care (Sabater Miriam et al., 2025). When working with vulnerable populations, cultural safety must be emphasized and practiced (Mkandawire-Valhmu, 2018). Cultural safety explores the impact of the various societal components that contribute to the inequitable power balances between vulnerable and dominant groups and consciously acknowledge the ways in which vulnerable people and communities experience disparities in economic, educational and healthcare structures. The goal is for those who are considered vulnerable to receive access to services and resources that do not further dehumanize and compromise their well-being (Mkandawire-Valhmu, 2018).

Marginalized Groups

The ideology of superiority and inferiority—as mentioned earlier—is a contributing factor in how the U.S society reinforces groups of people being marginalized (Stepney, 2022). Marginalization refers to specific groups of people being excluded or hindered from accessing opportunities, resources, and rights that are granted to the dominant group(s) (Stepney, 2022). These opportunities also include the financial stability that precludes economic trauma, housing uncertainty, structural violence and the discriminant presumptions helping professionals tend to make when vulnerable populates have diverse, yet intersectional deficits.

Vulnerable populations are also marginalized because they are constantly met with microaggressions, harassment, discrimination and unfair/unequal treatment based on a feature of their identity that is considered undesirable in social environments consumed by privilege (Stepney, 2022). Consequently, people of marginalized groups struggle navigating in a world in which they are facing mistreatment in a multitude of ways, increasing the likelihood of psychological, emotional, and physiological disruptions to their emotional well-being, distress and loneliness (Verissimo et al., 2021).

There are people of racial and cultural identities that have been historically marginalized, which reinforces the notion that they have less worth than those who are considered privileged. Furthermore, these historically marginalized identities experience intergenerational trauma, with an early and repetitious introduction to mistreatment in educational systems.

Black and Hispanic Students

The United States public school system was designed to provide access to a free, quality education for all students, but structural barriers have presented extreme challenges for certain student demographics. Black and Hispanic students, who have represented a large percentage of the student population enrolled in public schools, have not only faced a high level of discrimination, but have also experienced inequities that has hindered opportunities for successful outcomes. From elementary schools, where students could excel through gifted education, to high school options of taking honors, AP and dual enrollment courses, Black and Hispanic students have faced restrictions that has led to the underrepresentation of marginalized students in courses of high rigor (Young et al., 2024).

The immediate consequences, including negative learning experiences, are seldom considered as the antecedent that results in higher drop-out rates for marginalized students. However, the long-term consequences of marginalization in public schools is evident through lower percentage of college graduates, wage disparities, limited employment options, and harsh living conditions and weakened health (Blanden et. al., 2023). Black and Hispanic students are more likely to be diagnosed with a learning disability or deficient in the English language, and less likely to recommended for advanced opportunities (ASCA, 2018). Even in schools where the opportunity to take advantage of accelerated courses, Black and Hispanic students are less likely to register in advanced courses because of teacher implicit bias (Anderson, 2023). Historically and currently, Black and Latinx students in U.S. public schools have experienced racial and implicit bias in a way that has been detrimental to their academic achievement, college and career readiness, and overall mental health (Rutledge & Smith-Durkin, 2025).

When reflecting on the impact of economic trauma, one must consider the early exposure racially marginalized experience in school systems. The systemic racism Black, Hispanic, and other racial minoritized groups face excludes these groups from opportunities that could increase generational wealth, provide equitable access to healthcare and a lifestyle that could lead to longevity (Stopforth et al., 2022). However, there are educational policies designed to condone exclusionary practices, promote harsh disciplinary measures and biased decision-making from those put in positions to maintain wealth and privilege (Chittom & Walter, 2024). The marginalization of Black and Hispanic students in education is synonymous with the denial of basic human rights, and it's direct impact on our economy reinforces economic trauma and structural violence (Rafa, 2019).

LGBTQ+ Populations

Black and Latinx students/adults are not the only populations impacted by societal and systemic discrimination. Poor mental and behavioral health among school aged children has substantially affected—and been affected by—school settings, with very little mental health resources, yet 1 in 3 suicide-related behaviors were transpired by a student identified as lesbian, gay, bisexual and questioning (LGBTQ+) (Verlenden, 2024). Additionally, 9% of LGBTQ+ students reported being disciplined for their sexual identity. The discriminant behaviors targeted towards the LGBTQ+ population extends itself beyond the school setting, as the higher rates of mental health disorders, substance abuse, suicide and reported experiences of hate crimes are also attributed to the various denial of their civil rights (Ernstmeyer & Christman, 2022).

Members of the LGBTQ+ community also experience higher rates of poverty (22%) in comparison to their straight counterparts (16%), experience lower pay wages (4% for LGBTQ+ men and 13% for LGBTQ+ women), and higher unemployment rates (22%) as well (HRC, 2022). This, coupled with the research on LGBTQ+ populates and medical insurance, is a prime example of how economic trauma and structural violence detrimentally impact marginalized groups.

It is documented that healthcare settings discriminate against LGBTQ+ people, which is a compromise to their physical health (Mirza & Rooney, 2018). The fear of being unable to take care of one's basic needs while being discriminated against for one's sexual identity can increase the likelihood of the refusal to seek medical care, while suffering from psychological distress (Mirza & Rooney, 2018). Considering the blatant disparities between LGBTQ+ and non-LGBTQ+ people, it should be no surprise that anyone who is racially minoritized and part of the community faces even more discriminant practices—pushing them further into poverty and trauma (HRC, 2022).

INTERSECTIONALITY

Intersectionality refers to the multiple overlapping social identities that shape the experiences people have (Bauer et al., 2025). People can identify by race and gender, sexual identity and ableness, age and socioeconomic status, and/or anything that one believes impact the way they are viewed, as well as the way they view the world (Osman, 2019). All humans have multiple identities that can either dictate the amount of influence and power one has, or illustrate the compounded inequities marginalized populations face at the discriminant standards designed to keep people oppressed. Women and people of color face obstacles in the workforce, including wage gaps, that are heightened when these demographics lack the adequate education to pursue careers that yield a higher income (Niles & Harris-Bowlsbey, 2016).

While women and people of color are two groups that have been marginalized in the United States, the level of oppression black women have suffered is far greater. Black women have been stereotyped in a way that is comparable to white women and black men, but unique in that both groups have not experienced the level of discrimination black women have faced (Rosenthal and Lobel, 2016). The stereotypical portrayals, such as "mammies," "sapphires," and "jezebels," are viewed from a sexual, professional, and health standpoint as unattractive, masculine, poor, and uneducated (Rosenthal and Lobel, 2016). These beliefs perpetuate the racial and gender inequalities that black women have suffered—and forced to accept as the norm—in spaces such as school, healthcare, and work. Additionally, the long-term suffrage women of color endure as caregivers and victims of gender and racial discrimination perpetuates intergenerational trauma (El-Khalil et al., 2025). Women of color face mistreatment that results in psychological warfare that is then passed on to their children through exposure and reactions towards hardships, furthering the structural violence and economic trauma they are struggling to escape (El-Khalil et al., 2025).

LABOR EXPLOITATION

Labor exploitation can be defined as an approach to reinforce a capitalist system of economic growth through various forms of inequalities based on social class (Swidler, 2018). Labor exploitation is rooted in the philosophical ideals of Karl Max, who believed that a fraction of workers produce good to benefit the working class, and a larger portion of the produced goods go to the elitist class of society that do not participate in any form of labor, but benefit greatly from the labor performed (Kurz & Salvadori, 2023). The concept of labor exploitation commenced with acts of primitive accumulation, slavery and housework, but has now been replaced with normalized harsh conditions that entail wage workers receiving less wages for work that is conveniently considered responsibilities outside of the wage hours (Swidler, 2018).

This can range from employers staying on the clock until the next shift workers arrive, checking emails after hours, on weekends and during vacation, or even finishing paperwork outside of scheduled work hours (Swidler, 2018). The loophole in labor exploitation benefits employers, at the detriment of employees. This immoral practice further disenfranchises employees and puts them at greater risk of experiencing economic trauma, and it further marginalizes those of lower socioeconomic status. Additionally, there are two major problems concerning labor exploitation today: 1) there are weak labor policies in the South that result in wage theft and discriminatory practices and 2) both documented and undocumented immigrant workers are the most vulnerable populations of workers in the United States (Childers, 2023; Anderson & James, 2025).

Southern Economic Development Model

Rooted in racism dated back to the 17th century—in result of the Transatlantic slave trade to justify enslaving African and forcing them to inhumane labor, poor conditions and mistreatment (Osman, 2019)—the Southern Economic Development model was designed as a tactic to maintain access to cheap labor performed by Black people after the ending of slavery (Childers, 2023). This tactic entailed a mutually beneficial agreement between Southern politicians and wealthy businessmen to attract more businesses in the South by enforcing low wages and taxes, minimal labor protection laws, and minimal regulations against businesses (Childers, 2023).

Consequently, Mississippi, Louisiana, Alabama, Tennessee and South Carolina do not enforce a state minimum wage, despite there being a federal minimum wage of $7.25 per hour (Childers, 2023). Additionally, this model has had an adverse effect on the labor market in the south, as economic health across the South is low, and child poverty is up 20.9% (Childers, 2023).

Undocumented & Documented Immigrant Workers

While the economic development model of the South was designed to further marginalized Blacks, it was also designed to benefit from exploitative labor performed by Brown people as well (Childers, 2023). Undocumented workers make up 4.9% of the U.S. Workforce, representing 41.9%, 27.2% and 18.6% of home health aides, personal care aides and all occupations, respectively (Anderson & James, 2025). Additionally, as largely represented immigrant workers are in low wage positions, they are even largely victims of labor exploitation through the suspicious of wage theft (Anderson & James, 2025). Low wages coupled with challenging work conditions yield increased risks of workplace fatality (Anderson & James, 2025). More alarming is the disproportionate percentage of immigrant women who represent 87.2% of home health aides and 79% of personal care aides, while representing 46.9% of the U.S. workforce (Anderson & James, 2025).

The implications associated with having intersectional marginalized identities—gender and culture—while being exploited on the job are psychologically harmful to immigrant women, as they are less likely to report wage theft out of fear of deportation and further mistreatment, while being retraumatized through economic disparity (Anderson & James, 2025).

HOUSING INSECURITY

There is a strong correlation between income and housing, as low wage earners and victims of labor exploitation are also more likely to experience housing insecurity (Chun et al., 2023). Defined Paredes et al. (2024) as living space that is either overpopulated, unsafe, unaffordable or lacks unmet housing needs (p 2), housing insecurity made a negatively large impact on Black and Latinx populations at the height of Covid-19 (Chun et al., 2023). Roughly 20.5 million people experienced job losses due to the pandemic, and research demonstrated that overall, Black and

Latinx workers suffered immensely, as they generally had less savings and was less prepared for a global economic crisis (Chun et al., 2023).

However, there is growing concern regarding the housing status of older Black and Latinx adults, as 1 out of 3 adults over the age 65 experience at least one form of housing insecurity, but nearly 3 out 4 Black and Latinx adults over the age of 65 experienced at least one form of housing insecurity (Paredes et al., 2024). Some of the indicators associated with housing insecurity among older adults can be attributed to cognitive impairment, frailty—such as disability or injury—income, and poor neighborhood conditions, to name a few (Paredes et al., 2024).

The trials older adults face being susceptible to homelessness reveal an undertone of concern about the incessant cycle economic trauma presents. Vulnerable and marginalized people experiencing discrimination in schools, healthcare, workplace and other places are not only likely to experience home insecurity as older adults, but they are also likely to perpetuate intergenerational trauma and structural violence (Hargrave et al., 2024). Furthermore, these unfortunate circumstances are social drivers of poor physical, mental and psychological health (Kirkbride et al., 2024). Poor health and poor life experiences sustain poverty-stricken lives for the vulnerable and marginalized.

POVERTY

Poverty is a social and intersectional concept used to describe income deprivation (Clark et al., 2020; Foss-Kelly et al., 2017). Poverty is often categorized by thresholds or through statistics, with alarming details pertaining to who is impacted the most by poverty. In 2021, the U.S. determined the poverty line to consist of an individual income below $12,880, or below $26,500 for a family of 4 (Office of Disease Prevention and Health Promotion; 2023). Women, African American, people with disabilities, and those with intersecting marginalized identities experience poverty at higher risks than their counterparts (Clark et al., 2020), noting the profound social determinants of health associated with poverty (Ballo & Tribe, 2023; Foss-Kelly et al., 2017). The negative stereotypes regarding women, black people and people with disabilities are reinforced for poverty-stricken groups, as it is assumed that they are lazy, uneducated and/or poor work ethic (Foss-Kelly et al., 2017); in fact, there are mental health challenges that reinforce a harmful repetitive cycle of impoverishment for the vulnerable groups of people most afflicted by poverty.

Marginalized groups impacted by poverty are capitulated by distress, mental health risks, mortality, schizophrenia and generational poverty (Ballo & Tribe, 2023; Clark et al., 2020). These health implications are magnified when individuals have marginalized intersecting identities (Foss-Kelly et al., 2017). For individuals who suffer long-term from poverty, there is a less likelihood of overcoming these constraints because they lack the resources required to take care of their mental health, which would lead to greater success in other areas. Their mental state is reinforced by their current circumstances, creating a vicious negative perception of self (Foss-Kelly et al., 2017). Poverty is not just a negative circumstance some people undergo, it is a compromise to one's survival, as food, housing and limited access to resources creates a constant source of worry with consequential outcomes, such as economic trauma and structural violence (Ballo & Tribe, 2023).

FINANCIAL PRECARITY

The financial insecurity people face at the discriminant hands of poverty is tantamount to the uncertainty of one's financial future—even when employed. Financial precarity is defined as the constant worry over one's financial status (Meuris & Gladstone, 2023). The interlocking oppression between labor exploitation and financial precarity can cause extreme distress on marginalized people because people who are concerned about their financial stability tend to remain employed at a job due to economic dependency (Meuris & Leana, 2018).

People of vulnerable and marginalized identities are often expected—or forced—to work low-wage earning jobs that are not enough to cover all of their living expenses; this constant state of uncertainty pertaining to one's financial needs can impair cognitive abilities and result in emotional suppression, which is correlative to an employee's work performance (Meuris & Leana, 2018).

As prices for necessities such as food and housing continue to soar, the constrains and harmful experiences marginalized populations heighten. Social determinants of health—racism, addiction, inaccessible mental health resources, malnutrition, and interpersonal violence—will additionally be misperceived to negatively stereotype those most affected by financial precarity (Whittle et al., 2020).

CONSIDERATIONS

Employment exploitation, economic instability and housing disparity carry a range of physical, social and psychological trauma including chronic stress, anxiety, impaired decision making, reduced self-regulation, consumption of unhealthy food, lack of adequate exercise and other unhealthy behaviors, such as substance abuse, violence and self-harm (Williams & Etkins, 2021). There are negative biological effects associated with these outcomes, such as inflammation, premature aging, compromised functioning of one's immune system and infections (Jones et al., 2025).

Given the mental health implications that parallel vulnerable populations afflicted by employment, economic and financial strains, attention must also be given to children of impoverished families (Edgar et al., 2025). The systemic structure of US public schools is rooted in racism, trauma and inequities (Rutledge & Susko, 2023). US public school implemented strategies and policies that further marginalized minorities and provided less opportunities to close the achievement gap (Kholi et al., 2017).

Cultural awareness is a necessity when addressing the needs of marginalized students whose existence in the very setting that is reinforcing marginalization is rooted in trauma (Rutledge & Susko, 2023). This also includes recognizing when biases are taking place and actively addressing the concerns on behalf of your students to create safe spaces for them to learn and be prepared for life after school. Without this awareness, counselors and educators will only perpetuate the systemic barriers that are embedded in US schools and other areas of a child's life.

THE ROLE OF A COUNSELOR

The level of trauma vulnerable populations is exposed to and experience at the inequitable and harmful discriminant practices is both overwhelming and alarming. Trauma cannot be avoided; it can only be addressed. Additionally, the response to trauma varies by person, perceived impact and duration (Duffey & Haberstroh, 2020). Ratts et.al. (2016) encapsulates some of the conceptions that are key in acknowledging the multi-faceted components that values, embraces and supports the awareness of vulnerable and marginalized groups. A counseling professional should be intentionally inclusive, cognizant of barriers that impede on the appropriate and accurate representation of a marginalized group, and actively committed to developing strategies that are indicative of the advocacy of those in need. Cultural awareness is a necessity when addressing the needs of marginalized and vulnerable populations because it provides a deeper knowledge of the trauma they are constantly subjected to, existing in systems that reinforce marginalization (Rutledge & Susko, 2023). Counselors should engage in care that "consider intersectionality of identities that define systems of inequalities" (O'Hara et. al., 2021)

TRAUMA-INFORMED CARE

Given the many effects associated with employment, economic and housing strains, in addition to the mass percentage of vulnerable populations traumatically impacted by at least one of the barriers, it is important for counselors to consider practices that are culturally sensitive and competent to the diverse needs of those impacted by insecurity. Trauma-informed care requires mental health professionals to have a level of compassion for the different components that marginalize groups of people, instead of reinforcing it through preconceived thoughts about the actions, appearances and feelings of people.

Trauma-informed care is an approach that requires mental health professionals to understand the barriers and trauma individuals have faced, anticipate traumatic responses, possess the ability to respond to the issues in a gentle and non-judgmental manner, and be able to apply that understanding with a modified approach to meet the diverse and vulnerable needs of those who experienced trauma (Edgar et al., 2025).

Trauma-formed care also requires mental health professionals to be flexible in how services are designed and delivered, as trauma survivors may not be ready to fully engage in the healing process, may be guarded, feeling disempowered (Edgar et al., 2025). Establishing trust and allowing individuals to choose the pace in which they undergo healing and treatment are some key indicators that an individual may be receptive to the process. However, trauma-informed care requires a level of cultural sensitivity, competence and awareness to the types of traumas individuals face, as well as the impact one's marginalized identity(ies) may have reinforced within their traumatic experiences (Edgar et al., 2025). While this framework serves as the foundation for traumatic response, applying this framework with a cultural lens will strengthen the approach used to support vulnerable populations.

Relational Cultural Theory as a Trauma-Informed Approach

Relational-Cultural Theory (RCT) emphasizes mutuality, openness and connectivity as tenets of a healthy relationship between people. Additionally, the cultural aspect of RCT provides an awareness of "cultural privilege" and sheds light on the aspects of societal values that emphasize separation amongst people, compromising the human growth in totality (Jordan, 2024). Empathy is the core of traumatic responses. This reaffirms the relevance of RCT as a core theoretical approach for providing prevention and intervention for anyone afflicted by an event or experience that has a detrimental impact on his or her life.

Understanding that authenticity and mutual empathic connections—tenets of RCT—are the skills that can enhance or harm the healing process is what feels familiar as a counselor education (Duffey & Haberstroh, 2020). The relational aspect feels familiar because of the neurobiological effects human connections has on people experiencing any form of trauma. Relational connectedness can heal and empower people to recover from distress and create a new normal (Duffey & Haberstroh, 2020).

Additionally, assessing an individual's risk and threat parallels one's connectedness to another person, and this is equally essential—as well as familiar—as a mental health professional (Edgar et al, 2025). RCT, empathy and human connectedness are not just therapeutic skills; these approaches are measures mental health professionals can take to ensure safety and care for vulnerable populations (Duffey & Haberstroh, 2020). Moreover, these approaches are sensitive to the circumstances vulnerable and marginalized populations experience due to the economic trauma and structural violence imposed on them (Duffey & Haberstroh, 2020).

ECONOMIC JUSTICE

Economic disparity exists because there are people who believe they are of a superior group, and to remain that way, other people must receive less (Singh, 2025; Stigiltz, 2017). This connotation is reinforced through a faulty capitalist system meant to denigrate the existence of other humans, based on their appearance, ability and/or identity. Unfortunately, this system has created a mass of people incapable of thriving, as the lack of financial equity has created health concerns that not only impair and shorten their quality of life, but perpetuates dysfunction, lack of safety, and generational trauma (Stigiltz, 2017). Furthermore, it jeopardizes the economic stability of our country when the larger portion of the U.S. population is uneducated, incapable of contributing to our labor force market—making us less advanced and competitive in the global economy market—and unprotected (Singh, 2025).

The most soluble resolution is the promotion and advocacy of economic justice. As a nation, America can achieve economic justice by first eliminating the concept that individualized wealth is acceptable (Tolstoy, 2023). Creating a large wealth gap between vulnerable and marginalized groups also creates a divide in societal values, as well as a lack of considerations for social issues that negatively impact the less fortuned (Tolstoy, 2023). Programs such as Diversity, Equity & Inclusion (DEI), affirmative action and equal employment opportunities (EEO) not only provides employment opportunities to diverse workers, and decreases the poverty gap, but it also provides a more diverse work setting that consists of diverse set of skills—enhancing the overall performance of an organization (Pink-Harper et al., 2017).

A more diverse workforce results in a more work-friendly environment that increases job, retention, job satisfaction and a positive workplace culture (Pink-Harper et al., 2017). Considering vulnerable populations and people with marginalized identities already have a history of working above their pay, the negative stereotypes about the work ethic and abilities of those historically oppressed can be debunked, and more attention can be placed on the awareness of social issues that range from poverty to environmental change (Pink-Harper et al., 2017; Tolstoy, 2023).

CALL FOR ACTION

The exertion marginalized people and communities suffer from the multitude of inequalities invoked by U.S. societal standards is often misclassified as resilience (Williams & Etkins, 2021). Unfortunately, this perception overlooks and undermines the level of loneliness, mental health challenges and real life struggles marginalized people face daily (Jones et al., 2025). Labor exploitation, poverty, housing insecurity and financial precarity are all perpetuated by structural, discriminant behaviors designed to hold people in a constant cycle of oppression, and this is a public concern (Bauer et al., 2025; Keast et al., 2025; Verissimo et al., 2021).

It is important for counselors of diverse backgrounds to work together and create a continuum of care for all populations. Each type of counselor brings a unique strength and consideration for clients that collaboratively will enhance the lives of vulnerable and marginalized populations. Specifically creating a continuum of care will decrease barriers that make healthcare, economic resources, housing and mental health and educational services less accessible or less quality (Mehrotra & Swami, 2018).

Additionally, counselors should be advocating for the diverse needs of vulnerable and marginalized people through policy reform (Baker, 2025). Counselors can work in or alongside community-based organizations geared towards providing social services for those in need, assess the level of needs, and evaluate the capacity of needs through data collection (Reid et al., 2022). This leads to the reporting the gaps and inequities that must be met to decrease the public health concerns that negatively impact the members of impoverished communities and force the government to change the structure of systems that continuously marginalized the disadvantageous (Reid et al., 2022)

CONCLUSION

Economic trauma associated with employment, housing and financial instability are rooted in racist practices, undermines vulnerable and marginalized populations, and reinforces inequalities that are perpetuated by biased, societal norms. These disparities are also reinforced throughout education, healthcare and the legal system, emphasizing structural discrimination that is need of reform (Mkandawire-Valhmu, 2018). Vulnerable groups, namely Black Americans, documented and undocumented immigrants, LGBTQ+ people, elderly people, and children of impoverished homes face higher risks of psychological, emotional and physical trauma that can result in dire health conditions, feelings of disempowerment, loneliness, and loss of hope (Stepney, 2022).

Trauma-informed care is a strong approach for meeting the diverse needs of vulnerable people and communities based on its premise of understanding, flexibility and awareness (Edgar et. al., 2025). However, trauma-informed care with a cultural lens can equip mental health professionals with cultural competency and sensitivity necessary for working with vulnerable populations who've repeatedly experienced trauma (Duffey & Haberstroh, 2020). By working with vulnerable populations using a trauma-informed approach with a relational and cultural theoretical lens, individuals can feel empowered to recover from their trauma, increase a sense of hope, and work alongside mental healthcare professionals to remove systemic barriers that hinder equality for all.

Case Vignettes

Case Vignette # 1

Vera, a Mexican-born woman living in America with her three children, is having a hard time coping with life after separating from her children's father. Vera's oldest child Carlos, 26, lives at home with his girlfriend; Vera often relies on Carlos to help out with her 16-year-old son, Jose and 13-year-old daughter, Olivia. Vera does not speak English and works as an hourly server at a local diner during evening hours. When Vera gets off of work at the diner, she has enough time to try and get her younger two children up to go to school, and transition to her second job as a cashier at the local supermarket. However, Vera's middle son has not been going to school daily, and she does not have a working vehicle to take her youngest daughter to school.

Vera receives phone calls and letters in English about her children's attendance and grades, but does not understand what the consequences of her children missing school—despite her oldest son's explanation. Since Vera works non-salaried jobs, she does not have insurance or sick days. Vera called off from work after receiving a phone call from Olivia's school counselor that Olivia threatened to kill herself. Vera received resources of local places to take Olivia for an evaluation, but Vera can't afford to take her to a therapy center because without insurance, an evaluation is $300 and weekly sessions are $150 per hour. With Medicaid, Vera can take Olivia to see a therapist for $15 per session, but Vera does not know how to apply for Medicaid to receive health insurance and/or food stamps—now that the finances that were once contributing to the home has reduced significantly.

Vera has now lost a full day of pay at the supermarket and her supervisor has now reduced her work hours from 40 hours to 15 hours out of spite that Vera called off at the last minute. Vera now has to figure out how to make up the wages lost within the next two weeks, when the rent is due, and if she doesn't get Olivia seen by a therapist within the next three days, the school will contact Social Services to report child neglect. Jose's recent suspension from fighting in school has led to him becoming more aggressive at home, and she is constantly in fear that he is going to either report her for being an illegal citizen or physically harm her. Vera is sad, scared and frustrated.

Questions for Consideration

1. Given Vera's circumstances, which action takes priority, and what actions must be addressed later?
2. Did Vera's supervisor violate any labor laws after reducing her work hours? Can Vera prove this potential violation?
3. What possible ways is Vera's work schedule causing intergenerational stress?
4. How might a therapist work with Vera to address her growing concerns and needs regarding Olivia's mental health, housing and financial stability?
5. Does Olivia and/or Jose's schools have an obligation to assist Vera with her challenges? In what ways can they help?

Case Vignette # 2

Kiyah, 42, returned to her hometown to live with her 67-year-old mother after escaping an abusive relationship with the father of her 10-year-old daughter, Kimmie, and unborn son. Upon returning home, Kiyah and her mother argue weekly about Kiyah finding work and "getting out of her space" despite the fact Kiyah is 34 weeks pregnant, jobless, and slated to be on maternity leave soon. The stress is too great for Kiyah, and she decides to move into a homeless shelter with her daughter. A week later, Kiyah enrolls Kimmie at the local school, where Kimmie is having a hard time adjusting. Meanwhile, Kiyah gives birth to a premature baby boy who remains hospitalized for several weeks.

In between traveling to the hospital, Kimmie's school, and the shelter, Kiyah's finds her belongings are constantly missing. Additionally, the shelter told Kiyah she has ten weeks to find a job, as there is a waiting list of pregnant women seeking shelter's resources. Kiyah's phone is now turned off, so she is not receiving phone calls about Kimmie's reluctance to do schoolwork, eat, or participate. Kimmie is also being teased about her hygiene and attire. Kiyah eventually finds a job as a secretary at an auto dealer, but she constantly receives unwanted romantic propositions from married salesmen. Kiyah is trying her best to politely decline in fear of losing her job, but the advances are overwhelming. Kiyah must also secure housing before she is removed from the shelter.

Kiyah is feeling the weight of not having support for her children, her strained relationship with her mother, and her inability to help Kimmie with school. Her son is slated to be released from the hospital soon, and daycares are full. The most affordable apartment Kiyah can find would consume 75% of her monthly income, leaving her unable to pay for safe childcare. Kiyah enters a counseling center in tears, requesting to speak with someone on staff about her concerns.

Questions for Consideration:

1. What systemic barriers does the shelter create for Kiyah, a woman who does not have secure childcare for premature infant?
2. What trauma and/or financial stress could Kiyah's mother be dealing with that contributed to her hostility towards Kiyah?
3. How might the behaviors of Kiyah's colleagues be viewed as exploitation of Kiyah's circumstances?
4. As the mental health therapist, what challenges would you address first and why?
5. What resources could you provide for Kiyah and her children?

Case Vignette # 3

Nassim, a 23-year-old Muslim born male from Iran, has been homeless for the last two years. After coming out to his father as bisexual during his sophomore year in college, his father stopped paying his tuition and discontinued all communication with Nassim. To adjust to his new responsibilities—paying for college and housing—Nassim became a residence hall director and worked at the student café during the day. Nassim struggled managing the responsibilities of two jobs while attending school. To alleviate some stress, he decided to attend a nearby college party one Friday night. After having one drink, Nassim became very disoriented and passed out. He woke up to a man sexually assaulting him and was unable to fight off his attacker. Nassim was too afraid and embarrassed to report the assault, so he kept the assault to himself.

Every day Nassim replayed the assault in his head, and he tried going to the counseling center at his college—despite his cultural views about counseling. Nassim left the counseling center in tears after reviewing the intake paperwork and noticing the questions about sexual identity and history of abuse. Nassim tried his best to live "a normal life" but was fired from his residence director position for punching a male in the face who he mistook for his assaulter, as well as his café position when he was caught stealing food. Nassim eventually stopped going to class because he had nowhere to live and no money for food and transportation. After dropping out of school, Nassim tried to keep a job, but he would either quit or get fired for his angry outbursts, late arrival at work, or insubordination.

After being fired from his fifth job, Nassim went to a bar without any money to afford a drink. Nassim ordered a few drinks and tried to leave the bar without paying. The bartender tried to stop Nassim, and Nassim attacked the bartender until the bartender became unconscious. Law enforcement came to arrest Nassim; he became increasingly irate and began yelling "rape". Law enforcement brought Nassim to the hospital to speak with a crisis worker, and Nassim refused to speak in English. The crisis worker found a colleague who spoke native Farsi, and this crisis worker was able to begin the assessment.

Questions for Consideration:

1. In what ways is Nassim's intersectional identities marginalized? Does his father's disownment further marginalize Nassim?
2. What does Nassim's perception of the intake assessment say about the American process for counseling services? How can the paperwork be modified to be more welcoming of diverse clients?
3. What are some potential reasons Nassim was only willing to speak in his native language after being arrested?
4. Are there any missed opportunities for culturally competent, trauma-informed interventions that could have prevented Nassim's current circumstances?
5. What internal biases might a trauma-informed therapist possess when working with a client like Nassim?

REFERENCES

American School Counselor Association (ASCA). (2018). *The School Counselor and Equity for All Students*. Author.

Anderson, K. P. (2023). Biased Opportunities: The Role of Implicit and Explicit Bias in Advanced Placement and Dual Enrollment. *Educational Evaluation and Policy Analysis*, *46*(4), 735–763. DOI: 10.3102/01623737231192487

Anderson, S., & James, R. (2025). *4 charts on Immigrant Worker Exploitation in America*. Inequality.org. https://inequality.org/article/charts-immigrant-worker-exploitation/

Baker, J. (2025). *The overlapping roots of Mental Health Disparities: Poverty, racism, and trauma as Social Determinants - Behavioral Health News*. Behavioral Health News. https://behavioralhealthnews.org/the-overlapping-roots-of-mental-health-disparities-poverty-racism-and-trauma-as-social-determinants/

Ballo, E., & Tribe, R. (2023). Therapeutic work with clients living in poverty. *The International Journal of Social Psychiatry*, *69*(4), 1043–1050. DOI: 10.1177/00207640221139798 PMID: 36609182

Bauer, K. L., Eskew, S., Tung, G., Leiferman, J. A., Fort, M. P., McManus, B. M., & Johnson-Koenke, R. A. (2025). Marginalization and Intersectionality in Adults' Relationship to Society Explain Increasing Loneliness: A Critical Realist Lens on Thematic Narrative Inquiry. *International Journal of Qualitative Methods*, *24*, 16094069251346264. Advance online publication. DOI: 10.1177/16094069251346264

Blanden, J., Doepke, M., & Stuhler, J. (2023). Educational inequality. In E. A. Hanushek, S. Machin, & L. Woessmann (Eds.), *Handbook of the Economics of Education* (pp. 405-497). (Handbook of the Economics of Education; Vol. 6). Elsevier B.V. https://doi.org/DOI: 10.1016/bs.hesedu.2022.11.003

Bunch, L., & Ketema, H. (2025). *Health insurance coverage in the United States: 2024*. Census.gov. https://www.census.gov/library/publications/2025/demo/p60-288.html

Childers, C. (2023). *Rooted in racism and economic exploitation: The failed Southern Economic Development Model*. Economic Policy Institute. https://www.epi.org/publication/rooted-in-racism/

Chittom, L., & Walter, A. (2024). *Zero-tolerance policies in schools: Overview.* EBSCO. https://www.ebsco.com/research-starters/education/zero-tolerance-policies-schools-overview#about-the-author

Chun, Y., Roll, S., Miller, S., Lee, H., Larimore, S., & Grinstein-Weiss, M. (2023). Racial and Ethnic Disparities in Housing Instability During the COVID-19 Pandemic: The Role of Assets and Income Shocks. *Journal of Economics, Race, and Policy, 6*(2), 63–81. DOI: 10.1007/s41996-022-00109-5 PMID: 36474600

Clark, M., Ausloos, C., Delaney, C., Waters, L., Salpietro, L., & Tippett, H. (2020). Best Practices for Counseling Clients Experiencing Poverty: A Grounded Theory. *Journal of Counseling and Development, 98*(3), 283–294. DOI: 10.1002/jcad.12323

Duffey, T., & Haberstroh, S. (2020). *Introduction to crisis and trauma counseling.* American Counseling Association.

Edgar, N. E., MacLean, S. E., Jormand, M., Paranjkhoo, P., & Hatcher, S. (2025). Designing a trauma informed service to deliver trauma therapy with people experiencing homelessness: A qualitative study. *BMC Health Services Research, 25*(1), 1350. DOI: 10.1186/s12913-025-13428-8 PMID: 41074101

El-Khalil, C., Tudor, D. C., & Nedelcea, C. (2025). Impact of intergenerational trauma on second-generation descendants: A systematic review. *BMC Psychology, 13*(1), 668. DOI: 10.1186/s40359-025-03012-4 PMID: 40597246

Ernstmeyer, K., & Christman, E. (2022). *Nursing: Mental Health and Community Concepts.* Open Resources for Nursing (Open RN). Chippewa Valley Technical College.

Foss-Kelly, L. L., Generali, M. M., & Kress, V. E. (2017). Counseling Strategies for Empowering People Living in Poverty: The I-CARE Model. *Journal of Multicultural Counseling and Development, 45*(3), 201–213. DOI: 10.1002/jmcd.12074

Hargrave, A. S., Garcia, C. M., Lightfoot, M., Handley, M. A., Weeks, J., Olsen, P., Knight, K. R., & Kushel, M. B. (2024). "We Remember the Pain": A qualitative study of intergenerational trauma among older adults experiencing homelessness in the HOPE HOME study. *Journal of Social Distress and the Homeless, 33*(1), 103–111. DOI: 10.1080/10530789.2022.2080793 PMID: 38948456

HRC. (2022). *The wage gap among LGBTQ+ workers in the United States.* https://www.hrc.org/resources/the-wage-gap-among-lgbtq-workers-in-the-united-states#:~:text=Economic%20Disparities%20Faced%20by%20the,its%20basic%20necessities%20and%20resources

Jones, M. N., Elliott, K., Sherman, S. N., Falade, E., Clark, R. L., Lipps, L., Hill-Williams, L., Williams, C., Copeland, K. A., Beck, A. F., Unaka, N., Burkhardt, M. C., & Corley, A. M. S. (2025). "Racism Happens Every Day, All the Time": Black Families' Outpatient Experiences of Racism Across a Large Pediatric System. *Academic Pediatrics*, *25*(1), 102566. Advance online publication. DOI: 10.1016/j.acap.2024.08.011 PMID: 39191371

Jordan, J. V. (2024). *The development of relational-cultural theory*. Jean Baker Miller Training Institute. https://www.wcwonline.org/JBMTI-Site/the-development-of-relational-cultural-theory

Keast, R., Lengyell, M., Finnigan, C., Brown, J., & Jay, M. (2025). Barriers to Mental Health Care for Low-Income Clients As Perceived By Counsellors. *Journal for Social Action in Counseling and Psychology*, *17*(1), 2–21. DOI: 10.33043/r23873x5

Kirkbride, J. B., Anglin, D. M., Colman, I., Dykxhoorn, J., Jones, P. B., Patalay, P., Pitman, A., Soneson, E., Steare, T., Wright, T., & Griffiths, S. L. (2024). The social determinants of mental health and disorder: Evidence, prevention and recommendations. *World Psychiatry; Official Journal of the World Psychiatric Association (WPA)*, *23*(1), 58–90. DOI: 10.1002/wps.21160 PMID: 38214615

Kurz, H. D., & Salvadori, N. (2023). Marx's concept of "exploitation" and the problem of measurement. *Journal of Economic Behavior & Organization*, *212*, 887–896. DOI: 10.1016/j.jebo.2023.06.016

Lewis, R. K., Martin, P. P., & Guzman, B. L. (2022). COVID-19 and vulnerable populations. *Journal of Community Psychology*, *50*(6), 2537–2541. DOI: 10.1002/jcop.22880 PMID: 35567541

Mehrotra, S., & Swami, N. (2018). Looking Beyond Distress: A Call for Spanning the Continuum of Mental Health Care. *Cureus*, *10*(6), e2815. DOI: 10.7759/cureus.2815 PMID: 30128219

Meuris, J., & Gladstone, J. (2023). Contextual Inequality in the Performance Costs of Financial Precarity. *Journal of Management*, *50*(3), 014920632311531. DOI: 10.1177/01492063231153136

Meuris, J., & Leana, C. (2018). The Price of Financial Precarity: Organizational Costs of Employees' Financial Concerns. *Organization Science*, *29*(3), 398–417. DOI: 10.1287/orsc.2017.1187

Mirza, S. A., & Rooney, C. (2018). *Discrimination prevents LGBTQ people from accessing health care - centerforamericanprogress*. Center for American Progresss. https://www.americanprogress.org/article/discrimination-prevents-lgbtq-people-accessing-health-care/

Mkandawire-Valhmu, L. (2018). *Cultural Safety, Healthcare and Vulnerable Populations: A Critical Theoretical Perspective* (1st ed.). Routledge., DOI: 10.4324/9781315708706

Niles, S., & Harris-Bowlsbey, J. (2016). *Career development interventions in the 21st century* (5th ed.). Pearson.

O'Hara, C., Chang, C. Y., & Giordano, A. L. (2021). Multicultural Competence in Counseling Research: The Cornerstone of Scholarship. *Journal of Counseling and Development*, *99*(2), 200–209. DOI: 10.1002/jcad.12367

Office of Disease Prevention and Health Promotion. (2023). *Poverty*. Poverty - Healthy People 2030. https://odphp.health.gov/healthypeople/priority-areas/social-determinants-health/literature-summaries/poverty

Osman, J. (2019). *Navigating intersectionality: how race, class, and gender overlap*. Enslow Publishing. https://ebookcentral.proquest.com/lib/jmu/detail.action?docID=5733748

Paredes, L. G., Wang, Y., Keene, D. E., Gill, T. M., & Becher, R. D. (2024). Population-based estimates of major forms of housing insecurity among community-living older Americans. *Journal of the American Geriatrics Society*, *72*(12), 3773–3783. DOI: 10.1111/jgs.19167 PMID: 39229863

Pink-Harper, S. A., Davis, R. S., & Burnside, R. (2017). "Justice for all": An examination of self-identified LGBT job satisfaction in the US federal workforce. *Canadian Journal of Administrative Sciences*, *34*(2), 182–197. DOI: 10.1002/cjas.1420

Rafa, A. (2019). *The Status of School Discipline in State Policy*. Education Commission of the States. www.ecs.org/the-status-of-school-discipline-in-state-policy

Reid, K., Odusanya, A., Lawrence, W., & Hastings, J. (2022). Commentary: An Equitable Approach to Serving Structurally Marginalized Communities. *Family & Community Health*, *45*(4), 215–217. DOI: 10.1097/FCH.0000000000000345 PMID: 35985021

Rosenthal, L., & Lobel, M. (2016). Stereotypes of Black American women related to sexuality and motherhood. *Psychology of Women Quarterly*, *40*(3), 414–427. DOI: 10.1177/0361684315627459 PMID: 27821904

Rutledge, M., Cameron, E., & Susko, J. (2023). *School Counselors as Antiracist and Social Justice Advocates. Foundations of school counseling: Innovation in professional practice*. Springer Publishing., DOI: 10.1891/9780826187536.0001

Rutledge, M. L., & Smith-Durkin, S. D. (2025). Antiracist School Counseling Advocacy Framework. *Professional School Counseling, 29*(1), 2156759X251340047. Advance online publication. DOI: 10.1177/2156759X251340047

Sabater Minarim, D., Morgan, K. M., Buckley, K., Riviere, P., Ochoa, C., Deshler, L. N., Duran, E. A., Mehtsun, W. T., Rose, B. S., & Banegas, M. P. (2025). Racial and Ethnic Disparities in Perceived Healthcare Discrimination and Health Outcomes: Racial and Ethnic Disparities in Perceived Healthcare Discrimination. *Journal of General Internal Medicine, 40*(11), 2548–2557. DOI: 10.1007/s11606-025-09627-y PMID: 40447985

Singh, R. P. (2025). Promoting Social and Economic Justice in Black Communities in the Current Anti-DEI Climate. *Societies (Basel, Switzerland), 15*(10), 280. DOI: 10.3390/soc15100280

Sparks, G., Lopes, L., Montero, A., Presiado, M., & Hamel, L. (2026). *Americans' challenges with health care costs*. KFF. https://www.kff.org/health-costs/americans-challenges-with-health-care-costs/

Stepney, S. (2022). Multicultural and diversity perspectives in art therapy: Transforming image into substance. .DOI: 10.1016/B978-0-12-824308-4.00010-7

Stopforth, S., Kapadia, D., Nazroo, J., & Bécares, L. (2022). The enduring effects of racism on health: Understanding direct and indirect effects over time. *SSM - Population Health, 19*, 101217. DOI: 10.1016/j.ssmph.2022.101217 PMID: 36091297

Swidler, E. (2018). Invisible Exploitation: How Capital Extracts Value Beyond Wage Labor. *Monthly Review (New York. 1949), 69*(10), 29–36. https://doi.org/ DOI: 10.14452/MR-069-10-2018-03_2

Tolstoy, A. (2023). Culture and Economic Justice in America. *Sustainability and Climate Change, 16*(1), 83–94. DOI: 10.1089/scc.2022.0066

Verissimo, A. D., Henley, N., Gee, G. C., Davis, C., & Grella, C. (2021). Homelessness and discrimination among US adults: The role of intersectionality. *Journal of Social Distress and the Homeless, 32*(1), 1–15. DOI: 10.1080/10530789.2021.1935650

Verlenden, J. V., Fodeman, A., Wilkins, N., Jones, S. E., Moore, S., Cornett, K., Sims, V., Saelee, R., & Brener, N. D. (2024). Mental health and suicide risk among high school students and protective factors—Youth Risk Behavior Survey, United States, 2023. *MMWR Supplements*, *73*(4), 73. DOI: 10.15585/mmwr.su7304a9 PMID: 39378246

Whittle, H. J., Leddy, A. M., Shieh, J., Tien, P. C., Ofotokun, I., Adimora, A. A., Turan, J. M., Frongillo, E. A., Turan, B., & Weiser, S. D. (2020). Precarity and health: Theorizing the intersection of multiple material-need insecurities, stigma, and illness among women in the United States. *Social science & medicine (1982)*, *245*, 112683. DOI: 10.1016/j.socscimed.2019.112683

Williams, D. R., & Etkins, O. S. (2021). Racism and mental health. *World Psychiatry; Official Journal of the World Psychiatric Association (WPA)*, *20*(2), 194–195. DOI: 10.1002/wps.20845 PMID: 34002496

Young, J., Edosomwan, K., & Young, J. (2024). Advanced Placement and Black High School Students: A Logistical Regression of College Persistence Factors. *Journal of Urban Learning, Teaching, and Research.*

Zieff, G., Kerr, Z. Y., Moore, J. B., & Stoner, L. (2020). Universal Healthcare in the United States of America: A Healthy Debate. *Medicina (Kaunas, Lithuania)*, *56*(11), 580. DOI: 10.3390/medicina56110580 PMID: 33143030

Chapter 3
Religious/ Spiritual Harm and Trauma-Informed Care:
Abuse and Trauma Within Our Sacred Heart

Lois Curry-Catanese
http://orcid.org/0000-0001-8076-6855
Walden University, USA

ABSTRACT

The Pew Research Center (2018) recorded that 8 out of 10 individuals endorse a religious and/or a spiritual identity. Religious/ spiritual abuse is defined as the "mistreatment of an individual through mental or physical means by weakening, undermining, distorting, or decreasing their spiritual integrity." R/S abuse can result in various forms of trauma that distort one's image of God or a higher power and spiritual identity. Purity culture at its core posits that an individual's moral worth, particularly for women, is inextricably tied to their sexual "purity"—defined as a total absence of sexual thought, desire, or action outside of heterosexual marriage. The act of spiritual bullying can be observed in the extreme form of conversion practice. Ongoing and repetitive traumatic events of any kind can lead to long-term psychological and physiological consequences in addition to a potential spiritual crisis. Clinicians, health care providers, and spiritual caregivers can offer effective trauma-informed care

DOI: 10.4018/979-8-3373-8597-6.ch003

INTRODUCTION

The Pew Research Center recorded that eight out of ten individuals endorse a religious and/or a spiritual identity. With 89% of the American population identifying as "religious and spiritual"; while 27% stating that they were "spiritual but not religious" (Pew Research Center, 2018). An individual can be both religious and spiritual, they are not mutually exclusive of one another. With the majority of the global population identifying as religious and/ or spiritual they often cite that their belief and faith was a source of coping and resilience. Papaleontiou-Louca (2025) points out that the two, *religiosity* and *spirituality*, are different in their *function* and *context* with the understanding that the "sacred" is what binds the two together. Our religious identity is grounded in the development of these teachings. It is through the religious practices that we develop a "relational spirituality" with God (Ellis et al., 2022).

Religion established within institutions and traditions aims at promoting inner faith, unity with humanity and God (Papaleontiou-Louca, 2025). Within our religiosity we then develop faith which is the basis of spirituality. Ellis et al. (2022) identified that while there may still be some debate between the definition of religion and spirituality, there is a consistent agreement that "spirituality" can be defined as "the search for the sacred" while engaging in the religiosity of communities and institutions (p. 213). Spirituality creates a sense of purpose in life, connection to a higher power (God, Allah, etc.), and in the practice of religiosity there is a connection with a faith community. So, the function of religion is to achieve a specific goal (physical, psychological, social), while the function of spirituality is to search for the sacred (Papaleontiou-Louca, 2025). This search for the sacred has a foundation laid in the development of spiritual faith. The connection between spirituality, religiosity, and morality are closely linked to each other despite the different meanings the terms are often used interchangeably (Papaleontiou-Louca, 2025).

Papaleontiou-Louca (2025) believed that the development of spirituality and religiosity is an integral part of humanity. We, as humans, begin our religious journey as children. Being brought up under the guidance of our parents and their teachings on belief, obedience, prayer, and faith in God. Erikson (1964) suggested that the virtues of trust and faith served as the foundation of hope. And certain developmental theorists (Kohlberg, 1981; Piaget, 1929) discounted the need for spirituality in children, Fowler (1981) and Papaleontiou-Louca (2025) identified that spiritual faith development throughout the lifespan of an individual was vital to their meaning and purpose in life. They identified that spirituality has a powerful impact in life and it is beneficial to mental health. Over the years psychological problems have increased and have become one of the biggest health challenges in the world (Papaleontiou-Louca, 2025). With the increase of depression, anxiety, worry, suicidal ideation and suicide/ homicide actions in global societies religion and spirituality seem to be essential in reducing risk factors that contribute to psychological distress (Du, 2024). The experiences of religion and spirituality are an important aspect of many individuals around the world. Religion offers moral order, learned competencies, and social connections which are necessary to cope with life's hardships and tragedies (Du, 2024).

So, individuals who endorse *intrinsic* religiosity and spirituality have better mental health, while those that are not authentically engaged in their religious and spiritual beliefs suffer mor depression, anxiety and a lower sense of well-being (Papaleontiou-Louca, 2025). This *extrinsic* religiosity aims to gain social benefits and is more pathological (manipulative, selfish, superficial, controlling) in orientation. What if individuals, in the practice of religiosity and spirituality, encounter abuse and trauma? Religious/ Spiritual (R/ S) abuse and trauma can create damage not only to an individual's mental health or their physical well-being but to their sense of purpose and existence in the world thus creating a spiritual crisis harm (Ellis et al., 2022).

RELIGIOUS/ SPIRITUAL ABUSE AND HARM

Definition

Ellis et al. (2022) cited Johnson and VanVonderen (1991) as defining religious/ spiritual abuse as the "mistreatment of an individual through mental or physical means by weakening, undermining, distorting, or decreasing their spiritual integrity." This type of R/S abuse can result in various forms of trauma that distort one's image of God or a higher power and spiritual identity that translates into barriers of mistrust, unhealthy personal boundaries, and self-harm (addictions, suicidal ideations). Within the abusive R/S community, the leader uses their position of power by misusing religious texts to create an unhealthy submission and/ or obedience to manipulate and control a person who is seen as weak.

The perpetrator of R/S abuse and trauma has a false sense of authority, which they deem is God-given, to diminish one's sense of self resulting in psychological, physiological, and spiritual harm. Through lies, double-talk (gaslighting), hypocrisy, and other forms of demeaning or devaluing behaviors the perpetrator sanctifies hatred, bigotry, aggression and discrimination (Ellis et al., 2022; Papaleontiou-Louca, 2025). This misuse of power or using God (or higher power) to control or induce fear in others is exploitive whether the R/S abuse is intentional or unintentional (Ellis et al., 2022).

R/S abuse causes trauma that mirrors the symptomatology of posttraumatic stress (PTSS) as defined by the criterion outlined in *The Diagnostic and Statistical Manual of Mental Disorders, Fifth Edition, Text Revision (DSM-5-TR)* as published by the 2022 American Psychiatric Association (APA). Trauma is defined by the American Psychiatric Association Diagnostic and Statistical Manual of Mental Disorders, Fifth Edition, Text Revised, Section 43.8 (APA DSM-5TR, 2022) as an event that includes an "actual or threatened death, serious injury, physical or sexual violence, combat exposure and natural disaster" (Section 43.8, APA DSM-5TR, 2022). While standard PTSD usually stems from a single, discrete event, complex PTSD stems from "prolonged, repeated trauma within a captive relationship." In a high-control religious setting, "captivity" isn't always physical; it is psychological and spiritual.

However, a unique aspect of R/S trauma is the focus of the abuse being a form of "moral injury" and interpersonal violence (Ellis et al., 2022; Jones et al., 2022). Even with a C-PTSD diagnosis, some classifications of trauma have been clearly defined, while other events that are experienced as *traumatic* are not and they are considered *stressors* (Gradus and Galea, 2023). The religious trauma that is experienced by an individual or group of individuals can create pervasive psychological harm that through long-term exposure can undermine the mental health and spiritual well-being (Jones et al., 2022). The result of the R/S abuse causes a rigid belief that God is impersonal, indifferent, unforgiving, hostile, punitive and/ or threatening, that inevitably has negative effects on the psychological and physiological health of an individual (Ellis et al., 2022; Papaleontiou-Louca, 2025).

The detrimental impact on an individual's spiritual development can have an adverse effect on meaning making, sense of purpose, connection and belonging, as well as their faith, moral, and ethical standards (Kvarfordt & Herba, 2018). The sense of not having a safe place or the betrayal of the sacred that causes conflicting perceptions of God or a higher power who is supposed to heal is now the cause of your pain can create permanent hypervigilance. This could lead to a deep sense of soul-weariness.

RELIGIOUS TEACHINGS & BELIEFS: PURITY CULTURE, HOMOSEXUALITY

According to Oakley et al. (2018) 70% of adults in the United Kingdom reported that they felt manipulated by their current church and even a higher percentage endorsed feeling controlled by their church in the past. The participants shared that the church used scripture to control them and that created mistrust in the church and eventually a distrust in God. There are specific populations (Catholicism, Evangelical, Southern Baptist) that percentage rates of R/S abuse are even higher. A frequently identified form of R/S abuse and trauma appears in the practice of "purity" expectations. According to Ott (2025) purity culture was associated with white evangelical circles in the 1990s and at its core, it posits that an individual's moral worth, particularly for women, is inextricably tied to their sexual "purity"—defined as a total absence of sexual thought, desire, or action outside of heterosexual marriage. This deep preoccupation with controlling and restricting sexuality created emotional and spiritual guilt, inner conflict, depression, and suicidal ideations (Du, 2024).

The main tenet of the purity culture posits that sexual purity equates to moral and spiritual virtue. Along with the belief that a "pure body" can be exchanged for a divinely ordained marital relationship. Frequently fear-based rhetoric, shame, and other tactics (pledges, political propaganda) have been employed. The connection of the purity culture and the political right have spurred an ideology that a woman's body belongs to a man for "possession" in the adage of "your body, my choice" indicating that women have no right to choice for anything. Thereby establishing a belief system of conforming women's bodies as property (Ott, 2025).

This sexual subversion has been linked to sexual violence encompassing a wide variety of behaviors, attitudes, and beliefs. As Gottfried et al. (2014) has pointed out this form of "institutional violence" goes beyond just individual acts but encompasses political leadership that advocates the use of fear, coercion, threats, trafficking, and other such physical and emotional violence that is being deemed as acceptable. Purity culture with its link to "rape culture" is more than a social preference; it is a systemic framework that often results in significant psychological injury (Ott, 2025; Gottfried et al., 2014).

These physical and emotional abusive practices are often perpetrated by leaders that are seen as charismatic or representatives of God. However, they employ narcissistic tendencies of gaslighting, stonewalling, silence, devaluing, and discarding to manipulate the most vulnerable of populations. The narcissist is preoccupied with their own power, status, prestige and superiority of being on top (Ward, 2011). Ward (2011) goes on to suggest that the narcissistic leader lives under the illusion that God has bestowed upon them the idea that they are untouchable and entitled to be served. This range of behaviours and attitudes constitutes *spiritual bullying* (Ward, 2011).

The act of spiritual bullying can be observed in the extreme form of conversion practice. In a study conducted by Simmons (2017) current and former members of The Church of Jesus Christ of the Latter-Day Saints (LDS), reported abuse due to identifying with the LGBTQ+ community (as cited by Ellis et al., 2022). Of the 95% LGBTQ+ population, at least 86% endorsed meeting the criteria of posttraumatic trauma and/ or stress-related symptoms. Jones et al. (2022) examined the various practices of sexual conversion and gender suppression experienced by LGBTQA+ populations. The ideology of conversion therapy is to heal the "sexual brokenness" of an individual through coercive, controlling, and abusive techniques (Jones et al., 2022).

These conversion tactics produce heightened rates of suicidal ideations, increased substance usage, homelessness, poor mental health and spiritual abandonment. The negative experiences of spiritual practices, grief over the loss of a supportive religious community, and damage to their spiritual identity, LGBTQA+ members endorsed the symptomology of posttraumatic stress disorder (PTSD), complex – posttraumatic stress disorder (C-PTSD), guilt and shame that is strongly associated with moral injury (Jones et al., 2022). A moral injury diagnosis is applicable to the LGBTQA+ communities because it meets the three criteria that describes moral injury. That criterion is (a) an act that violates what is considered right; (b) violates the self; (c) and the event occurs in a high stakes' situation (Jones et al., 2022). The perpetrated act of transgression impacts ones deeply held belief and forces an individual to choose between core parts of themselves as they are being forced to change or suppress their sexual orientation or gendered identity.

Members of the "purity culture" and LGBTQA+ communities, along with other individuals that suffer emotional or sexual abuse by religious/ spiritual leaders incur a second harm from the religious populace (Ellis at el., 2022; Jones et al., 2022). This harm can be experienced in direct accusation from the religious community that the individual is lying, and denying the offence by the religious leader, thereby ostracization of the injured person.

RELIGIOUS & CULTURAL COMMUNITY

Religion and spirituality are important factors that contribute to mental and physical health. From early childhood on, effectively inculcating individuals with moral and spiritual development was left up to parents, teachers, cultural and religious communities to affirm the importance of such values (Papaleontiou-Louca, 2025). Those values included telling the truth, obeying, helping and respecting others, kindness, acting responsibly, and finally, inspiring and encouraging others to do the same (Gregg et al., 1994 as cited by Papaleontiou-Louca, 2025). Papaleontiou-Louca, (2025) pointed out that this does not mean that all religious organizations are associated with positive outcomes. The role of religious communities in victim blaming, minimizing, marginalizing and isolating the "victims" result in re-traumatizing the individual or group (Ellis et al., 2022). This secondary form of trauma inflicts psychological, physical, social, and spiritual harm (Ott, 2025). Impairment and rupture to an individual's safety and sense of belonging manifests deep sorrow, grief, damage to their spiritual self-concept, meaning or life purpose, and experience (Jones et al., 2022).

The grief that is associated with the actual R/S abuse and trauma is compounded by the loss of one's spiritual community. The interconnectedness of social and cultural within the religion is what binds all participants. R/S abuse is multilayered and multifaceted in its abuse in which it significantly violates physical, psychological, and spiritual boundaries (Ward, 2011). In a relationship that is meant to create trust, empathy, openness, a sense of belonging and purpose, R/S abuse and trauma endorse the psychological effects of depression, anxiety, and negative coping styles resulting in risky sexual behaviors, body shaming, eating disorders, self-harm, and suicidal ideations (Ellis et al., 2022). The negative impact on an individual's spiritual identity creates a feeling of disconnection with God, skepticism, and distrust in religious communities.

The antidote to R/S abuse and trauma is to provide experiences of healing and spiritual transformation through adopting a new spiritual identity (Ellis et al., 2022). Vetting a therapist who is familiar with R/S abuse and trauma, outside of knowing how to treat generalized anxiety or depression, needs to understand the triggers and symptoms. Therapists also need to be familiar with Religious Trauma Syndrome (RTS) which encompasses the symptoms of C-PTSD (Winell, 2011 as cited by Singh et al., 2024). The other important factor in vetting a therapist for the treatment of R/S trauma is that they must be able to suspend their own religious or spiritual beliefs to validate the person's anger towards God.

The next section will address the clinical implications that can assist an individual in recovery and healing from R/S abuse and trauma while developing a new and fulfilling spiritual identity. An in-depth study conducted by Drew et al. (2022) explored the level of comfort and discomfort among practitioners. While in her book, *Trauma-Informed Spiritual Care*, Danielle Hansen (2024) outlines the interventions required for safety, meaning, reconnection, and justice. Other researchers (Lucchetti et al., 2021; Perry, 2024, Kress et al., 2018) contribute to the R/S abuse and trauma literature by explaining the connections between religiousness, spirituality, mental health and a feminist approach to post-traumatic growth within the clinical setting.

CLINICAL IMPLICATIONS & TRAUMA-INFORMED CARE

The study of spirituality and health is growing in examining the relationship and clinical interventions of treating various mental health disorders such as depression, anxiety, PTSD and C-PTSD, even suicidal ideations (Lucchetti et al., 2021; Du, 2024). In a research study, Drew et al. (2022) conducted a survey of 52 clinicians across various fields (LCSW, LPC, LMFT) and discovered that 15-25% of clinicians confirmed a level of discomfort with discussing religion and spirituality with their clients. That is significant in that 89% of Americans admitted to believing in God or a higher power and conservatively 27-33% of adults have experienced religious and spiritual trauma. As Drew et al. (2022) pointed out, awareness of religion and spirituality in a clinical setting is becoming more prevalent.

For this reason, the assessment of a client's religious and spiritual belief system is paramount in providing treatment interventions. Inquiring into a client's development of a faith, religious, and spiritual identity can provide useful insight into the starting point of R/S abuse and trauma. An individual's cultural framework shapes their belief and value system in establishing positive or negative coping skills with others, self, and God, especially within a diverse population of clientele (Oxlander & Parrish, 2018). Clinicians can then begin to assist their clients with healing the ruptured feelings of disconnection with God, evaluate their client's skepticism, and distrust in the religious communities that perpetrated their abuse and subsequent trauma.

UNDERSTANDING R/S TRAUMA: A FEMINIST APPROACH TO SELF-AWARENESS

Counseling theories are increasingly advocating for the usage of relational-cultural theory (RCT) in promoting a healthy relationship with individuals who have experienced any sort of traumatic event like R/S abuse and trauma (Kress et al., 2018). The history and background of the relational-cultural theory stems from the work of Miller (2012) who wrote the text, *Toward a New Psychology of Women*. Then with the help of other scholars like Jordan (2019) they went on to conduct research, write and present papers, as well as form the Stone Center.

Jordan (2024) went on to write a paper on the mutual effects of empathy in relational-cultural therapy. This style and approach are steeped in the foundational beliefs that as humans we all desire connection, empathy, and mutual respect for a growth-fostering relationship. It is through a growth-fostering relationship that a sense of trust, safety and well-being are formed (Jordan, 2019; Jordan, 2024). When R/S abuse and trauma occur, it destroys the foundational trust and safety of a person.

It is important to point out that not every individual reacts or develops symptoms related to a traumatic event. In part, reactions to a traumatic event are subjective, even when they occur within a sociocultural or historic context (Kress et al., 2018). However, RCT can be a useful approach to providing intervention to an individual or group that has experienced religious/ spiritual trauma because of the nature of the interpersonal and intrapersonal relationships. Women, more than men, tend to endorse higher levels of trauma-related stress both physically and psychologically because they place a higher value on relationships.

This is especially true when it comes to R/S abuse and trauma among the religious communities that practices conversion therapy and demands purity in young women. These beliefs and practices are embedded in a much wider system of symbolic, institutional, and political power (Ott, 2025). It is critical to challenge those damaging beliefs and practices through relational and trauma-informed therapy which educates and advocates for the re-defining sense of trust and respect for each other, as well as self.

An RCT tenet addresses disconnection, self-blame, and shame that is associated with the dogma of purity culture and conversion therapy. With an emphasis on self-empathy, awareness, and understanding to the connection of the traumatic event and their experiences a relational-cultural intervention can set about assisting clients with repairing and rebuilding a foundation for interpersonal and intrapersonal relationships. That means developing a treatment plan that addresses a person's connection and disconnection; explores relational expectations; and fosters mutuality, empathy, and shared power within the counseling relationship (Kress et al., 2018).

RESILIENCE, SPIRITUAL IDENTITY, FORGIVENESS & HEALING

As counselors broach the aftermath of R/S abuse and trauma there needs to be a re-evaluation as to the expectations and responsibilities of what constitutes "*spiritual care*" within the agency of professional practice (Hansen, 2024; Ott, 2025). Clinicians who receive little or no training on the occurrences of religious trauma risk harming the client further (Jones et al., 2022). By being more aware and actively engaged with a client's experiences through education, and understanding of the tenets of purity culture and the queer theories surrounding LGBTQA+ conversion practices, a clinician can assist in establishing trust and safety (Ellis et al., 2022). Thereby encouraging openness about the survivors' spiritual harm experienced by R/S abuse thus leading to resilience through recovery and healing.

Judith Herman (1997) wrote a book entitled *Trauma and Recovery*, in it she discusses that trauma comes in many forms and it has become part of the human experience. She also described a three-stage model of recovery and healing that incorporates safety, opportunities to process, and encouragement to reconnect with their religious communities (Herman, 1997 as cited by Hansen, 2024). That "safety" is associated with not only physical and psychological components but spiritual as well. When a person experiences safety, they feel that they can trust others and themselves to be unconditionally accepted for who they are. To be "spiritually" safe involves allowing the beliefs and values of an individual to practice in whatever religious manner they chose without shame of who they are in human form. Spiritual safety is one reason a person can comprehend their abuse and cope with their trauma as they engage in the process of healing.

Trauma recovery requires three components: (a) meaning making, (b) reconnection, and (c) resolution (Hansen, 2024). The important part in establishing *meaning making* is remembering the trauma and grieving what was lost. There are two forms of meaning making that are either *global* or *situational*. Global meaning making is the way a person orients themselves with the world around them. In that context of global meaning there exists embedded beliefs and spirituality. Situational meaning making has to do with how a person assesses a particular event and then derives meaning from it. Hansen (2024) points out that embedded beliefs within a traumatic event can create a spiritual crisis of meaning. The integration process requires bringing together all the conflicting parts into a whole. This process is observed in *posttraumatic growth*.

Posttraumatic growth (PTG) is different from resilience, and it can be divided into five domains (Hansen, 2024). Those domains include: (a) appreciation for life, (b) awareness of new possibilities, (c) new ways of relating to others, (d) awareness of personal strength, and (e) changes and growth in spirituality. In regard to R/S abuse and trauma to facilitate healing, posttraumatic growth (PTG) decreases the mental health symptomology while constructing meaning (Perry, 2024). The Association for Spiritual, Ethical, and Religious Values in Counseling (ASERVC) emphasizes the importance of therapists recognizing their client's R/S beliefs (or absence thereof), along with their worldviews (ASERVC, 2024). Recognition of an individual's R/S abuse and trauma is imperative to recovery and healing (Ellis et al., 2022). A therapist must differentiate between R/S abuse; spiritual wounding and harm; adverse religious experiences and trauma (Perry, 2024).

Perry (2024) stated that the aftermath of R/S abuse has a profound effect on an individual's psychological, physiological, and spiritual well-being. Clinicians can support the client by helping them identify the red flags of high-controlling religious organizations. This is a vital step in deconstructing and managing the "*shame spiral*" that is associated with R/S abuse. That shame spiral is linked to old thought patterns that were engrained into a person through the practice of purity or the attempt at LGBTQA+ conversion. By recognizing the triggers, a clinician can provide the client with grounding techniques such as the "*observer*" technique that challenges the programmed thought of "I am a sinner," to "I am noticing a feeling of guilt." This creates a distinction between the indoctrination rhetoric and the reality of what is happening at the moment.

While examining the psychological effects of R/S abuse and trauma, increasing the client's understanding of the physiological symptoms that they may be experiencing is important as well (Kress et al., 2018). The disconnection that the client feels can be repaired by incorporating grounding techniques that include the somatic of "5-4-3-2-1" this incorporates the identification of senses through seeing, feeling, hearing, smelling, and tasting. Clinicians can also introduce meditation, yoga, and body tapping to reconnect the client to the here and now.

It is also important to allow, even encourage, the client to grieve the loss of certainty, community support, and self-identity. The unmet expectations and the reality of skewed relational dynamics are significantly impacted by R/S abuse. Therefore, clinicians need to empower their client to foster self-empathy and compassion, while *reparenting* their own self-identity with new relational strategies (Kress et al., 2018). This process can be accomplished through three areas: (a) *recognition* – naming the abuse, (b) *relaying* – exploring the trauma, and (c) *redefining* – transformation of spirituality (Perry, 2024). The most powerful therapeutic tool can be found through storytelling and narrative sharing to work through this PTG process (Lee et al., 2016). Clinicians, helping professionals and religious communities can foster a safe space and essential spiritual dialogs by demonstrating genuine empathy, cultural curiosity, and spiritual sensitivity (De Vynck et al., 2023). It is essential for professionals to remain reflective and aware of their own personal bias in order to prevent inadvertently imposing personal beliefs onto their clients (Zaeske et al., 2024).

In addition to the clinician developing a better understanding of R/S abuse and trauma to assist the client, clinicians can work towards educating the community (Ellis et al., 2022). As of 2019, an organization called the *Religious Trauma Institute* (https://www.religioustrumainstitute.com) became a resource for survivors, and clinicians to collaborate with the religious community to discuss the signs and symptoms of R/S abuse (Ellis et al., 2022). It is important for clinicians to engage in self-evaluation and reflection, while seeking out proper supervision when treating a client who is a survivor of R/S abuse and trauma.

CONCLUSION

Advocacy and Social Justice

Clinicians, health care providers, and spiritual caregivers can offer effective trauma-informed care and restorative justice provides the final transformation (Hansen, 2024). Restorative justice is a philosophical approach to communication through a variety of formats, such as group conferences, victim-offender mediation, and circle processes to promote empathy, agency, and discernment. The process of restorative justice takes a long time and commitments from the victim and offending party while demanding deep introspection (Hansen, 2024). Ongoing and repetitive traumatic events of any kind can lead to long-term psychological and physiological consequences in addition to a potential spiritual crisis (Kress et al., 2018). People who experience religious/ spiritual abuse and trauma experience a sense of betrayal, powerlessness, stigmatization and ostracization. The philosophy of restorative justice and trauma-informed spiritual care is to incorporate empathy, compassion, active listening, active listening, reflectiveness, the use of silence and open-ended questions to create an overall understanding of a client's religious and spiritual abuse (Hansen, 2024). Practitioners must posses these core competencies to facilitate recovery and healing.

REFERENCES

American Psychiatric Association. (2022). *Diagnostic and statistical manual of mental disorders* (5th ed., text rev.)., DOI: 10.1176/appi.books.9780890425787

Association for Spiritual, Ethical, and Religious Value in Counseling (2024). *Competencies for Addressing Spiritual and Religious Issues in Counseling*. Alexandria: Association for Spiritual, Ethical, and Religious Value in Counseling https://aservic.org/

De Vynck, E., Boynton, H. M., & Burns, V. F. (2023). Pulled from the shorelines in search of spacious spirituality: Journeys of spiritual distress, resilience and post-traumatic growth for women for evangelical Christian backgrounds in a Canadian context. *Religions*, *14*(9), 1193. DOI: 10.3390/rel14091193

Drew, D., Banks, B., & Joseph, R. (2022). Religion and spirituality in clinical practice: An exploration of comfort and discomfort among practitioners. *Social Thought*, *41*(1), 104–120. https://psycnet.apa.org/doi/10.1080/15426432.2021.1994099

Du, L. J. (2024). The associations between religiosity and resilience when individuals are challenged by risk factors of suicide and mental illness. *Frontiers in Public Health*, *12*, 1442248. DOI: 10.3389/fpubh.2024.1442248 PMID: 39145184

Ellis, H. M., Hook, J. N., Zuniga, S., Hodge, A. S., Ford, K. M., Davis, D. E., & Van Tongeren, D. R. (2022). Religious/spiritual abuse and trauma: A systematic review of the empirical literature. *Spirituality in Clinical Practice*, *9*(4), 213–231. DOI: 10.1037/scp0000301

Erikson, E. H. (1964). Inner and outer space: Reflections on womanhood. *Daedalus*, •••, 582–606.

Fowler, J. W. (1981). *Stages of faith*. Harper & Row.

Gottfried, A. W., Gottfried, A. E., Bathurst, K., Guerin, D. W., & Parramore, M. M. (2014). Socioeconomic status in children's development and family environment: Infancy through adolescence. In *Socioeconomic status, parenting, and child development* (pp. 189–207). Routledge.

Gradus, J. L., & Galea, S. (2023). Moving From Traumatic Events to Traumatic Experiences in the Study of Traumatic Psychopathology. *American Journal of Epidemiology*, *192*(10), 1609–1612. DOI: 10.1093/aje/kwad126 PMID: 37218615

Hansen, D. T. (2024). *Trauma-informed spiritual care: Interventions for safety, meaning, reconnection, and justice*. Fortress Press. DOI: 10.2307/jj.12949092

Jones, T. W., Power, J., & Jones, T. M. (2022). Religious trauma and moral injury from LGBTQA+ conversion practices. *Social science & medicine (1982), 305*, 115040. https://doi.org/Top of FormDOI: 10.1016/j.socscimed.2022.115040

Jordan, J. V. (2019). Relational-cultural theory: the power of connection to transform our lives. *Journal of Humanistic Counseling, October 2017, 56,* 228-243

Jordan, J. V. (2024). Relational–cultural therapy. *(3rd Ed).* American Psychological Association. Bottom of FormJohnson, D. W. and VanVonderen, J. (1991) *The subtle power of spiritual abuse*. Bethany House Publishers DOI: 10.1037/0000411-000

Kohlberg, L. (1981). *The psychology of moral development*. Essays on moral development. Harper & Row.

Kress, V. E., Haiyasoso, M., Zolden, C. A., Headley, J. A., & Trepal, H. (2018). The use of relational-cultural theory in counseling clients who have traumatic stress disorder. *Journal of Counseling and Development*, *96*(1), 106–114. https://psycnet.apa.org/doi/10.1002/jcad.12182. DOI: 10.1002/jcad.12182

Kvarfordt, C. L., & Herba, K. (2018). Religion and spirituality in social work practice with children and adolescents: A survey of Canadian practitioners. *Child & Adolescent Social Work Journal*, *35*(2), 153–167. DOI: 10.1007/s10560-017-0513-5

Lee, H., Fawsett, J., & Demarco, R. (2016). Stroytelling/ narrative theory to address health communication with minority populations. *Applied Nursing Research*, *30*, 558–560. DOI: 10.1016/j.apnr.2015.09.004 PMID: 27091254

Lucchetti, G., Koenig, H. G., & Granero Lucchetti, A. L. (2021). Spirituality, religiousness, and mental health: A review of the current scientific evidence. *World Journal of Clinical Cases*, *9*(16), 7620–7631. DOI: 10.12998/wjcc.v9.i26.7620 PMID: 34621814

Miller, J. B. (2012). *Toward a new psychology of women*. Beacon Press.

Oakley, L., Kinmond, K., & Humphreys, J. (2018). Spiritual abuse in Christian faith settings: Definition, policy and practice guidance. *Journal of Adult Protection*, *20*(3-4), 144–154. DOI: 10.1108/JAP-03-2018-0005

Ott, T. (2025). Purity cultures and the ideology of 'bodies as property'as form of sexual violence. *Theology and Sexuality*, *31*(1-3), 54–73. DOI: 10.1080/13558358.2025.2525613

Oxlander, H. K., & Parrish, D. E. (2018). Integrating clients' religion/ spirituality in clinical practice: A comparison among social workers, psychologists, counselors, and nurses. *Journal of Clinical Psychology*, *74*, 680–694. DOI: 10.1002/jclp.22539 PMID: 29023713

Papaleontiou - Louca, E.Papaleontiou - Louca. (2025). Spirituality and religiosity in the developing person. *Journal of Beliefs & Values*, *46*(1), 15–46. DOI: 10.1080/13617672.2023.2267924

Perry, S. L. (2024). *Religion for realists: Why we all need the scientific study of religion*. Oxford University Press. DOI: 10.1093/oso/9780197672549.001.0001

Piaget, J. (1929). *The child's conception of the world*. Harcourt, Brace.

Ward, K. (2011). *Is religion dangerous?* Lion Books.

Zaeske, L. M., Dye, A. R., Spadoni, S., Strothkamp, R., Kane, M. L., Ridgway, K., Dugan, A. J., Patterson, T. P., McEathron, S. R., & Cole, B. P. (2024). Addressing harm from adverse religious/ spiritual experiences in psychotherapy: A scoping review. *Practice Innovations (Washington, D.C.)*, *9*(1), 1–18. https://psycnet.apa.org/doi/10.1037/pri0000237. DOI: 10.1037/pri0000237

Chapter 4
Cumulative Relational Trauma in Long-Term Role Engulfment:
A Trauma-Informed, Operationalizable Framework Using the Dual-Track Emotional System

Eva Yifan Li
http://orcid.org/0009-0009-7396-3565
University of Pittsburgh, USA

ABSTRACT

Trauma-informed care has matured around acute events but remains under-theorized for the chronic relational deprivation accumulating in long-term family systems, where adults perform functional roles for decades while their emotional identity becomes progressively unseen. This chapter argues such under-recognition constitutes cumulative relational trauma. It introduces the Dual-Track Emotional System, which distinguishes a functional responsibility system from a personal emotional system and traces how dominance of the first attenuates the second. A heuristic illustration from the literature shows how role engulfment, identity attenuation, and relational deprivation converge in one individual over time. The chapter centers both the role-strained adult and the unseen primary partner, who carries their own betrayal trauma. The framework is operationalized through an assessment protocol, clinical heuristics, organizational implementation suggestions, and reflective-practice guidance. Ethical accountability and intersectional awareness frame the application, with attention to misuse risks.

DOI: 10.4018/979-8-3373-8597-6.ch004

I. INTRODUCTION

Trauma-informed care has matured rapidly over the past three decades. The field now offers shared principles (SAMHSA, 2014), a clear empirical base for the impact of acute and complex trauma (Herman, 1992; van der Kolk, 2014), and increasingly well-developed organizational frameworks for safety, trustworthiness, choice, collaboration, and empowerment. Yet most trauma-informed protocols still presume identifiable events. The acute assault, the combat exposure, the early-life abuse, the disaster: these provide the conceptual templates around which assessment and intervention are organized.

A different kind of trauma is less well theorized. It is not produced by a single event. It is produced by years, sometimes decades, of being structurally present and emotionally unseen inside an ostensibly functioning relational system. An adult fulfills the role of spouse, parent, provider, caregiver, household manager, and emotional regulator for others. The family looks stable from the outside. Bills are paid. Children are raised. The marriage endures. Yet over time, the person inside the role loses contact with a dimension of self that exists apart from what they sustain for others. The erosion is slow. It is rarely framed as harm. It almost never produces a presenting complaint marked "trauma."

This chapter takes that erosion seriously as a trauma-informed concern. It argues that chronic emotional under-recognition inside long-term role-based functioning is a form of cumulative relational trauma: not a moment of rupture but a slow attenuation of subjective identity under sustained role demand. To support clinical and institutional engagement with this pattern, the chapter introduces the Dual-Track Emotional System, a conceptual framework distinguishing two interrelated but psychologically distinct identity processes—a functional responsibility system (the self organized around social role, obligation, and external performance) and a personal emotional system (the self organized around recognition, affective resonance, and subjective presence). The chapter traces how the first track can come to dominate the second over the course of an adult life, and how that dominance accumulates as relational trauma.

One downstream manifestation of this attenuation is extradyadic emotional attachment in mid-adulthood, in which a person experiences sudden emotional recognition outside the primary relationship and finds it difficult to disengage. This pattern is sometimes treated by clinicians as moral failure, sometimes as relational pathology, sometimes simply as a problem to be solved through behavioral correction. This chapter resists those readings without endorsing the behavior. Extradyadic attachment is approached here as one observable expression of an underlying process. It is neither the only expression of that process nor a behavior the framework recommends. The unseen primary partner, who has often endured the same structural conditions and may also have been emotionally deprived, is taken seriously as a person whose experience constitutes its own form of relational trauma—an explicit corrective to the asymmetric attention this topic often receives.

The chapter proceeds in seven parts. Section II locates the work in the relevant literatures: trauma-informed care, role strain, emotion regulation, adult attachment, betrayal trauma, and intersectional analysis. Section III describes the conceptual approach, including the use of a heuristic illustration and the scope of the chapter's claims. Section IV develops the Dual-Track Emotional System and illustrates it through the example of A and B, then turns directly to the experience of the unseen partner. Section V is the operational core of the chapter: a trauma-informed assessment protocol, clinical decision heuristics, organizational implementation suggestions, and reflective practice for practitioners. Section VI addresses ethical accountability and intersectional application, including explicit misuse risks. Section VII concludes and identifies directions for empirical work.

II. LITERATURE REVIEW

2.1 Trauma-Informed Care: From Acute Events to Cumulative Relational Deprivation

Modern trauma-informed care rests on the recognition that exposure to violence, abuse, neglect, and disaster shapes psychological functioning across the life course (Herman, 1992; van der Kolk, 2014). The U.S. Substance Abuse and Mental Health Services Administration (SAMHSA, 2014) consolidated the field around four assumptions—realize, recognize, respond, and resist re-traumatization—and six guiding principles: safety; trustworthiness and transparency; peer support; collaboration and mutuality; empowerment, voice, and choice; and cultural, historical, and gender issues. These principles now anchor practice across mental health, social work, education, and increasingly healthcare and human resources.

The dominant operational template, however, still tilts toward identifiable events. Screening tools ask whether a client has experienced specific occurrences. Treatment models address symptoms tied to those occurrences. Complex trauma literature has extended this work to capture chronic interpersonal harm in childhood (Herman, 1992), and a growing literature on betrayal trauma (Freyd, 1996) names the specific psychological injury produced when harm comes from a person on whom one depends. These extensions matter. They have not yet, however, fully addressed what happens inside long-term adult role systems that look from the outside like ordinary functioning marriages and ordinary functioning families, but inside of which an individual's emotional identity is steadily attenuated under role demand.

This chapter takes that pattern as its central concern. It treats prolonged emotional under-recognition inside a functional relational structure as a form of cumulative relational deprivation that produces trauma-relevant outcomes: identity erosion, regulatory depletion, attachment activation, and—in some cases—the kinds of behaviors and decisions that bring people into clinical contact long after the underlying injury has set in.

Empirical work in adjacent areas supports the clinical seriousness of this pattern. MacIntosh's (2024) pilot study of Developmental Couple Therapy for Complex Trauma demonstrates that trauma-informed couple interventions can produce meaningful improvement in trauma symptoms, emotion regulation, and attachment-related anxiety without requiring structural dissolution of the relationship, suggesting that functional stability and emotional repair are not mutually exclusive clinical aims. Longitudinal observational research on marital interaction (Gottman & Driver, 2005) provides a different angle on the same pattern: couples who ultimately divorced responded to one another's bids for emotional connection at a rate of approximately 33%, while couples whose marriages endured responded at approximately 86%. The sustained non-response to emotional bids inside an outwardly intact marriage is, in effect, a quantitative trace of the chronic emotional deprivation this chapter takes as its central object. Read together, these literatures suggest that the deprivation pattern is both clinically tractable and observable in interaction, even when it has not been formally named as a trauma-relevant concern.

2.2 Role Strain, Role Engulfment, and Identity Attenuation

Sociology has long described the structural pressures of multiple-role occupancy. Adults routinely inhabit overlapping roles—spouse, parent, provider, caregiver, emotional anchor, household manager—and the demands of those roles regularly exceed available resources (Thoits, 1991; Simon, 1995). When demands chronically outpace resources, role strain becomes a sustained background condition rather than an episodic challenge.

Kroger (2007) describes role engulfment as the far end of this process: a single dominant role gradually crowds out other dimensions of identity, until the self organizes almost entirely around what the person does for others rather than who they are. The shift is rarely dramatic. It accumulates through years of choosing relational stability over personal expression, through the steady prioritizing of performance over presence. The functional self stays competent and visible. The emotional self does not disappear, but it becomes harder to locate inside the relational structures of daily life.

Two features of this literature are worth marking. First, role engulfment is identity-level, not merely behavioral. It changes how a person relates to themselves, not only what they do. Second, the conditions that produce it are structural. Gendered divisions of caregiving and emotional labor, occupational demands, cultural scripts about responsibility, and the absence of institutional supports for chronic emotional load all push individuals toward the functional pole (Hochschild, 1983/2003; Umberson et al., 2006). The strain is personal in experience and systemic in origin.

2.3 Emotion Regulation and Interpersonal Co-Regulation

Adults regulate emotion both intrapersonally and through close relationships (Gross, 1998; Zaki & Williams, 2013). Partners co-regulate one another's affect; the perceived availability of a caring other is itself a regulatory resource. Research on emotional labor inside marriage shows that this co-regulatory load is often unevenly distributed, with one partner shouldering disproportionate responsibility for emotional containment (Hochschild, 1983/2003; Umberson et al., 2006). Over time, that asymmetry depletes the carrying partner. The person who has spent years stabilizing others may find that their own affective experience is rarely received in turn.

Two implications follow. First, regulatory depletion is not a private failure of coping; it is the predictable downstream of a particular relational arrangement. Second, when intrapersonal resources are exhausted and interpersonal recognition is unavailable inside the primary relationship, regulatory pull toward other relational contexts is not anomalous. It is what the system does.

2.4 Attachment Dynamics in Long-Term Adult Relationships

Adult attachment theory provides the working vocabulary for understanding how early caregiving experiences shape adult expectations of closeness (Bowlby, 1969/1982, 1988). Securely attached adults can tolerate both closeness and distance; insecurely attached adults oscillate. In long marriages, anxious–avoidant pairings often produce a pursuer–distancer dynamic in which moves toward closeness are met with withdrawal, generating cycles of approach and retreat. These dynamics are well-mapped at the level of interaction.

What attachment theory has historically said less about is how these dynamics intersect with chronic role demand across decades. The attachment system does not switch off when the marriage settles into routine. It continues to track, often outside awareness, whether the person is being seen. When recognition is persistently absent, attachment activation may begin to seek it elsewhere—not as betrayal in the moral sense, but as a system doing what attachment systems do (Mikulincer & Shaver, 2016). The clinical challenge is that the same activation can be either an opening for repair or a slide into harm, and the framework available to the practitioner often does not distinguish well between them.

2.5 Betrayal Trauma and the Limits of Existing Infidelity Frameworks

Infidelity research has generated useful descriptive findings—prevalence, predictors, correlates—but has been shaped by an evaluative frame that treats extradyadic involvement primarily as moral failure or relational pathology (Glass & Wright, 1985; Atkins et al., 2001; Allen et al., 2005; Mark et al., 2011). The frame is not wrong about consequences. It is incomplete about process, and it has tended to obscure the experience of the person who is betrayed.

Freyd's (1996) betrayal trauma theory provides the corrective. Harm inflicted by a depended-upon person produces a distinctive psychological injury that the more general trauma frameworks do not fully capture. The primary partner of someone engaged in extradyadic emotional attachment is not simply a person experiencing relational disappointment. They are a person whose central attachment object has, in fact, withdrawn affective availability and committed it elsewhere. The injury is real, and it is properly named.

Two important nuances follow. First, betrayal trauma frames the primary partner's experience as deserving the same trauma-informed seriousness as the experience of the role-engulfed partner. Second, attention to betrayal trauma sharpens what is at stake in any framework that explains extradyadic attachment: the framework must not become a tool for rationalizing harm. The chapter returns to this point repeatedly.

2.6 Intersectional Dimensions of Role Strain and Emotional Deprivation

Role engulfment, emotional suppression, and identity attenuation are not evenly distributed. They are produced and intensified by the intersecting conditions of gender, race, class, culture, and sexuality (Crenshaw, 1989; Collins, 2000). Gender norms in many cultural contexts assign emotional labor disproportionately to women, increasing their structural exposure to role engulfment inside traditional marital arrangements (Hochschild, 1983/2003; Umberson et al., 2006). Cultural scripts equating masculinity with emotional restraint intensify suppression among male partners. Collectivist cultural contexts may normatively prioritize family function over individual emotional expression, shaping how the functional–emotional split is experienced and expressed. Class constrains access to therapy, paid support, and respite, deepening deprivation without offering legitimate channels for recognition. Race and migration histories add further layers of structural strain, including the demands of cultural translation and the cumulative weight of discrimination.

An intersectional reading is not an optional overlay on this framework. It is part of the diagnostic substance. Two clients reporting identical surface symptoms—chronic depletion, feeling unseen, a recent emotional attachment outside the marriage—may be located in radically different structural positions, and competent practice requires attending to both the individual's psychology and the conditions that shaped it.

2.7 What Is New Here: Distinguishing the Dual-Track Emotional System from Adjacent Concepts

Several existing concepts share territory with the Dual-Track Emotional System without doing the same work. It is worth stating the distinctions clearly.

Compartmentalization and splitting describe defensive processes by which a person keeps incompatible affective states or representations apart. The Dual-Track frame is structural, not defensive. The two tracks are not split-off contents of a fragile self; they are domains of identity organization. Both tracks remain integrated into the same self; what shifts over time is the asymmetric expression of each.

The emotional–sexual infidelity distinction (Glass & Wright, 1985) classifies extradyadic involvement by content. The Dual-Track frame does not classify infidelity. It describes the underlying identity process within which extradyadic attachment, when it appears, can be made legible. The process can be present in many people who never engage in extradyadic involvement at all.

Finkel's suffocation-of-marriage thesis argues that contemporary marriages are asked to deliver more psychological goods than any single relationship can sustainably provide. The Dual-Track frame is compatible with this argument but operates at a different level. Suffocation describes the structural mismatch between marital demand and marital capacity. The Dual-Track frame describes the intrapsychic correlate of prolonged role-based functioning regardless of whether the marriage in question is overburdened in Finkel's sense.

Parallel attachment models in adult attachment literature describe the existence of multiple attachment figures—parents, partners, close friends—across the lifespan. The Dual-Track frame is not primarily about multiple figures. It is about two tracks of self-experience within one person, only one of which can be activated through a given relational context at a given time.

What is new in the Dual-Track Emotional System is the integration. It holds role strain, regulatory depletion, attachment activation, and identity attenuation as facets of a single process unfolding inside one person across time. It is offered not as another diagnosis to be added to the inventory, but as a clinically usable map of cumulative relational trauma in role-engulfed adults—one that can be operationalized for assessment, intervention, organizational practice, and reflective work.

2.8 Research Gap: Toward an Integrated, Operationalizable Framework

The existing literatures converge on a problem. Role theory shows how prolonged demand attenuates the self. Emotion regulation research shows how relational depletion produces regulatory pull toward other contexts. Attachment theory shows how unmet recognition activates the attachment system. Betrayal trauma theory shows the injury sustained when a depended-upon other withdraws. Intersectional analysis shows whose lives bear the heaviest structural exposure. None of these literatures, on its own, gives the practitioner an integrated way to assess, name, and respond to cumulative relational trauma inside long-term role engulfment. None offers a usable set of decision heuristics for cases in which the surface presentation is an extradyadic emotional involvement but the underlying process is identity attenuation.

The remainder of this chapter develops such an integrated, operationalizable framework, with explicit attention to the unseen partner and to the misuse risks that any such framework carries.

III. METHODOLOGY

3.1 The Vignette as Heuristic Illustration

The case of A and B presented in Section IV is a constructed heuristic illustration, not a real couple, not a single client, and not a composite drawn from the author's own clinical caseload. It is built to render the conceptual framework concrete: the mid-career professional whose marriage has settled into a functional steady state; the unexpected workplace meeting; the slow build of emotional recognition; the rhythm of approach and withdrawal; the partner at home who is not in the room. Each of these elements is recognizable from the published clinical and theoretical literature on long-term partnership, role strain, and adult attachment (Hochschild, 1983/2003; Kroger, 2007; Mikulincer & Shaver, 2016; Perel, 2007); the vignette synthesizes those patterns into a single illustrative example so that the abstract distinctions of the Dual-Track framework can be followed in narrative form.

This use of constructed illustration has an established place in conceptual and theoretical scholarship across psychology, social work, and clinical education (Fishman, 1999; Stake, 2005). Its function is pedagogical and analytic rather than evidential. It allows a framework to be developed at the level of pattern rather than individual occurrence, which is appropriate when the goal is theory development rather than empirical claim. It also makes pedagogically transparent that the vignette's role is to clarify the framework, not to substantiate it.

Narrative inquiry traditions (Clandinin & Connelly, 2000) and case-based reasoning in clinical training (Schön, 1983) provide further grounding. Both treat the structured description of a case as a legitimate form of disciplined knowledge work, distinct from but in productive relationship with statistical and experimental traditions. The Dual-Track framework as developed here is intended to be tested, refined, and revised through subsequent empirical work, including the studies identified in Section VII.

3.2 Scope, Standpoint, and Limits of Generalization

Several limits should be named explicitly.

First, this chapter does not report human subjects research. No IRB review was sought or required, because no individual data are analyzed and no real client material is presented. The vignette of A and B is constructed for illustrative purposes from the published literature, and should not be read as case evidence.

Second, the framework is therefore conceptual, not empirical. The claims advanced are claims about how a particular pattern can be usefully named, assessed, and worked with—not claims that the pattern operates in any specific frequency in any specific population. Empirical work testing the framework's components—the assessment protocol, the decision heuristics, the relationships among role engulfment, regulatory depletion, and downstream outcomes—remains to be done, and Section VII identifies specific directions for that work.

Third, the author writes from the standpoint of a social work scholar engaging the published literature on trauma-informed care, adult attachment, role theory, and clinical ethics. The chapter is offered as a conceptual contribution that synthesizes these literatures into an integrated framework usable by trauma-informed practitioners. It is not offered as a report of independent clinical practice, and the operational components in Section V are presented as proposed tools to be examined, refined, and validated by clinicians and researchers with the relevant practice experience and empirical methods.

Fourth, the framework is offered as a tool for trauma-informed practitioners and researchers, not as a self-application instrument for the general public. Several features of the framework—including the language of cumulative relational trauma and the explicit attention to unmet emotional recognition—can be misappropriated as justifications for behavior the framework does not endorse. Section VI returns to this risk in detail.

IV. THE DUAL-TRACK EMOTIONAL SYSTEM: CONCEPTUAL FRAMEWORK

4.1 The Functional Responsibility System

The functional responsibility system organizes identity around social role and structural obligation. It is the dimension of self constructed through what the person sustains: spouse, parent, provider, caregiver, household manager, professional. Its psychological work is regulatory and stabilizing. It maintains predictability, continuity, and external order. It learns, over years, to dampen emotional expression that might destabilize the systems it sustains.

This track is not a problem in itself. It is, in fact, the basis on which families function, children are raised, and partnerships endure across decades. Its appropriate development across adult life is part of what allows adults to be reliable to one another. The trouble begins when its development crowds out the development of the other track.

4.2 The Personal Emotional System

The personal emotional system organizes identity around recognition rather than performance. It is the dimension of self that wants to be perceived—not for what it sustains, but for what it feels. It tracks attunement, resonance, and affective presence. It needs to be received, not only to receive.

This track does not disappear when the functional system dominates. It persists, often quietly, as an internal experience of being incompletely known. It is the dimension that registers what role engulfment costs, even when the person cannot yet articulate the cost. When this track has been chronically under-engaged for years, its sudden reactivation in a new relational context can feel disproportionate to what has actually occurred. It is not disproportionate; it is overdue.

4.3 Coexistence, Imbalance, and Dynamic Regulation

The two tracks are not in inherent conflict. Under conditions of reciprocal emotional availability inside the primary relationship, both develop in parallel and remain integrated. What produces the patterns described in this chapter is asymmetric development over time: years of functional reliability with declining emotional reciprocity.

The imbalance generates a predictable dynamic. The functional system continues to perform. The emotional system continues to need recognition. The need is not extinguished by being unmet; it accumulates. In some people the accumulation produces depression, in others somatic symptoms, in others a turn inward and a quiet narrowing of expressive range. In some it produces, eventually, an unexpected encounter in which long-dormant recognition activates rapidly, and a person who has been quietly competent for twenty years finds themselves unable to step away from a conversation that has nothing to do with their functional life.

When that activation happens, the functional system does not vanish. It remains alert, and it reasserts itself. The result is a rhythm of approach and withdrawal in which the activated emotional track and the consolidated functional track each press their claim. This is not pathology in a clinical sense. It is two systems doing their work simultaneously inside a person whose architecture has become asymmetric. Reading the rhythm as ambivalence misses the structure. It is not that the person is unsure of what they feel. It is that they are organized by two systems with non-identical priorities.

4.4 Case Illustration: Developmental Origins and Emergence (A and B)

A and B are introduced here as a heuristic illustration, with all the limits described in Section III.

When they met they were both in their early forties, both more than a decade into long-term marriages, both leading capable working lives in overlapping professional fields. Their first contact was at a work meeting. Nothing in the encounter was unusual in social terms. What both noticed, almost immediately, was the absence of effort in being understood. The work conversation continued, and underneath it ran a parallel current of mutual recognition: each could read the other's fatigue, restraint, and unspoken pressure inside the formal setting.

Their developmental histories had produced complementary architectures. A had grown up with early relational experiences in which her emotional expression was recognized and at least sometimes received. She developed strong affective attunement (Siegel, 2012) and a regulatory capacity that served her well across professional and family roles. Over the years, however, that capacity had calcified into a one-way function. She was consistently the regulator, rarely the recipient of recognition. Her emotional system worked. It was not being met.

B had grown up in an environment that rewarded responsibility and punished emotional exposure. He had built a high-performing functional self organized around self-discipline, reliability, and structural control. His emotional system had not been extinguished by this development; it had been managed (Gross & John, 2003). His pattern had aspects of fearful–avoidant attachment in the adult attachment literature (Mikulincer & Shaver, 2016): an underlying wish for closeness held in check by acquired regulatory caution.

When A and B met, A's attunement perceived in B what B had spent decades not showing. B's quiet emotional depth, when met by A's reception, became available in a way that was structurally rare in his life. Their connection developed slowly, over about two years, mostly as conversation and presence rather than as a project of relational restructuring. Neither tried to remake the other's life. Neither tried to fold the other into their respective functional system.

The rhythm of the connection was not linear. Periods of genuine emotional opening were followed by withdrawal, with B as the primary driver of the oscillation. Each move toward A activated his personal emotional system; each subsequent withdrawal represented his functional responsibility system reasserting its long-consolidated regulatory priority. The attachment did not extinguish in the withdrawals. It persisted underneath them. A's pattern was structurally different: she remained more emotionally steady, able to hold uncertainty without requiring resolution, in part because her own functional system did not feel acutely destabilized by the connection. Her stability was not only a personal trait. It was a structural condition that made the parallel track possible at all.

The dynamic between A and B is presented here for one analytic purpose: it makes the operation of the Dual-Track Emotional System concrete. The functional and emotional tracks coexisted in both individuals. The connection allowed the emotional track to be activated without immediately collapsing the functional track. The activation was, in a clinically meaningful sense, a reactivation: a return of a dimension of self that had been steadily attenuated over years of role engulfment inside their respective long-term marriages.

The reactivation does not, by itself, tell us what either person should do.

4.5 The Other Side of the Track: Centering the Unseen Partner

The case of A and B is incomplete on the page in the way that such cases are almost always incomplete in clinical attention: the primary partner of A and the primary partner of B are not in the room. They have not consented to being characters in a framework about emotional reactivation. They are likely, in fact, themselves carrying cumulative relational trauma of their own. A trauma-informed treatment of this material must center their experience directly, not as an ethical footnote but as a substantive part of the framework.

Three points are worth stating plainly.

First, the primary partners are not background. They are people whose attachment systems are organized around the very people whose emotional availability is being committed elsewhere. Freyd's (1996) betrayal trauma theory names the specific injury produced when harm is delivered by a depended-upon other. The primary partner of an adult engaged in extradyadic emotional attachment is not experiencing ordinary relational disappointment. They are sustaining attachment-level injury from the person on whom their attachment is organized. This injury is real even when the extradyadic relationship has not become sexual. It is real even when the partner does not yet know consciously that the configuration has changed. The relational atmosphere shifts; the unspoken withdrawal of emotional availability is perceived, often before it is named.

Second, the role engulfment described in Section IV is not unique to A and B. Their respective primary partners are also embedded in long-term role-based functioning. The household runs, the children are raised, the bills are paid, and in many such households the partner who is not the focus of clinical attention has been quietly carrying their own version of the same erosion. The framework that explains A's emotional deprivation also, in many cases, explains the deprivation of the person across the table from A at dinner. To use the Dual-Track frame as if it identified one party in the marriage as the truly suffering one is to misuse it.

Third, the framework explicitly does not warrant ongoing relational harm. It is offered to help clinicians understand a process. It is not offered to license its continuation. A practitioner who hears a client describe a years-long extradyadic emotional involvement and validates it as "emotional self-preservation" without engaging the parallel reality of the primary partner is not practicing trauma-informed care. They are practicing a partial reading of one party's pain at the cost of another party's well-being. This is the failure mode the framework most needs to guard against, and the operational sections that follow are constructed with that risk in view.

Centering the unseen partner has several practical implications taken up in Section V: the assessment protocol asks directly about the experience of others affected by the client's relational situation; the clinical heuristics include explicit guidance against using the framework to rationalize harm; the organizational guidance treats systemic supports as relevant to both partners in a marriage, not only the one whose suffering happens to be in the room.

V. OPERATIONALIZING THE FRAMEWORK

The book in which this chapter appears foregrounds operationalization: the translation of trauma-informed principles into concrete, usable practice across systems. This section offers four operational components: a trauma-informed assessment protocol for long-term role strain (5.1); clinical practice guidelines and decision heuristics (5.2); organizational and institutional implementation (5.3); and reflective practice guidance for practitioners (5.4). None of these is a validated instrument. They are structured, usable tools intended to be adapted by competent practitioners and refined through empirical work.

5.1 A Trauma-Informed Assessment Protocol for Long-Term Role Strain

The protocol is organized as a semi-structured interview across six assessment domains. It is intended for use after rapport is established and after the practitioner has explained the rationale, including the explicit framing that experiences in long-term role-based functioning can be assessed in trauma-informed terms even when they have not been previously named that way. The protocol does not produce a score. It produces a clinical formulation.

Practitioners should adapt the language to the client's cultural and linguistic context, and should pace the protocol over more than one session when material is heavy. The protocol assumes the practitioner is also attentive to the safety, voice, and choice of the client throughout, in keeping with SAMHSA (2014) principles. Table 1 presents the six domains, what each assesses, and sample prompt questions for use in clinical interview.

Table 1. Six-domain trauma-informed assessment protocol for long-term role strain

Domain	What the domain assesses	Sample prompt questions
1. Role architecture	The structure of roles the client carries, their duration, and the resources available to sustain them	"Walk me through the roles you hold day to day. How long have you been carrying each of these? Where do you feel you have support; where do you feel you are mostly alone in the work?"
2. Identity attenuation	The extent to which the client experiences a gap between the functional self they enact and a subjective self that feels less visible to them	"When was the last time you felt clearly like yourself, not in a role? What dimensions of you do you feel are not currently being seen anywhere in your life? If you set down all your responsibilities for an afternoon, what do you imagine would surface?"
3. Emotional recognition history	The pattern, across time, of being emotionally seen inside the primary relationship	"When you are struggling, where do you take that? When was the last time you felt your partner perceived something you were feeling without you having to point at it? Has this changed over the course of the relationship?"
4. Regulatory load and depletion	The cumulative regulatory work the client is doing for themselves and others, and signs of depletion	"Whose feelings are you tracking in a typical day? Who tracks yours? What does your body do when you are at the end of a hard week? How recoverable does that feel?"

continued on following page

Table 1. Continued

Domain	What the domain assesses	Sample prompt questions
5. Activation outside the primary system	Whether emotional activation has begun to seek expression in other relational contexts, and how the client understands it	"Have you noticed yourself looking forward to interactions outside the marriage in a way that feels new? Are there relationships in which you feel more like yourself than you do at home? How do you make sense of that?"
6. Impact on others	The client's awareness of and engagement with the experience of others in the relational system, including the primary partner and any children	"How is your partner doing? What do they know about your inner state? If we asked them to describe the relationship, what do you think they would say? How are the children placed in all this?"

The sixth domain matters in trauma-informed practice. Clients in role engulfment are often so depleted that the only experience available to them is their own. The protocol intentionally surfaces the others in the system without making the client defensive about doing so. The aim is not to challenge or accuse; the aim is to bring the people in the system into shared view so that clinical work proceeds with their presence honored.

Practitioners should treat the protocol as generating hypotheses rather than answers. Two domains scoring as severely depleted may indicate cumulative relational trauma; the same pattern may also reflect a major depressive episode, an undiagnosed health condition, or an acute external stressor. The protocol is a way of looking, not a way of concluding.

5.2 Clinical Practice Guidelines and Decision Heuristics

The following heuristics are offered as guidance for clinicians working with clients whose presentations include features of the pattern described in this chapter. They are framed as practice-level orientations rather than rules.

1. Name the process before naming the behavior. Where extradyadic emotional involvement is part of the presentation, attend first to the underlying process of role engulfment and identity attenuation. Beginning with the behavior tends to recapitulate the moral frame the client already inhabits and forecloses the more useful clinical work.
2. Hold the framework as descriptive, not prescriptive. The Dual-Track Emotional System describes a pattern. It does not recommend any specific relational outcome. It is not a permission slip for the continuation of an extradyadic relationship; it is also not a verdict in favor of immediate disclosure or termination. The decision is the client's, and the clinician's role is to support reflective decision-making.

3. Keep the unseen partner in the room. Across sessions, return to the experience of the primary partner. Use the assessment protocol's sixth domain repeatedly, not only at intake. The clinical risk is silent erasure: the partner who is not present becomes, over time, less imaginatively real to the work. Counteract that with deliberate attention.
4. Distinguish the activation from the action. The activation of the personal emotional system in response to a new context is a piece of clinical information. It is not by itself an indictment or a justification. The pertinent therapeutic work is what the person does with the activation: whether it becomes a window onto unmet needs that could, in some cases, be addressed within the primary relationship; whether it becomes a sustained extradyadic involvement with its own consequences; whether it becomes information that helps the person face that the primary relationship is no longer viable. Each of these paths is real. None is foreclosed by the framework.
5. Name betrayal trauma when it is present. If the client's primary partner is aware of the extradyadic involvement, or eventually becomes aware, the partner is sustaining betrayal trauma in the sense described by Freyd (1996). This is a clinical reality, not a moral judgment. The framework's intelligibility does not soften this fact, and competent practice will not present it as if it did.
6. Slow the work. Decisions made under acute activation often serve neither the client nor the others in their system. Cumulative relational trauma has built up over years; sustainable response is not built in days. Where the institutional setting permits, the clinician's pacing should resist pressure toward premature resolution.
7. Know when to refer. The framework supports individual therapy with one party. It does not substitute for couples therapy with both partners present, and it does not constitute family or systemic intervention. When the situation calls for couples work, or for work with the children, or for legal or financial consultation, the clinician should refer.
8. Engage your own consultation. Material of this kind activates clinicians. Reflective practice, consultation, and supervision are not optional features of competent work in this territory.

A brief illustration of the heuristics at work may make their application more concrete. Consider a hypothetical client, M, a 47-year-old hospital administrator with two adolescent children and an 18-year marriage. M presents with insomnia, low-grade depression, and recent involvement in a sustained emotional connection with a colleague. The novice clinical instinct may be to begin with the connection itself: clarify its boundaries, advise on disclosure, address the behavior. The heuristics above suggest a different opening. Begin with the architecture: what M is carrying, for how long, with what support, and against what kind of recognition deprivation at home. The emotional connection becomes a piece of clinical data inside that fuller picture, not the headline. The pacing of the work, the framing of decisions, and the eventual options M considers all look different when the underlying process is named first. This is the work the framework supports.

5.3 Organizational and Institutional Implementation

The framework points beyond the individual clinical encounter to the systems inside which long-term role engulfment is produced and sustained. Trauma-informed institutional response involves three layers.

In healthcare systems, primary care and behavioral health integration provide a natural site for early identification. Long-term role strain produces patterned somatic and affective findings—chronic fatigue, sleep disturbance, persistent low-grade depression, increasing alcohol use—that often arrive at primary care long before they arrive at a therapist's office. Brief screening for sustained role load and recognition deprivation, embedded inside ordinary visits, can route adults toward appropriate support before the trauma has consolidated into a relational crisis. Such screening should be designed in consultation with patients and with trauma-informed clinicians, and should follow the SAMHSA (2014) principles around choice and non-retraumatization.

In employee assistance programs (EAPs) and human resources contexts, the operational implication is the development of supports for the chronic, low-visibility emotional load of working adults across the life course. The standard EAP frame, oriented around acute episodes, is not well calibrated for the slow accumulation this chapter describes. Concrete steps include: making short-course reflective groups available to mid-career employees; training managers in trauma-informed supervision so that role load is named rather than only assumed; providing genuine, non-stigmatized routes into therapy that protect confidentiality; and recognizing caregiving leave and recovery time as workforce needs rather than personal indulgences.

In community mental health and social service systems, the operational task is the recognition of cumulative relational deprivation as a presenting concern in its own right rather than as a soft preamble to more easily codable diagnoses. Intake protocols can incorporate the assessment domains in Section 5.1. Group programs can be developed around chronic role strain and identity attenuation, particularly for caregivers of children, of older parents, or of disabled family members. These programs need not be deficit-framed. The most usable framings name the strength involved in long-term role-based functioning and create space for the dimensions of self that the work has crowded out.

Across all three layers, a trauma-informed systems orientation requires explicit attention to who is left unsupported by current arrangements. Adults of color, working-class adults, immigrant adults, and adults in caregiving labor are typically under-served by the existing EAP and behavioral health infrastructure, often precisely the populations whose structural role load is heaviest. Operationalizing the framework at the systems level means designing for, and with, these populations rather than assuming that supports developed for higher-resource patients will scale down.

5.4 Reflective Practice for Practitioners

Trauma-informed work with this material is not technique-only work. It activates the clinician. Practitioners who themselves are deep into mid-career role engulfment may find their own systems engaged by the client's material in ways that warrant explicit reflection. The following practices are offered as supports.

Maintain a reflective journal that includes, at least monthly, attention to two questions: where in my current life am I primarily inhabiting the functional track, and where am I being seen as a person rather than as a role? The aim is not therapeutic self-disclosure; it is to keep the practitioner's own architecture visible to them.

Use peer consultation deliberately. Cases involving extradyadic emotional involvement frequently invite splitting in the consultation room as well as in the client's life. Consultation groups in which one client is consistently rendered as the suffering protagonist and the absent partner is consistently rendered as the obstacle are doing the splitting they should be helping clinicians notice. Structure consultation so that the unseen partner is brought into the discussion deliberately.

Sit with the limits of the framework. The Dual-Track model is a useful map. It is not the territory. When the framework appears to be explaining everything, the practitioner should treat that as a signal to slow down, not as evidence of the framework's power.

Tend to one's own intersectional location. The clinician's gender, culture, class, race, and relational status shape what they hear in this material and what they overlook. Reflective practice means engaging those locations explicitly rather than assuming neutrality.

A clinician new to this material may also find it useful to develop a working personal vocabulary for the rhythms the framework describes. The shift from "an affair" to "an extradyadic emotional involvement inside a long-term pattern of role engulfment" is more than a phrasing change. It alters what the clinician listens for in intake, what they record in notes, and what they organize the work around. Such vocabulary is not jargon for its own sake. It is the practical equipment for keeping the framework usable across cases.

VI. ETHICAL ACCOUNTABILITY AND INTERSECTIONAL AWARENESS

6.1 Ethical Tensions in Applying the Framework

The application of the Dual-Track Emotional System raises a distinctive ethical tension. The framework asks clinicians to take seriously the suffering of role-engulfed adults whose surface lives look functional, including the dimension of that suffering expressed through extradyadic emotional involvement. It is meaningful precisely because it does not begin from a moralizing posture toward the behavior. The risk is that, in not beginning from moralism, it can drift into the opposite posture: the validation of a client's experience to the exclusion of the experience of others affected by the same situation.

Three commitments hold this tension. The framework names a process; it does not justify outcomes. The framework centers one party in clinical attention because clinical attention is necessarily focal; it must, simultaneously, hold others in the room imaginatively. The framework supports the client's reflective decision-making; it does not lobby for any specific decision, including continuation, disclosure, or termination of the extradyadic involvement.

6.2 Comparative Ethics: Harm Relative to What Alternative?

A second dimension of ethical accountability concerns what clinicians are implicitly assuming when they frame the parallel emotional bond purely as harm to be eliminated. A systemic, trauma-informed reading invites a different question: harm relative to what alternative? In cases where the functional marital structure has become so identity-consuming that one or both partners have lost contact with their own emotional life, the available pathways are rarely binary. Full relational transparency may precipitate family dissolution, with real consequences for children who are structurally dependent on an intact household. Continued emotional suppression—role performance without any emotional track at all—may preserve the outward structure while accelerating internal depletion, raising the risk of clinical depression, somatic illness, parental disengagement, and the further erosion of the self as a felt subject. Esther Perel (2007) has argued that long-term partnership generates a structural tension between domestic functionality and the felt sense of being an emotionally alive subject; the parallel emotional bond is not always the source of that tension, but sometimes a downstream sign of it.

A harm-reduction framing, familiar from trauma-informed work in adjacent fields, treats such situations as requiring a comparative rather than absolute calculus. The parallel emotional bond, in this systemic view, sometimes functions as the lesser cost: it allows the individual to remain a functioning parent and partner precisely because some portion of their subjective self has been returned to them. Research on parental emotional depletion (Mikulincer & Shaver, 2016) suggests that caregivers who lack access to their own emotional regulation resources are less able to provide the sensitive, attuned caregiving that children require for secure attachment. A parent who has begun to feel alive again may, paradoxically, be a more present parent. This observation does not resolve the ethical complexity. It deepens it. But ethical accountability, properly understood, requires the clinician to hold this complexity rather than resolving it prematurely through the imposition of a culturally dominant moral script.

This reframing also engages a meaning-centered understanding of adult development. Frankl (1959/1984) argued that the capacity to find meaning—to experience one's life as pointing toward something—is a fundamental psychological need, and that its absence constitutes a form of existential suffering as debilitating as any clinical disorder. When adults in role-engulfed long-term partnerships describe a parallel emotional bond as the first experience in years of feeling genuinely seen, or of sensing that their existence matters beyond its instrumental function, they are describing the restoration of meaning-making capacity. A trauma-informed ethical stance requires that this restoration be taken seriously as a clinical and human reality—not as a justification for deception, but as a datum that enlarges the field's understanding of what has been lost in chronic role engulfment and what recovery might require. Holding this account alongside the betrayal trauma framework of Section 4.5 is the actual work of ethical accountability in this material: not the resolution of the tension between the two, but its competent, non-collapsing maintenance across cases.

6.3 Holding Multiple Affected Parties in View

Section 4.5 took the unseen partner seriously as a subject of cumulative relational trauma in their own right. That commitment shapes ethical practice across the work. Three operational implications follow.

First, language matters. Describing the primary partner exclusively in functional terms—"the husband," "the wife," "the marriage"—while describing the extradyadic involvement in emotional terms—"the connection," "the recognition"—frames the situation asymmetrically before any analysis has begun. Practitioners should listen for and resist this asymmetry in their own speech and writing.

Second, children are persons in the system. The cases this chapter addresses frequently involve adolescents and adults' minor children who have not chosen the emotional configuration of their parents and whose welfare is part of any responsible decision. The framework does not adjudicate decisions about disclosure to children, custody, or family structure. It does mark the children as present.

Third, the framework should not be applied in contexts of coercion, abuse, or power asymmetry in the primary relationship without explicit attention to those dynamics. A client describing emotional deprivation may also be describing controlling or abusive treatment by the primary partner. Conversely, a client describing emotional deprivation may be the partner whose chronic withdrawal has been the primary driver of the very deprivation they now report. The framework does not adjudicate these realities by itself. The practitioner must.

6.4 Intersectional Application: Gender, Culture, Class, Race

Intersectional analysis is part of the framework's substantive content, not an add-on. Several specific clinical implications follow.

Gendered exposure to role engulfment is real and patterned (Hochschild, 1983/2003; Umberson et al., 2006). Women in heterosexual marriages, particularly those carrying disproportionate caregiving and emotional labor, are structurally over-exposed to the conditions the framework describes. Clinicians should expect this asymmetry in caseloads and should resist treating it as coincidence.

Cultural context shapes both the experience and the expression of emotional deprivation. Collectivist family scripts may foreground duty in ways that further normalize the functional pole and stigmatize the emotional one. Clinicians working across cultural contexts should not impose individualist therapeutic frames on clients for whom those frames are themselves an additional pressure. The framework can be applied across cultural contexts, but its language and its operational tools should be adapted accordingly.

Class shapes access. The supports recommended in Section 5.3 are unevenly available. A trauma-informed and intersectionally aware application of the framework engages structural advocacy as part of clinical practice, not as a separate political activity.

Race intersects all of the above. The cumulative relational load carried by adults of color in contexts shaped by discrimination is not a separate domain from the role engulfment described in this chapter; it is one of its compounding conditions. The framework's operationalization should attend to that compounding directly rather than treating race as a demographic variable.

LGBTQ+ adults, adults in non-monogamous relational configurations, and adults whose family structures do not match dominant scripts encounter the patterns the framework describes in their own forms. The framework's language—two tracks of identity inside one person under role demand—translates across these contexts, but the assessment protocol and decision heuristics should be applied with attentiveness to the specific structural conditions of the client's life.

6.5 Limits of the Framework and Misuse Risks

The framework has several specific misuse risks worth naming.

It can be used to intellectualize behavior the user wishes to continue. A client who reads parts of this chapter may arrive in session articulating "Dual-Track Emotional System" language as a justification for ongoing extradyadic involvement they have chosen not to disclose. The framework's job in that moment is not to support the justification but to help the client engage what they have not yet engaged.

It can be used to pathologize ordinary marital ambivalence. Not every long marriage is characterized by role engulfment and identity attenuation. Many adults in long marriages are simply navigating the ordinary unevennesses of partnership. The framework is calibrated to a specific cumulative pattern. Over-application is a misuse.

It can be used to displace responsibility onto the primary partner. The framework explains the conditions under which one party's emotional system becomes attenuated. It does not entail that the primary partner has caused this attenuation, and it should not be deployed to construct the primary partner as the antagonist of the case.

It can be deployed by practitioners as a self-narrative. Practitioners who recognize aspects of their own lives in the framework should engage that recognition in supervision and personal therapy, not by reading their own situations through their clients' material.

It can be reduced to a single explanation for a wide range of presentations. Adults in long-term partnerships present with many forms of distress that do not reduce to the pattern this chapter describes: chronic medical conditions, addiction, grief, financial precarity, undiagnosed neurodivergence, the slow accumulation of unaddressed conflict. The framework is not a master key. When it does not fit, it should be set down and a different lens picked up.

These risks do not invalidate the framework. They mark the limits within which it should be used. Section VII returns to the empirical work that would let the field refine those limits more precisely.

VII. CONCLUSION AND FUTURE DIRECTIONS

Trauma-informed care has been built largely around events. This chapter has argued that the field's operational toolkit needs to extend to a category of cumulative relational deprivation that does not look like trauma from the outside:

chronic emotional under-recognition inside long-term role-based functioning. The Dual-Track Emotional System has been offered as a conceptual framework for that work, distinguishing the functional responsibility system (the self organized around obligation) from the personal emotional system (the self organized around recognition) and tracing how their asymmetric development over years produces identity attenuation, regulatory depletion, and—in some cases—the relational dynamics that bring people into clinical contact.

Three commitments have run through the chapter. The first is operational: assessment protocol, clinical heuristics, organizational implementation, and reflective practice have been described in sufficient concrete detail that competent practitioners can begin to use them. The second is ethical: the unseen primary partner has been centered as a person whose betrayal trauma is real, and the framework has been explicitly bracketed against use as a rationalization for ongoing harm. The third is intersectional: the structural conditions that produce role engulfment have been named, and the practice implications across gender, culture, class, race, and family configuration have been written into the framework rather than appended to it.

The framework should also remain modest about what it is. It is conceptual and clinical, not empirical. It rests on patterns observed in clinical and supervisory contexts, not on systematic data. Several lines of empirical work would strengthen it. Mixed-methods studies could examine how the assessment domains in Section 5.1 perform in practice across diverse populations. Longitudinal designs could test whether sustained dominance of the functional track predicts the downstream outcomes the framework anticipates. Couple-level research could explore how the primary partner's experience tracks alongside that of the role-engulfed partner. Implementation research in EAP and primary care settings could examine whether early identification routes adults toward effective supports before relational crises consolidate. Cross-cultural work could test the framework's portability and identify the adaptations required for its use in different contexts.

One closing observation belongs in the chapter rather than in a separate phenomenological section. Adults in long-term role engulfment often describe their experience as an ordinary one, even though it is steadily costing them something. They live the same days, fulfill the same responsibilities, occupy the same houses. From the outside nothing breaks. From the inside, a dimension of the self has been quietly missing for a long time. Trauma-informed care, applied to this terrain, does not require that the structure of life be overturned. It requires that the dimension of self that has been missing be brought back into clinical, organizational, and institutional view—not as a private matter for the role-strained adult alone, and not at the cost of the partner who has been beside them all along, but as a shared concern for the systems that ask adults to carry what they carry.

REFERENCES

Allen, E. S., Atkins, D. C., Baucom, D. H., Snyder, D. K., Gordon, K. C., & Glass, S. P. (2005). Intrapersonal, interpersonal, and contextual factors in engaging in and responding to extramarital involvement. *Clinical Psychology : a Publication of the Division of Clinical Psychology of the American Psychological Association, 12*(2), 101–130. DOI: 10.1093/clipsy.bpi014

Atkins, D. C., Baucom, D. H., & Jacobson, N. S. (2001). Understanding infidelity: Correlates in a national random sample. *Journal of Family Psychology, 15*(4), 735–749. DOI: 10.1037/0893-3200.15.4.735 PMID: 11770478

Bowlby, J. (1982). Attachment and loss: Vol. 1. *Attachment* (2nd ed.). Basic Books. (Original work published 1969)

Bowlby, J. (1988). *A secure base: Parent-child attachment and healthy human development.* Basic Books.

Clandinin, D. J., & Connelly, F. M. (2000). *Narrative inquiry: Experience and story in qualitative research.* Jossey-Bass.

Collins, P. H. (2000). *Black feminist thought: Knowledge, consciousness, and the politics of empowerment* (2nd ed.). Routledge.

Crenshaw, K. (1989). Demarginalizing the intersection of race and sex: A Black feminist critique of antidiscrimination doctrine, feminist theory, and antiracist politics. *University of Chicago Legal Forum, 1989*(1), 139–167.

Fishman, D. B. (1999). *The case for pragmatic psychology.* New York University Press.

Frankl, V. E. (1984). *Man's search for meaning* (Rev. ed.). Washington Square Press. (Original work published 1959)

Freyd, J. J. (1996). *Betrayal trauma: The logic of forgetting childhood abuse.* Harvard University Press.

Glass, S. P., & Wright, T. L. (1985). Sex differences in type of extramarital involvement and marital dissatisfaction. *Journal of Sex Research, 21*(4), 361–387.

Gottman, J. M., & Driver, J. L. (2005). Dysfunctional marital conflict and everyday marital interaction. *Journal of Divorce & Remarriage, 43*(3–4), 63–77. DOI: 10.1300/J087v43n03_04

Gross, J. J. (1998). The emerging field of emotion regulation: An integrative review. *Review of General Psychology, 2*(3), 271–299. DOI: 10.1037/1089-2680.2.3.271

Gross, J. J., & John, O. P. (2003). Individual differences in two emotion regulation processes: Implications for affect, relationships, and well-being. *Journal of Personality and Social Psychology, 85*(2), 348–362. DOI: 10.1037/0022-3514.85.2.348 PMID: 12916575

Herman, J. L. (1992). *Trauma and recovery: The aftermath of violence—from domestic abuse to political terror.* Basic Books.

Hochschild, A. R. (2003). The managed heart: Commercialization of human feeling (20th anniversary ed.). University of California Press. (Original work published 1983)

Kroger, J. (2007). *Identity development: Adolescence through adulthood* (2nd ed.). Sage.

MacIntosh, H. B. (2024). Developmental couple therapy for complex trauma: A pilot study of treatment outcomes. *Journal of Marital and Family Therapy, 50*(2), 411–432.

Mark, K. P., Janssen, E., & Milhausen, R. R. (2011). Infidelity in heterosexual couples: Demographic, interpersonal, and personality-related predictors of extradyadic sex. *Archives of Sexual Behavior, 40*(5), 971–982. DOI: 10.1007/s10508-011-9771-z PMID: 21667234

Mikulincer, M., & Shaver, P. R. (2016). *Attachment in adulthood: Structure, dynamics, and change* (2nd ed.). Guilford Press.

Perel, E. (2007). *Mating in captivity: Unlocking erotic intelligence.* HarperCollins.

Schön, D. A. (1983). *The reflective practitioner: How professionals think in action.* Basic Books.

Siegel, D. J. (2012). *The developing mind: How relationships and the brain interact to shape who we are* (2nd ed.). Guilford Press.

Simon, R. W. (1995). Gender, multiple roles, role meaning, and mental health. *Journal of Health and Social Behavior, 36*(2), 182–194. DOI: 10.2307/2137224 PMID: 9113142

Stake, R. E. (2005). Qualitative case studies. In Denzin, N. K., & Lincoln, Y. S. (Eds.), *The Sage handbook of qualitative research* (3rd ed., pp. 443–466). Sage.

Substance Abuse and Mental Health Services Administration. (2014). *SAMHSA's concept of trauma and guidance for a trauma-informed approach (HHS Publication No. SMA 14-4884)*. U.S. Department of Health and Human Services.

Thoits, P. A. (1991). On merging identity theory and stress research. *Social Psychology Quarterly, 54*(2), 101–112. DOI: 10.2307/2786929

Umberson, D., Thomeer, M. B., & Lodge, A. C. (2006). Intimacy and emotion work in lesbian, gay, and heterosexual relationships. *Journal of Marriage and Family, 77*(2), 542–556. DOI: 10.1111/jomf.12178 PMID: 25814771

van der Kolk, B. A. (2014). *The body keeps the score: Brain, mind, and body in the healing of trauma*. Viking.

Zaki, J., & Williams, W. C. (2013). Interpersonal emotion regulation. *Emotion (Washington, D.C.), 13*(5), 803–810. DOI: 10.1037/a0033839 PMID: 24098929

KEY TERMS AND DEFINITIONS

Cumulative Relational Trauma: The psychological injury produced by prolonged emotional under-recognition inside an ongoing relational system, accumulating across years rather than arising from a discrete event, and producing trauma-relevant outcomes including identity attenuation, regulatory depletion, and attachment activation. Dual-Track Emotional System. A conceptual framework that distinguishes two interrelated identity processes within the same person—the functional responsibility system and the personal emotional system—and describes how their asymmetric development across adult life produces the patterns of role engulfment, identity attenuation, and downstream relational behavior addressed in this chapter. Functional Responsibility System. The dimension of identity organized around social role, obligation, and external performance; the self constructed through what the person sustains for others. Personal Emotional System. The dimension of identity organized around recognition, affective resonance, and subjective presence; the self that needs to be perceived rather than only to perform.

Role Engulfment: The process by which a single dominant role gradually crowds out other dimensions of identity, leaving the person organized almost entirely around what they do for others rather than who they are (Kroger, 2007). Identity Attenuation. The progressive thinning of subjective self-experience under sustained role demand, in which the emotional self does not disappear but becomes increasingly difficult to locate inside the structures of daily life. Emotional Reactivation. The renewed external expression of a previously under-engaged personal emotional system, typically occurring when a relational context offers recognition that has been chronically absent. Betrayal Trauma. The distinctive psychological injury produced when harm is delivered by a person on whom one depends, particularly relevant to the experience of primary partners of adults engaged in extradyadic emotional involvement (Freyd, 1996).

Trauma-Informed Care: An approach to service delivery grounded in awareness of trauma's prevalence and impact, organized around the principles of safety, trustworthiness and transparency, peer support, collaboration and mutuality, empowerment and choice, and attention to cultural, historical, and gender issues (SAMHSA, 2014). Intersectional Application. The clinical and institutional practice of attending to how gender, race, class, culture, sexuality, and family configuration shape both the production of role engulfment and the resources available for its address (Crenshaw, 1989; Collins, 2000).

Chapter 5
Trauma Induced by Psychology Training:
Programs Harm Disabled and Neurodivergent Students

Christine E. Hagion-Rzepka
http://orcid.org/0009-0001-5212-1774
California Southern University, USA

ABSTRACT

This chapter identifies layers of systemic oppression of disabled and neurodivergent students and psychology trainees, using a trauma-informed lens. It focuses on disability-related discrimination; ableist microaggressions by faculty and clinical supervisors; ableistic program design; and exclusionary expectations. Twelve short case studies illustrate recurrent practices imposing trauma upon a vulnerable population by those in power, exercising unjust privilege and disability prejudice. It examines politics behind the resulting institutional betrayal. Ethical and legal issues are highlighted, as a disability-related social justice issue. It portrays the depth and breadth of the problem within clinical training sites and academic programs, deepening understanding through a justice-oriented lens. It discusses institutional resistance to inclusion of disability and neurodiversity, which perpetuate inequity. The chapter offers implementable changes to deconstruct discriminatory and exclusionary existing structures, while upholding rigorous standards that are equitable and accountable.

DOI: 10.4018/979-8-3373-8597-6.ch005

INTRODUCTION

Trauma-informed care has been a buzzword in community care and mental health policy, but it is not practiced toward students in the educational system for professional training in psychology and clinical mental health counseling.

Those who are shaping the workforce of future mental health practitioners—including counselor educators, supervisors, clinical training directors, faculty and directors of academic training programs—have often viewed trauma-informed practice solely through the lens of the end-user: the client, or the patient, only. What has frequently been forgotten in this training paradigm is that those who are the future providers (i.e., the graduate students being trained to provide such care) may be survivors themselves of various forms of trauma. Programs of high quality will recognize this to some degree, and will hopefully provide resources for these students and trainees to deal with their countertransference, to address vicarious trauma, and prevent burnout in such cases.

However, there are frequent experiences during the training itself that induce trauma upon the students and trainees in graduate programs, often the result of misused power by those in positions of evaluative authority. This is particularly true for disabled and neurodivergent students.

Purpose

This chapter will address the systemic barriers faced by disabled and neurodivergent students and trainees within clinical mental health training programs, using a trauma-informed lens. Not only will it present the relevant research, but it will also provide anecdotal evidence in twelve case studies to forcefully illustrate the need for improvement to make our clinical mental health training programs more inclusive and welcoming to all, regardless of ability status.

How This Chapter is Organized

This chapter is organized into seven parts, and uses a trauma-informed lens to examine the systematic and structural barriers for disabled and neurodivergent people. *Conceptual Foundations* (Part I), covers definitions, the concept of disability as a social identity and its complexities when expanded to the neurodivergent population, and disability as an element of diversity that is often not included in most discussions on diversity, equity, inclusion, and belonging. This section will briefly cover how accommodations are one of the things distinguishing disabled and neurodivergent people from other minority groups and the programming provided to them. It will also briefly discuss the intersections between disability and other minority group identities.

Uncovering the Layers of Systemic Oppression (Part II), identifies eight elements affecting the full inclusion of disabled and neurodivergent people in society as well as in graduate training for psychology. It covers 1) disability prejudice and 2) discrimination, 3) ableism, 4) ableist microaggressions, 5) the erasure of people with disabilities, 6) disproportionality within clinical mental health training programs, 7) complications and misunderstanding of the need for accommodations, and 8) lack of necessary accommodations.

Disability Accommodations (Part III) addresses the accommodations process, accommodations in academia, and examples of formal and informal academic accommodations, and how the power differential intersects with disability in seeking accommodations, workplace accommodations in clinical training, and how accommodations are an issue of equity for disabled and neurodivergent trainees.

Case Studies of Ableism in Action (Part IV), includes four case studies in academia, four case studies in clinical training, and four case studies of trauma imposed upon PWDN in both academic and clinical training sites. The practical training as a dual component of professional psychology education will be described, and legal and ethical issues are identified for all cases presented.

Analyzing the Psychological Complexities of These Case Studies (Part V), examines the concept of institutional betrayal in both academia and in clinical training, including the weaponization of student expectations and codes of conduct and use of DARVO tactics. The section then covers the misuse of the gatekeeping function of psychology, politics behind institutional betrayal, and the potential involvement of the dark triad in disability discrimination, lack of awareness of disability laws, as possible causes of noncompliance, and a discussion of uneven power dynamics.

How the Psychology Training-to-Workforce Pipeline Can Improve (Part VI), Covers

the ABCs of disability inclusion, dissemination of disability research, adopting a trauma-informed and disability inclusive approach within the educational setting, recommendations to address the structural issues in academia and in clinical training, as well as within the profession overall.

APA's Public Policies Regarding Disability (Part VI), summarizes the many policy documents published by the American Psychological Association on issues of disability, including documents calling for disability inclusion, organizational commitment to the full participation of disabled psychologists, the unique concerns for disabled and neurodivergent interns and applicants, and future directions for the profession based upon the leadership of the foremost professional organization for psychologists.

I. CONCEPTUAL FOUNDATIONS

The Population of Interest in This Chapter

People With Disabilities are often referred to in the academic literature with the abbreviation, PWD. However, even that acronym leaves out a subpopulation of the people with disability, namely those who are neurodivergent.

Neurodivergence refers to those whose brain differs in some way from standard development, and may be attributable to congenital differences, developmental issues, injury, or infection. Thus, neurodivergence in itself has a wide possibility of presentations. Some of the conditions that fall under the umbrella term of neurodiversity include the following: Attention Deficit Disorder (with or without the Hyperactivity component), people on the autism spectrum, Sensory Processing Disorders (defined in the next paragraph), Tourette's Syndrome, and conditions previously called "learning disabilities," such as dyslexia, dyscalculia, dysgraphia, nonverbal learning disorders, auditory processing disorders, dyspraxia, and other nonspecific conditions that fall into this category (Fung, 2021). Some scholars also include Post-Traumatic Stress Disorder (PTSD) or Complex Post-Traumatic Stress Disorder (CPTSD), Bipolar Disorders, Fetal Alcohol Syndrome, and acquired or traumatic brain injury (TBI) in the list of neurodivergent conditions (Bolton, 2023).

According to Galiana-Simal et al., (2020), Sensory Processing Disorders fall into certain categories, including Sensory Modulation Disorder, with three subtypes (Sensory Over-Responsivity, Sensory Under-Responsivity, and Sensory Craving); Sensory-Based Motor Disorder (dyspraxia, postural disorder); and Sensory Discrimination Disorder (visual, auditory, tactile, taste/smell, position or movement, and interoception). All SPDs are neurodivergent conditions involving how sensory stimuli is processed within the brain. Some literature refers to people who are blind or low vision or those who are Deaf or hard of hearing as having sensory disabilities, which should not be misconstrued for the various forms of SPDs, which are neurodivergent but not physical conditions as are deafness and blindness.

This chapter will use the PWD acronym, using such only when speaking exclusively to those with disabilities, be they visible or invisible. However, neurodivergence itself is considered a disability for the purposes of obtaining services and accommodation, though many who are neurodivergent do not adhere to a disability identity. For maximum inclusivity, this chapter will adapt the use of PWD by adding an N, so that it will signify both people with disabilities or neurodivergence (PWDN).

Disability as an Identity in and of Itself

Bogart et al. (2017) point out that while a large percentage of our global population has a disability, a much smaller fraction of them identify as a disabled person (Watson, 2002). There are contextual factors that may impact whether or not a person chooses to "pass" as a nondisabled individual, among them being environmental factors such as stigma and social support, as well as the level of impairment (Bogart et al., 2017). Undoubtedly, for persons with visible disabilities, the calculus may differ, but for those with invisible disabilities, their impairment factors (identified by Bogart et al., 2017) as duration, noticeability, presence of congenital impairment, pain, severity, and total number of impairments) play a role, as well. In their research, the level of stigma as well as severity of the impairment were the most common factors that determined whether the disabled individuals int their study identified as being disabled or not (Bogart et al., 2017). Research has shown that a strong disability identity is protective in combatting the negative impact of exclusion, microaggressions, bullying and related trauma (Dunn & Burkaw, 2013).

Disability as an Element of Diversity

Disability, Equity, and Inclusion (DEI) programs have advanced in recent decades in both educational and employment settings, in order to increase plurality and cultural sensitivity. Moreover, many strive to promote equity, with a view to the end that groups which have been historically disadvantaged would enjoy the same level of attainment as those holding more privilege in our dominant society. In addition, some add a B to the acronym, as they seek to provide environments which promote a sense of belonging to those whose identities may have been excluded.

However, DEI(B) programs almost routinely exclude disability and neurodiversity, despite the disabled population being the largest of all minority groups. One in four persons in the United States has a disability (Tran et al. 2025), affecting roughly 30% of the American population (Bogart et al., 2026).

DEI programs have been hotly debated in recent years, with some who are not part of affinity or identity groups for people of color, or gender nonconforming individuals, or sexual minorities feeling excluded from the very programs which are intended to promote inclusivity.

Such criticisms also often claim that these affinity groups have been granted priority and have obtained positions because of their minority status, rather than by merit. On the other side of the equation, those promoting diversity, equity, and inclusion claim that these minority groups have been marginalized and those not a part of these affinity groups hold unearned privilege as a result.

This chapter will not review these issues as they have been extensively covered elsewhere, except with a nod to the notion that many who have been historically disadvantaged also report having experienced systemic oppression. This chapter will, however, address the issue of systemic oppression as it is experienced by disabled persons and those with neurodivergent conditions.

Accommodations: A Departure from the DEI(B) Norm

In other minoritized populations, such as Black, Indigenous, and People of Color (BIPOC), as well as sexual minorities and gender-nonconforming populations (LGBTQI+), there are specialized services specifically for these groups in most universities and private schools for professional psychology. Students enrolling in services for BIPOC or LGBTQI+ groups enjoy cultural diversity awareness days or months, themed events tailored to identity or affinity groups, minority scholarships, unique placement opportunities, and occasionally even separate graduation ceremonies. Many corporations have similar programs to promote diversity within their workforce along this same subset of people.

Conversely, PWDN generally have no such campus groups or unique programs to promote visibility, cultural awareness, or sensitivity in either college campuses, in corporations, private industry, or the public sector. One thing that makes the PWDN population unique is that many of its members require accommodations specific to their respective disability in order to obtain an education or to be successful in employment. The third section of this chapter will speak directly to accommodations.

Intersectionality

Moreover, in many educational or employment settings who do have DEI(B) programs, PWDN who also self-identify in one or more marginalized groups often must choose between programming for the other group (such as BIPOC or LGBTQ+ programs), in order to procure support services (McDonald et al., 2007). In some cases, PWDN who also happen to be persons of color, or are gender nonconforming, or are part of a sexual minority group, have been exposed to hostility and ostracizing behavior by those within the diversity organization who are not also disabled or neurodivergent themselves (McDonald et al., 2007).

The intersections between race, gender, sexual orientation and disability have long been overlooked in both education in general, and especially within psychology (Lund et al., 2023). For those wishing to learn more, Liasidou and Gregoriou's (2024) recent systematic literature review delves more fully into issues of intersectionality and disability in education. Wolbring and Nasir's (2024) scoping review of intersectionality—a hot topic of research in the last decade, found that less than

3% of the articles included disability within its discussion of intersecting identities. They concluded that even within the intersectionality-focused literature, disabled people are rarely included.

II. UNCOVERING THE LAYERS OF SYSTEMIC OPPRESSION

PWDN face systemic barriers that are unacknowledged and unaddressed. Many within the educational programs as well as the clinical training sites in which disabled and neurodivergent graduate students and trainees are placed are unaware of the issues that PWDN face in these settings. Some faculty, administrators, and clinical supervisors are more than willing to make adjustments to programs, assignments, and physical arrangements as necessary to ensure that all students—including disabled ones—can participate. But sadly, these are the exception rather than the rule.

Using the term "oppression" may seem to be strident and excessive when discussing the issues of exclusion, ostracization, discrimination, and harassment that many PWDN experience. Yet, as this chapter will demonstrate, there are indeed multiple barriers affecting disabled and neurodivergent graduate students and trainees that are not shared by the population of their peers who are nondisabled and neurotypical. These obstacles occur in both academia as well as clinical training, and while some are more easily managed, others can be downright traumatizing and soul-crushing (hence this chapter).

Prejudice is Common

It is often said that one cannot legislate morality. This is both unfortunate and true. Attitudes of prejudice are not illegal, but they precede the illegal acts of discrimination.

Many people are not even aware of their own implicit bias (Banaji & Greenwald, 2013), although there are now online tests to uncover them to bring them to one's attention (Implicit.harvard.edu). The Disability Implicit Bias Associations Test, developed by Harvard University, is one variation of such a test, to detect prejudice against persons with disabilities.

Discrimination is Illegal, But is Widespread

While discrimination based on race, gender, sexuality, religion, class, and disability are illegal—at least in the United States—those who are disadvantaged in some way due to being a member of a minority often face discrimination in one form or another. Likewise, issues of systemic oppression occur within psychology training programs or clinical placements. Nowhere is that experience of discrimination more prominent than in the disabled and neurodivergent population.

Ableism

The ABCs of ableism are: (1) *Attitudes* or negative emotional reactions, (2) *Behavioral* actions, and (3) *Cognitive* beliefs or ideologies (Nario-Redmond, 2024). These elements exist at the personal, interpersonal, and institutional levels and can have profound consequences affecting perceptions, relationships, and group power dynamics (Nario-Redmond, 2024). These ableist beliefs often result in the behaviors of microaggressions, and are described below.

Microaggressions

Microaggressions are "inadvertent expressions of bias embedded in daily actions" (Conover et al., 2017, p. 571). The evidence for the damaging effects of microaggressions (Williams, 2020) is mounting, as research on this topic has exploded over the last two decades. Much of the research on microaggressions centers on the interactions) between people of different racial groups. However, PWDN experience ableist microaggressions just as racial minorities do.

Ableist microaggressions sometimes result in disabled and neurodivergent students dropping out of education (Lett, 2018). Williams (2020), using longitudinal studies, documents that both psychological and physical harm result from the everyday experiences of discrimination. Olkin et al. (2019) indicate that microaggressions occur more frequently against those with invisible disabilities.

Erasure of People with Disabilities

In both daily life, as well as in academia and clinical training, there is a hesitancy to use the word "disability" (Andrews, et al., 2019). This often stems from nondisabled people being made uncomfortable by PWD, as well as lack of clarity on how to address disability without being offensive. In some respects, it is analogous to White people being uncomfortable if a Black person is around when issues of race arise.

While some people do hold negative stereotypes of disability, many are simply unaware and lack familiarity. Most are probably well-intentioned but simply ignorant. Some, on the other hand, are exploitative and hold disabled people in contempt. This may in part explain why some PWD with invisible disabilities may attempt to "pass" in society without disclosing their disability status (Bogart et al., 2017).

Disproportionalities in Clinical Mental Health Training Programs

Disabled and neurodivergent students are individuals with a stigmatized identities not only in society, but especially within professional psychology (Lund, 2018). Disabled individuals are more often attracted to the mental health professions than other disciplines, likely in part because they believe their ability to counsel others will be something they realistically can do, despite physical limitations. Yet in graduate training paradigms, expectations based upon able-bodied privilege and neurotypicality result in underrepresentation of disabled and neurodivergent providers in clinical practice.

Accommodations can be Complicated and are Often Misunderstood

The process of obtaining accommodations can be long and difficult in some cases. In others, where the educational institution or employer has well-developed systems in place, it can be a much smoother endeavor. Disclosure is a prerequisite of formal accommodations. The issues of accommodations will be addressed fully in a subsequent section.

Lack of Accommodations is Extremely Prejudicial (Not to Mention Illegal)

There are times when accommodations are too expensive or too impractical to be provided. This does happen, when one's disabilities are severe, but such instances are relatively rare, thankfully. More often, provided there is the political will to do so and an agreeable administration, there are ways to work out adjustments that are amenable to the person with a disability, and the removal of barriers provides an equitable environment.

Unfortunately, there are many who could provide accommodations, but choose not to do so. Often the excuse provided is that the accommodations are too expensive, when in fact the cost of the software, service, or renovation is one that could either be built into the budget or for which a grant might be applied. Frequently, funding for these items is often available, if the organization or institution is sufficiently motivated to find and allocate it.

In such cases, the lack of accommodations is not truly one where the agency or institution lacks the capability, but withholds the accommodation that could be otherwise provided. Intentional failure to provide accommodations is one of the most common forms of systemic oppression of disabled and neurodivergent students and trainees (Bumgardner, 2023).

III. DISABILITY ACCOMMODATIONS

There are many elements that determine whether or not a student or clinical trainee is able to obtain accommodations which will enable them to be successful in their education or to perform the essential functions of their job.

The Process of Obtaining Accommodations

Disability Must First be Known and Acknowledged

Many people who have a disability in one form or another and are legally eligible for accommodations may not identify as a person with a disability. Some may be unaware that accommodations are available, or know the process of obtaining them. There are others who do not know what type of accommodations they might need or what could be provided to them, but of which they are not aware. Additionally, only some disabilities are listed under the Americans with Disabilities Act (ADA) as being eligible for accommodations, and others that are not on the list can be excluded. Only recently were autism and intellectual disabilities added under the Americans with Disabilities Amendments Act of 2008 (ADAAA).

Diagnosis Required to Obtain Accommodations

The process of obtaining a diagnosis can be very onerous for some due to lack of access to medical or mental health providers (especially in some rural areas), affordability and insurance issues, and distrust of the medical profession (particularly for people of color, due to historical exploitation and deception). Another issue of access is transportation to the medical provider to obtain the necessary diagnosis, especially if one's condition is such that travel to the clinical facility is an extreme hardship either physically or financially. This is particularly true for some PWDN.

Some conditions are more amenable to diagnosis than others. Misdiagnosis is not an uncommon occurrence, and is often complicated by other factors such as age of presentation, as well as gender and race (Baughman et al., 2025). Additionally, some conditions are more easily diagnosable. Others are far less straightforward, be they medical or neurodivergent in nature. For example, women with fibromyalgia report multiple years prior to receiving a diagnosis. The methods of diagnosing this neurological condition were published in 1990 by the American College of Rheumatology, but this widespread pain is often misunderstood or not taken seriously by medical providers in other specialties.

Similarly, autism is frequently diagnosed in males, but is much less often recognized in females, as the symptom presentation can be quite different, unless the condition is severe (Nerenberg, 2020). Because females are socialized differently than males, with far more emphasis on being nice and getting along with others, girls are more often given to masking their neurodivergence in order to fit in. Consequently, females with autism tend to get diagnosed in their late 30s or 40s, with many having gone decades hiding their neurodivergence and not receiving services that could have greatly benefited them (Bargiela et al., 2016; Leedham et al., 2020.

Accommodations in Academia

In a larger college or university, many have their own department to ensure compliance with both the ADA and Section 504 of the Rehabilitation Act. Such offices coordinate accommodations requests from students, manage documentation from medical providers that substantiate the needs for services, and draft letters of accommodation. They may occasionally run interference for students when faculty members do not understand the unique needs of their individual students.

Educational Accommodations

Typical types of accommodations a student might require may include the ability to record lectures, having a designated note-taker, extra time on examinations or papers, and a distraction-free testing environment. A student with low vision visually impaired student may require seating up front in the classroom to either reduce distraction or to ensure the board is visible (applicable for in-person classes), books available in Braille or large-print format for those with visual impairments, or electronic books and articles that are amenable to screen readers on a computer. In particular, for blind or low vision students in clinical psychology, assessment instruments are most often not available in Braille or large-print formats.

A Deaf student might require an ASL interpreter in the classroom, or CART services (a real-time transcription of verbal communication onto a computer screen). A student with a hearing impairment attending an in-person class will require an understanding instructor and classmates who are willing to work collaboratively with them during discussions.

The types of accommodations required may is diverse, and the list of examples provided above is by no means exhaustive. However, for smaller institutions and private colleges, there is often not an Office of Disability or an ombudsman, and their ability to offer certain accommodations is often curtailed. For instance, a distraction-free testing environment on exams for students with disabilities is difficult to proctor if the institution does not have a Disability Services office.

Examples of Formal Academic Accommodations in Action

Test Proctoring

Attitudes of faculty toward students with disabilities can be problematic, and may require the advocacy of staff of the Disability Services Office to mediate between the student and the faculty member. An example of how they may facilitate these disputes follows:

> *At a large college, an instructor required that her class complete a handwritten essay in a Blue Book. One disabled student had tried at first to comply, but her carpal tunnel issues got so inflamed from having done so that she was in great pain for multiple days following the exam, and could not even hold a pencil for over a week. Thus, for subsequent exams, she requested the ability to type her responses into a computer instead.*
>
> *The faculty member balked at such a request, although the Disability Services Office indicated it was a simple procedure that was easily implemented. The faculty member remained skeptical, fearing that the student would cheat by looking things up on the internet to find the answers. The Disability Services Office assuaged the professor's fears by ensuring that the student would be observed by a staff member, the computer would not be attached to the internet, and all the student's belongings (including cell phones and other electronic devices) would be stored in a locked cabinet in a separate room during the examination. With these assurances, the student was allowed to take her examination on the computer and performed well.*

Extra Time on Exams

> *Extra time (time-and-a-half) on exams is a common accommodation for students with disabilities, especially for those who struggle with attentional issues from ADHD, PTSD, TBI, or chronic pain.*
>
> *One disabled student in a clinical psychology training program required testing in a distraction-free environment. She was pleasantly surprised when the staff member at her Disability Services Office at her graduate school locked the student's belongings in the office and escorted her to a private room with a desk, provided earplugs to block out any extraneous noises, and gave her two perfectly sharpened pencils with erasers. The staff member set the clock for the timed paper-and-pencil examination and exited the room, leaving the student*

to take the test in solitude. These accommodations enabled her to be extremely successful in passing her advanced statistics course.

The accommodations of test proctoring can be difficult to proctor at smaller institutions that lack the resources for a more robust Disability Services Office.

Services to Ensure that Hearing-Impaired Students Can Participate in Courses

Traditional methods of instruction, with the professor at the front of the classroom, work well for those who are able-bodied, but for persons with visual or hearing impairments, often these methods require adaptation.

In one private university, professors often spoke softly or did not project their voice in large classes. Many students thus had difficulty hearing them, and asked for the instructors to use microphones. Because the staff felt uncomfortable using them, this request was repeatedly denied. Several students complained, and after numerous years, finally the faculty relented, after receiving many course evaluations stating the need for amplification.

Students cannot be reasonably expected to do well on coursework if they are unable to hear the professor. Nor can they engage in discussions or answer questions if they cannot hear.

A hearing-impaired doctoral student enrolled at a small institution required CART services so that she could engage in classes. The university was unwilling to make this change, incorrectly assuming that if the student simply turned up her hearing aids, which would be sufficient. She was registered with the Disability Services Office, which did little to ensure that the accommodations needed and authorized were actually implemented. It was not until this student obtained legal representation and was in the process of filing a lawsuit against the university that the faculty finally complied and provided the CART services to which she was legally entitled.

Example of Informal Academic Accommodations in Action

Formal accommodations may not even be necessary, provided the faculty member or clinical supervisor does not hold prejudicial attitudes toward people with disabilities.

One disabled student in a clinical psychology program had difficulty walking, and approached her faculty member after he had announced a ten-minute break. She assured him she would return as quickly as possible after visiting the restrooms, but that due to her mobility issue, she could not ensure she could get back within that period of time. She asked that he not misinterpret her tardy return as a sign of disrespect but instead to be cognizant of her physical limitations. He responded positively and patiently, and asked her only to do her best.

This student was stunned the following week when the professor had taken the initiative to get the course location moved to a classroom closer in proximity to the facilities. This instructor responded with sensitivity and took pragmatic action on her behalf.

Of course, moving a class from one location to another may not be a practical solution in all academic institutions. This astute professor showed extraordinary sensitivity and agency.

How the Power Differential Intersects with Disability

There are, sadly, some in academia and in positions of evaluative authority such as clinical directors and supervisors who lack understanding of many elements of disability. Because of their positions of power, they are able to allow or—conversely, to restrict—the flow of necessary resources to disabled graduate students and trainees in clinical placements (practica, internships, post-doctoral fellowships, etc.).

Such resources might include accommodations, to which the student is legally entitled, and without which the student or post-doc may not achieve success in their chosen profession. Yet these accommodations, which are mandated by law in some cases, are often disallowed. Lack of accommodations presents as real a barrier to students as a concrete staircase would be to a person in a wheelchair. Two ways in which these resources are restricted by those in positions of power are the pressure to prove one's disability, and false presumptions that certain conditions are not real.

Pressure to Prove One's Disability

For those who have invisible disabilities, often they are not believed when they disclose and are expected to prove it. This is often the case for those who are neurodivergent.

One doctoral student with Sensory Processing Disorder had difficulty finishing an assignment in a required format and sought permission from her instructor to do the work in narrative rather than table form, which was denied. In some cases, it would have been an inappropriate request (i.e., if the student was in an accounting or financial services course that required the use of a spreadsheet). But in this instance, this student's request to complete it in an alternate format could have been easily adapted to accommodate her condition.

But not believing in the presence of a disability that is not visible also occurs with physically disabled individuals, as well.

One student disclosed to her professor in a virtual appointment that she had an intermittent mobility impairment, and when she finally met him during the in-person portion for the class, he stated, "well, you looked just fine over Zoom." Despite her previous disclosure, she was disbelieved.

In both circumstances, the behavior of the instructors showed a lack of understanding and humility. Both students were left with feeling "othered" and unwelcome in the learning community because of their disabilities.

False Presumptions that Certain Conditions are not Real

One graduate student was taught within the context of a psychology course that "fibromyalgia is not real." Her professor stated emphatically that it was "just a made-up condition, and that "it is all in someone's head."

When that graduate student who had been wrongly taught met another one who suffered greatly from fibromyalgia, the latter provided concrete medical literature on that neurological disorder and research to document its existence, and the former was convinced.

Unfortunately, there are many professors who disbelieve the presence of certain conditions that are well-documented in the research and the medical literature. Yet fibromyalgia is a disease affecting the central nervous system, which disproportionately affects women, and trauma survivors are much more susceptible to developing it, according to medical research. In fact, ICD-11, the diagnostic manual for medical and mental health conditions used around the world, has a diagnostic code (MG30.01, Chronic Widespread Pain) for fibromyalgia, (World Health Organization, 2019). It is a very real physiological condition, which causes chronic nerve pain, fatigue, and brain fog, among other symptoms If that opinionated faculty member had been the professor of the student with fibromyalgia, his prejudice might well have adversely influenced his treatment of her in the classroom.

Workplace Accommodations in Clinical Training

Because practicum trainees, internships, and post-doctoral fellowships are essentially on-the-job training settings, they fall under the same federal employment laws which prohibit discrimination and mandate reasonable accommodations. However, what may seem reasonable in one setting might not necessarily translate to another, as clinical training sites offer a wide variety of settings, including community mental health clinics, prisons and jails, school and college counseling centers, hospitals and medical environments, inpatient psychiatric facilities, day treatment in mental institutions, community outreach programs such as those to serve the unhoused, and rural health care. (Of course, this list is not exhaustive.)

Examples of Informal Accommodations in Action in Clinical Placements

Freedom to Perform Clinical Documentation Alternatively. Many disabled students require accommodations for clinical documentation, such as extra time to complete them. These requests are usually easily accommodated informally, if the clinical supervisor is understanding, agreeable, and sensitive to the unique needs of PWDN.

In a practicum site, a disabled trainee was having difficulty completing the documentation in the ten-minute period between clients. Because of her disability, she required the use of that time for self-care, and requested permission from her clinical supervisor to do the documentation in the afternoons, after seeing clients all morning. Her supervisor granted her request, and the trainee was successful in completing all necessary documentation, having been given the freedom to perform this essential task in a way that suited her disability.

Revision of Clinic Practices. In many clinical settings, guidelines are implemented to ensure safety of patients and staff, as well as to comply with governmental mandates. But many are based on ableistic standards.

In one clinic, an opioid replacement center in which patients obtained Methadone maintenance, SAMHSA regulations required that all medications be kept under lock and key, and thus clients were disallowed to roam the clinic without an escort. One intern with a mobility impairment requested an unofficial accommodation, seeking permission to have a member of the reception staff to accompany her clients to the therapy room on the days she was having difficulty walking. Her request was granted, and thus both clinician and site remained in compliance with the federal requirements.

Disabled Parking for Practicum Trainees

Many supervisors and staff at clinical sites lack the sensitivity to PWD and awareness of accessibility issues within their own facilities.

One practicum trainee with a mobility impairment had difficulty walking on a cold and overcast day because of prior musculoskeletal injuries. Her practicum director commented with disapproval, "I noticed you parked in the handicapped spots today."

"Yes," the trainee replied. "I put my handicap placard on the dashboard."

"Well, those spots are only for patients," the trainee was told.

From that day on, even though it caused her great pain and effort, this trainee parked much further away, even though she was legally entitled to use her handicapped placard and to park in front of the clinic. There was no understanding on the part of the clinic director that this trainee had just as much right to park there as one of the patients.

Accommodations as Equity

The purpose of accommodations is simple: to remove the barriers that are experienced by PWDN so that they can be as successful in either academia or employment (and clinical placements) as non-disabled or neurotypical people can.

In this respect, accommodations are adjustments made by the academic institution, the employer, or the clinical sites, to level the playing field for PWDN. This aim is similar in many respects to the DEI(B) principle of equity.

However, some professors and clinical staff feel that PWDN are getting special privileges, and may resist accommodations due to opinions that stigmatize disability. But removal of obstacles is an attempt to help a marginalized community enjoy the opportunities afforded to the nondisabled and neurotypical population. As Hagion-Rzepka (2023) notes: "equity is eclipsed by issues of access."

IV. CASE STUDIES OF ABLEISM IN ACTION

The following anecdotes have been shared with the author by a number of disabled graduate students and trainees. There are three basic sections: Ableism in Academic Settings (cases 1-4), in Clinical Placements (cases 5-8), and Trauma in Clinical Psychology Education and Training (cases 9-12).

The graduate students and trainees are all in the fields of clinical and counseling psychology, and they each related their encounters with trauma in the context of discrimination and lack of accommodations.

Their factual stories are being shared below with their knowledge and permission, presenting the pertinent information with the use of pseudonyms for all involved, but without superfluous details that would violate their confidentiality or make these individuals easily identifiable.

Ableism in Academic Settings

Case Study 1: Study Abroad Program

Freesia, a student with advanced arthritis, disclosed her intermittent mobility issues when inquiring about a study abroad program. Dr. Dracena assured her she would be accommodated.

Upon arrival overseas, Dr. Dracena and her classmates welcomed her joyously. However, after Freesia arose from a seated position and he witnessed her difficulty walking, his attitude changed drastically. Though previously friendly and supportive, Dr. Dracena became hostile and spoke sharply to Freesia on numerous occasions.

Consequently, her classmates followed his example, shunned her because of her mobility impairment, and refused to interact with Freesia. Since the planned group activities were inaccessible, she was repeatedly excluded. In addition, she was left alone in a foreign country for multiple days on a school-sponsored trip, for which Freesia taken out substantial student loans for a less-than-satisfactory academic program.

Legal and Ethical Issues in This Case. *The program claimed that the trip was accessible, without taking steps to follow through to ensure that students could participate fully regardless of ability status—all the while knowing beforehand about the unique needs of one of its attendees. This is a dereliction of duty, as well as false representation of the academic program. Potentially, it could be considered fraudulent, in that federal student loans were used to finance this study abroad trip (an important detail about which the school was previously aware), and the university was paid handsomely for a program that was inaccessible to the student who had enrolled in it. The APA ethics code requires that instructors do not practice unfair discrimination or harassment based on disability status, which both this professor and his students did in this case.*

Case Study 2: Unpredictability of Disability

Vinca, a student with Type 1 diabetes, had an insulin pump. She had previously undergone transplantation surgery, with fetal cells implanted in the pancreas because Vinca's islet cells ceased functioning. Because of her condition, she unexpectedly required hospitalization at times when Vinca's blood sugar spiked, despite close medical management.

She sought extensions on her coursework due to an inpatient stay, since the concrete walls in her hospital ward blocked all Wi-Fi capability, but Vinca's instructors balked when she cited the lack of connectivity with which to submit her assignments. Faculty refused to consider her medical emergency, demanding prior notice for extensions on papers. Thus, Vinca was often forced to take a zero on an assignment, necessitating the repeat of several classes.

The nature of Vinca's condition was such that she lacked physiological awareness of low blood sugar, quite dissimilar to most diabetics. Both the institution's disability office and faculty failed to provide reasonable accommodations for Vinca because her disability was not one that was easily foreseeable and often required adjustment in its medical management, even with her insulin pump. She sought representation to file a lawsuit against the university, alleging disability discrimination due to lack of appropriate accommodations.

Legal and Ethical Issues in This Case. *Section 504 of the Rehabilitation Code mandates reasonable accommodations in education. Moreover, the ADA covers all institutions—including private ones—and expands these protections beyond federal facilities. The university and its instructional staff, by insisting upon previous arrangements for extensions and ignoring the fact that the student's condition was by nature unpredictable, violated the ADA. In addition, the APA ethics code prohibits instructors engaging in discrimination based upon disability.*

Case Study 3: Issues of Accessibility at a Professional Conference

In one graduate class, students were required to participate in a weeklong professional conference. When registering for the convention, Camelia noted that she was a wheelchair user, a requested accommodations, and was told the venue was accessible. Travel and accommodations were arranged by the professor, Dr. Artemisia. Camelia required transportation from the hotel to the conference, which was held at a nearby university. Because of her motorized scooter, she was mostly autonomous, requiring help only to open doors to enter the breakout presentations.

Yet the design of the lecture hall for the plenary sessions was not conducive to audience members in wheelchairs. Each row of chairs was built with stadium-style seating, in a stepped arrangement, with only stair access. No accessible platform existed in the back for wheelchairs, and thus, Camelia was forced to sit in her scooter, in front of the first row. She had limited visibility of the slides as they were projected on the screen, painfully craning her neck throughout the keynote to view the visuals.

Afterward, Dr. Artemisia castigated her. He accused her of upstaging the speaker by sitting up front, and complained about the "annoying" noises Camelia's electronic scooter made, which he claimed distracted attendees from the presentation. He also exhibited visible frustration when her wheelchair batteries required recharging. Dr. Artemisia gave Camelia the lowest possible grade, all for things directly related to her disability.

Legal and Ethical Issues in This Case. *The conference venue was falsely reported as being accessible, and the convention planners should have investigated it* *onsite beforehand to ensure that claim prior to contracting with the facility. Failure to do so is a violation of both the ADA as well as Section 504 of the Rehabilitation Act, which mandate reasonable accommodations in education.*

Additionally, the architecture of the lecture hall was not something over which this student had any control. Holding the student accountable for a design flaw was unethical and violates the principle of nonmaleficence in the APA Ethics Code (APA, 2017). Moreover, there is a power differential between the professor and the student, and assigning her a lower grade because of her being a wheelchair user also violates the principle of nonmaleficence in the Ethics Code, as it is an intrinsic characteristic and should not be subject to lower marks. Furthermore, his microaggressions about her wheelchair violates the ethical principle of respect for persons. Because of the violation of the enforceable provision mandating nondiscrimination by instructors toward their students, the university—in addition to the individual professor—could be subject to an ethics complaint, which may damage the reputation of the institution.

Case Study 4: Public Shaming in a Large Professional Meeting

Daphne, a physically disabled doctoral student in clinical psychology, participated in a large professional meeting with many of her classmates and her professor, Dr. Maranta. This event was a required part of the curriculum, although it took place off-site, not at the campus.

During one social event, while others networked over drinks and hors d'oeuvres, Dr. Maranta (who perhaps had consumed alcohol at the event) began shouting at Daphne about her physical disability—and several other attendees stared at the loud, unnecessary disruption. Previously, he had demonstrated multiple acts of ableist microaggressions toward Daphne, and had become increasingly hostile toward her over time.

Legal and Ethical Issues in This Case. *This professor's behavior is not only unprofessional, but illegal and unethical, as well. Even though the event was not held on campus, because it was required as part of the curriculum, academic standards still apply. Since he was loud enough that others in attendance heard, when he shouted about her disability, this professor violated both the Family Educational Rights and Privacy Act (FERPA) as well as the ADA, which protect disabled students from unauthorized disclosures of disability status by faculty and school administrators. The APA ethical code forbids unfair discrimination or harassment of students, which was clearly done in this case, specifically due to her disability status. His public shaming of this woman violates the principles of respect for persons, in addition to the principle of nonmaleficence in the ethical code. Because of the violation of the enforceable provision that mandates nondiscrimination by instructors toward* *their students, an ethical complaint could be filed against both the school and the instructor, which may ultimately affect the university's accreditation status, as well.*

Practical Training as a Dual Component of Professional Psychology Education

Entry into clinical mental health as a profession is not just limited to scholastic preparation, but requires training programs such as those for clinical psychology at the doctoral level and clinical mental health counseling at the master's level. Thus, these occupations are distinct from many other fields in psychology (experimental psychology, social psychology, for example) in that they require practicum placements, internships, and in some cases, post-doctoral fellowships as well prior to national and state certification exams required in order to obtain licensure. This trajectory is not dissimilar to many other health professions.

Therefore, successful completion of many of these clinical placements in psychology is required prior to graduation. While a disabled student may receive educational accommodations at their institution, they must also navigate the vicissitudes of practical training, in which they often may require accommodations, just as they might in an occupational setting. Although these trainees are in a quasi-employee role, PWDN may not always have the same rights afforded them as would be applicable to those in traditional employment.

It is important to understand the trajectory of students in clinical psychology at the doctoral level and clinical mental health counseling:

academic coursework → practicum (clinical training) → internship → graduation

In order to move toward their degree procurement goals, one must first successfully pass their clinical placements. Unlike most on-the-job training, however, trainees' degree progress is dependent upon the accumulation of a certain number of clinical hours in direct provision of services in addition to patient documentation, clinical supervision, and a didactic component of the training site, along with administrative duties. If one completes their clinical placement and receives a less-than-satisfactory-report, their educational advancement may be stalled or halted entirely, despite years of earlier scholarly achievements.

This dilemma of course is not unique to disabled students, but applies to the total population of graduate students of psychology. Yet those with disabilities or neurodivergent conditions face similar obstacles in these training experiences that often exceed those in academia, which are far more well documented. This chapter is one of the few in the professional literature to elucidate such experiences.

Ableism in Clinical Placements

Case Study 5: Lack of Accommodations at Internship Ended Clinical Career

Aster, a doctoral student in clinical psychology, completed all the academic requirements to be eligible for her internship at a site affiliated with her university, and then experienced a freak accident. She survived, miraculously, but was left with a physical disability, and chronic pain. Because of her success in the program, her internship spot was left open until she had recovered sufficiently, and she looked forward to it with relish. However, her internship site could not supply the accommodations she required. Thus, Aster was prevented from providing therapy to clients and from accumulating the clinical hours needed to pass the internship in order to finish her program.

Aster had a previous working relationship with Dr. Hosta, the director at the training site, which was a clinic associated with the same educational institution where she had studied. Dr. Hosta was also a former instructor of hers. Since he was in a powerful position at the university and an influential theorist of great renown, Dr. Hosta was able to leverage that prestige to advocate on her behalf. He told the administrators at the educational institution for which he worked that *she* had not failed, but the system had failed *her,* and that Aster should still be allowed to graduate, although she did not have the internship experience required for the clinical degree. Dr. Hosta was successful in his advocating for her, and the university allowed her to graduate with a general psychology doctorate instead. Thus, Aster was ultimately able to secure a professorial position, but her career in clinical psychology was truncated.

Legal and Ethical Issues in This Case. *In this case, Aster was not provided with the necessary accommodations and thus was unable to complete her predoctoral internship. Therefore, she could not obtain the clinical hours necessary to be eligible for the licensing exam, and her dreams of a career as a clinical psychologist came to an abrupt end. The internship site did not comply with their legal obligation under the ADA, a failure for both the agency and the student. If it had not been for the vociferous advocacy and worldwide reputation of Dr. Hosta, however, Aster would not have been able to graduate at all. Of course, this situation caused undue stress upon her, even though she pivoted successfully. Yet many trainees in clinical psychology finance their graduate education with student loans, and the financial burden of the debt load imposed upon them is substantial. Several seek positions in clinical employment afterwards qualify for loan forgiveness as a result. Yet for those denied graduation due to lack of accommodations at clinical placements, they may consequently end up insolvent.*

Case Study 6: Accessible Entry Point Disallowed

Amaryllis, a master's student in clinical mental health counseling, required the use of a walker. At her practicum site, however, she was expected to enter from the front, despite the disabled parking being in the rear of the facility, as was push-button door access. Instead she was required her to ambulate around the very large building. Amaryllis had requested an exception, citing her mobility impairment and requisite use of an assistive device, but it was denied.

At the front, her entry was further complicated since Amaryllis had to hold the door open simultaneously while attempting to lean on her walker to navigate the narrow doorway, with her laptop bag hanging over her shoulder (because the site did not provide computers for clinical documentation). This daily difficulty was not only impractical; it could have resulted in damage to her walker or laptop, neither of which she could afford to replace. Fern, her supervisor, had repeatedly demonstrated her lack of sensitivity to issues of disability. Thus, the trainee was afraid to push the issue, fearing Fern would give Amaryllis a reduced score on her evaluation, and she was unwilling to take the risk of failing the required practicum, as it would affect her academically.

Legal and Ethical Issues in This Case. *The ADA requires that public buildings are accessible to persons with disabilities, but this does not apply to many private structures, which have been grandfathered in to allow exceptions for noncompliance. Moreover, many nonprofit organizations (through which several clinical training sites are situated) are small enough that these agencies are able to have exemptions from the federal mandate, resulting in numerous sites that disabled trainees find inaccessible. This trainee's training site, however, did in fact have an ADA-compliant entry point, yet her supervisor refused her access to it. This was a violation of the ethical requirement of competence, as this clinical supervisor's complete disregard of the student's mobility impairment was illustrative of a lack of competence with the disabled population. Moreover, this supervisor's actions violate the APA Guidelines for Clinical Supervision in Health Service Psychology by ignoring this element of diversity. Furthermore, this refusal impaired the supervisory relationship, creating one that felt neither safe nor respectful to the trainee, which also violates the supervisory relationship standard in the APA Guidelines. While the masters-level counseling program adheres to a different ethical code (the American Mental Health Counselors Association, rather than the American Psychological Association), the principles are the same with regard to clinical supervision.*

Case Study 7: Lack of Accommodations at Practicum Resulting in Non-Clinical Work

Marigold, a doctoral student with a hearing impairment, encountered a barrier at her practicum site. Their cordless phones were Bluetooth-enabled, but incompatible with the amplifier Marigold needed to pair with her hearing aids.

Her supervisors presumed headphones used by other employees would suffice, but these headsets were not designed for hearing-impaired people. The agency was unable to obtain this vital resource Marigold required to provide therapy for her clients. Fearing she would miss out on practicum experience at this site due to the expense, Marigold eventually purchased the technology for the accommodations she needed, costing her several hundred dollars.

Though Marigold was prevented from doing clinical work because accommodations were not supplied, she was given an alternate assignment, doing other supporting tasks that benefited the site. The agency ultimately obtained a grant resulting from her outreach, to provide far more effective client services. But she accumulated zero clinical hours during her practicum experience, making her much less competitive when the time came to apply for internship.

Additionally, the stress caused by the delay resulted in Marigold experiencing substantial health and mental health symptoms. She gained 15-20 pounds from "stress eating", but forced herself to finish, feeling she had no other choice. Because she was unable to do clinical work, she was assigned to do outreach instead. She was required to do her hours at night, often leaving the office after midnight and sometimes not until the early hours of the morning (3 or 4 am). Furthermore, as result of the lack of sunlight exposure, her Vitamin D levels measured at an 8; the normal range is 30-80. Consequently, her ability to heal from oral surgery was compromised. After 6 months' time at her practicum, Marigold recalls, "I was a dysregulated mess and [was] crying frequently. My husband dragged me to restorative yoga and meditation classes." After about a year of these modalities, her nervous system's ability to regulate was eventually restored.

Legal and Ethical Issues in This Case. *In this case, the student eventually provided the accommodations herself and was able to successfully complete her practicum training. Legally, the technology this trainee required should have been provided by the site as a reasonable accommodation under the ADA, although the law does allow for noncompliance if the cost is prohibitive. Because of the flexibility and cooperative relationship between the program staff and the trainee, she was able to complete her practicum successfully, although she did not get the clinical experience she had initially sought. This site fulfilled the ethical requirement to provide supervision free of discrimination, and supported this student with an alternative assignment that was mutually beneficial for both the trainee and the organization,* *despite it not being the exact function originally anticipated. However, they did not comply with the practicum contract in that the student was unable to perform clinical work, which was the sole purpose for the clinical placement.*

Case Study 8: For Accommodations Denied at Practicum

Dahlia, a doctoral student with a mobility impairment, experienced difficulty completing her clinical documentation at practicum because the site had 12 trainees but only four desktop computers. After client sessions, she headed toward a computer to complete her therapy notes, but Dahlia walked more slowly toward the desk than the able-bodied trainees, who would slip in faster than she could move. Dahlia approached this situation as a resource issue, asking Dr. Calathea, her clinical supervisor, for permission to complete clinical documentation at home. Her request was denied. Dahlia spoke of her disability as a factor in the reasoning for remote access, suggesting it would ensure timely notes, without addressing the other students' unprofessional behavior. He refused to consider the possibility.

Dr. Calathea later informed Dahlia her notes were late, and she again requested an accommodation to do notes remotely, specifically mentioning her disability. He would not relent. Shortly thereafter, Dr. Alocasia, the clinical director, casually asked Dahlia how she had been enjoying the practicum. She commented about the site's limited computers, which Dr. Alocasia acknowledged. Dahlia stated she had asked Dr. Calathea twice for reasonable accommodations to no avail, and reiterated a possible solution. Dr. Alocasia immediately granted consent, and the issue was resolved. But Dr. Calathea later lied on Dahlia's final evaluation, downgrading her because of what he deemed "late" clinical documentation despite Dr. Alocasia's implementation of an agreed-upon timeline for submission of clinical notes. Furthermore, Dr. Calathea falsely claimed that she had not requested accommodations.

Legal and Ethical Issues in This Case. *Like many clinical training sites, this small agency had a lack of resources that caused a substantial problem. However, the supervisor's refusal to consider reasonable accommodations, even with confidentiality protections, is a violation of the ADA. Moreover, his unwillingness to address the accommodations request—not once, but twice—constitutes discrimination, a violation of the APA Ethics Code. In addition, his doing so undermined the alliance between the two, which violates the supervisory relationship standard in the APA Guidelines on Clinical Supervision. Thankfully, the director recognized the jeopardy in which the community health clinic was being placed due to the behavior of the supervisor, and reversed his unethical and illegal decision. Yet he retaliated for the student going "over his head" in obtaining the accommodations he had denied, and penalized her unjustly. This action could have resulted in an ethical complaint against him with the state licensing board.*

Trauma in Clinical Psychology Education and Training

Many of the stories above of lived experience involving disabled and neurodivergent students did not have a clean resolution; even fewer had a positive outcome. Some might discount the hardships faced by the students and trainees in the previous section as simply a reflection of the difficulty and rigor of any doctoral program. Clearly, that would be an incorrect assumption. While doctoral programs are by nature designed to be challenging, the prejudice, discrimination, and lack of accommodation, were all directly related to disability. Thus, the difficulties were not equally spread across the entire population of graduate students, but was directed at one particular minority group—PWDN.

The anecdotal evidence presented in the next set of case studies goes a bit further, with aberrant issues related to noncompliance with disability protections and ethical standards in both academia as well as in clinical training.

Case Study 9: Supervisor Prejudice Against Neurodivergence in Clinical Placement

Jade enjoyed unusual success in his educational program, resulting in publications in two academic journals. Although demonstrating research potential and achievements, he struggled in his clinical placement. He disclosed his neurodivergent condition to obtain accommodations at his training site, a large private practice clinic owned and operated by a coalition of psychologists, including Dr. Ledebouria.

Upon hearing his request, Jade was emphatically told by Dr. Ledebouria, his supervisor, "you'll never be able to be a psychologist if you have ADHD!!" This statement was captured on an audio recording, along with a number of further personal insults made toward Jade by the supervisor.

Jade was unable to complete his placement, as a result of multiple other instances of discrimination. Despite having adequate proof of unlawful behavior, Jade eventually was forced to dropped his lawsuit against the psychological corporation because Dr. Ledebouria's legal maneuvering and delaying tactics drained the financial resources available to Jade and his family.

Legal and Ethical Issues in This Case. *The brazen disability discrimination faced by this student was substantial, and is an obvious violation of the ADA. Additionally, the evaluative authority of the supervisor was misplaced, as he incorrectly presumed that neurodivergence was a disqualifying factor in terms of entering the profession of psychology. This violates the principle of nonmaleficence in the APA Ethics Code, as well as the enforceable standard regarding supervisors providing respectful feedback and avoiding discrimination. Likewise, the powerful position of the well-resourced agency imposed undue burden on him financially as they de-*

fended themselves in court while his career ended. The agency could have been held accountable had an ethical complaint been filed against them with the state board of psychology, as could the individual supervisor. This could potentially endanger the supervisor's license to practice, as well as the business' ability to operate.

Case study 10: Disability Discrimination and Accommodations Refusal at Internship

Zinnia, an intern at mental health setting in an integrated medical clinic, was expected to complete her clinical documentation during her therapy sessions, as many physicians do during their appointments. Cognitive interference because of Zinnia's chronic pain caused difficulty with such task-switching. Moreover, Zinnia felt typing into a computer compromised the therapeutic alliance, and asked another provider whether this was an absolute requirement.

"No, it's more of a guideline," Zinnia was informed. Therefore, she completed her documentation outside therapy sessions, as she had done successfully at her three previous clinical placements. Zinnia disclosed this practice to Dr. Chia, her internship supervisor, who agreed, provided notes were completed in a timely manner.

But during Dr. Chia's vacation, Dr. Gasteria, the clinic director, reacted negatively during supervision when Zinnia mentioned completing her documentation after the therapy appointment. She confirmed that this informal accommodation was approved by Dr. Chia, explaining the effect her disability had on doing her clinical notes simultaneously during therapy.

"Not to be insensitive, but this is what we expect of interns," Dr. Gasteria said dismissively. In countless circumstances, she was unwilling to consider Zinnia's disability, although Dr. Gasteria was aware of it prior to accepting Zinnia into the internship. Zinnia had sought and was granted formal accommodations from the agency's corporate offices, which Dr. Gasteria refused to implement. As a result, she intended to fail Zinnia at her internship, due to Dr. Gasteria's insistence that all interns perform their work in a prescribed way, ignoring the fact that essential functions of the job were being performed in a timely manner. This led to adverse physical and emotional symptoms for Zinnia, who experienced concentration difficulties, sleeping problems, substantial increase in her physical pain levels, decreased motivation, depressive symptoms, and weight loss exceeding 20 pounds due to extreme stress. Despite these challenges, Zinnia was still expected to provide clinical care to her patients. In consultation, the APPIC ombudsman agreed the accommodations were reasonable, but did not hold the site accountable for providing them.

Legal and Ethical Issues in This Case. *The intern had disclosed the reason why her condition prevented her from completing the clinical documentation in the preferred way, and the supervisor's agreement with her was an informal accom-*

modation, which should have continued during her temporary absence. The ADA mandates reasonable accommodations in the workplace for persons with a disability; by providing a usable workaround, the intern was able to successfully perform the essential functions of the job to the standards of the site.

Moreover, the clinic director's refusal to honor the subsequent formal reasonable accommodations granted by her agency is a blatant violation of the ADA. Her actions violate the nonmaleficence principle of the APA Ethics Code. In addition, the enforceable standard regarding supervisors avoiding discrimination applies to the director, as well. In addition, her actions could subject both her and the agency to ethical complaints with the state board of psychology, potentially endangering the director's license to practice, and that of the organization. Furthermore, the intern could file a complaint with the APPIC board, jeopardizing the site's accreditation.

Case Study 11: Retaliation After Reporting Discrimination

Abelia faced discrimination by Dr. Tradescantia, a faculty member, while in her doctoral program. Abelia respectfully pushed back on his inaccurate judgments due to his prejudicial attitude toward her disability. Abelia tried, unsuccessfully, to placate her professor. Abelia filed a formal complaint against Dr. Tradescantia for violating the school's Anti-Discrimination Policy.

Subsequently, his disability prejudice influenced his grading. Despite Abelia passing the course, Dr. Tradescantia filed a complaint against her, falsely claiming she was unprofessional and resistant to feedback. Because clinical psychology programs in general have the expectation students will accept corrective input, the false allegation by Dr. Tradescantia fell under the student code of conduct. Abelia was subjected to a student disciplinary process, increasing her stress so significantly it further impacted her condition, leading to increased symptoms and reduced functionality. The doctoral program not only ignored her complaint about Dr. Tradescantia's discrimination, but the disciplinary committee put Abelia on an unnecessary course of corrective action.

She appealed, as the remediation plan was onerous and unrealistic, and did not take her disability into account. Abelia sought an accommodation on the grounds she was unable to comply with the corrective action plan due to her physical limitations, but her request was denied. The student disciplinary board refused to consider the role Abelia's disability played, claiming she was noncompliant with the remediation plan, and expelled her from the program. At each subsequent level of appeal, the committee reified their position, exhibiting confirmation bias by interpreting that Abelia's actions—following the institution's established protocol for grievance—constituted evidence of resistance to feedback.

Legal and Ethical Issues in This Case. *The professor's disability discrimination is a blatant violation of the ADA and Section 504 of the Rehabilitation Code. Because of the mischaracterization of this student by this instructor, her clinical program's disciplinary committee exercised an egregious lack of judgment without recognizing the nature of disability prejudice the student had experienced and the professor's obvious violations of federal law.*

Furthermore, the program's disciplinary committee misused their gatekeeping function to deny an otherwise-qualified doctoral candidate from entering the profession. By mistaking the student's advocating for her rights as a disabled student, the program labeled her with an inaccurate character judgment of being unwilling to accept feedback. This action could subject the institution to an ethical complaint, potentially impacting their accreditation status. Although the professor who practiced discrimination in the first place was not licensed, the members of the disciplinary committee were, and each of them could also be brought up on ethical complaints by the state Board of Psychology, if the student chose to pursue it.

Case Study 12: Disastrous Faculty Advice

Heather experienced significant ongoing disability discrimination at her internship. She tried to address the issues at multiple levels—first with her supervisor, then with the site director, and finally at the corporate level of the organization—but without success. Heather hired an attorney, planning to file a complaint with the Equal Employment Opportunity Commission (EEOC) against the training site.

During a regular check-in meeting with Dr. Kentia, her faculty advisor condemned Heather's legal action and strongly suggested she resign instead. He implied that filing a suit with the EEOC might negatively impact her future licensing application to the state board of psychology. Dr. Kentia promised to advocate on Heather's behalf and help find her another internship in order to obtain her degree. Against her better judgment, she did so, and subsequently her academic program dismissed her from the institution. Multiple appeals were unsuccessful, and Heather's career was aborted because of the unlawful disability discrimination at her internship. Heather was left with substantial student loans she was unable to repay, as she could not obtain employment in the field because she had not graduated.

Legal and Ethical Issues in This Case. *The disability discrimination the student faced at the site meant she was well within her legal rights to file with the EEOC. The faculty advisor was operating outside the scope of his competence, in giving what could be construed as legal advice. In addition, the faculty advisor's suggestion of resigning the internship was likely motivated by trying to salvage the school's reputation with the agency providing internship positions, rather than being concerned about the student's future. Thus, he was not acting in her best interest, as required* *by the APA ethics code for professors and advisors. Whether he was disingenuous or merely unsuccessful in later convincing the program's administration is unclear, and is a matter of speculation.*

However, the decision by this institution to dismiss the student from her academic program was atrocious, given that she took action based upon the flawed advice of her advisor, whom she had trusted. This instance is a travesty, and this injustice represents the conflicting interests of faculty, who must simultaneously serve the interest of the institution which employs them while endeavoring to coach students, whose tuition pays their salaries.

V. ANALYZING THE PSYCHOLOGICAL COMPLEXITIES OF THESE CASE STUDIES

The Concept of Institutional Betrayal

The term was first coined in 2014 by Smith and Freyd, referring to institutions (such as colleges, military institutions, or churches) that exacerbate the trauma of rape by their administrative responses to the reporting of the crime. This is an additional action, in which the institution itself either denies, excuses, or covers up for, the unethical or illegal act of one of its employees or other related parties, which has first committed an act against the student.

As applied here, institutional betrayal indicates that the institution (the college or university, professional organization, or the agency in which clinical placements for trainees), has betrayed the student or trainee or intern by allowing disability discrimination or noncompliance with federal law; cases 11 and 12 are clear examples of this phenomenon. In Lett's research, disabled students experiencing institutional betrayal suffered from anxiety, depression, and decreased self-esteem (Lett, 2018). Moreover, the institutional betrayal worsened the experience of ableist microaggressions against the disabled student (Lett, 2018). Disabled trainees report clinical supervision as the "worst part of training" to become a clinical psychologist (Olkin, 1999) due to circumstances like those recounted here.

Betrayal trauma involves harm by trusted others (Freyd et al., 2005). In many of the cases reviewed in this chapter, the betrayal trauma by faculty, supervisors, and institutions was a heart-wrenching element of what these trainees and interns endured. Moreover, Freyd et al.(2005) found evidence that individuals experiencing betrayal trauma resulted in depressive symptoms, anxiety, dissociation, as well as physical ailments.

Freyd et al. (2005) examined post-traumatic stress levels in research participants who had experienced low-betrayal traumatic events (e.g., such as natural disasters or vehicular accidents), as well as those who had experienced high betrayal experiences (betrayal trauma exposures such as abuse). Low-betrayal traumas are primarily fear-based (Freyd et al., 2005), and are the types of trauma exposures often considered in diagnosing PTSD. The Freyd et al. study proved that high-betrayal trauma experiences predicted greater trauma symptomatology: high-betrayal trauma and trauma symptoms (TSC) was higher (zero-order r = .48, semi-partial r = .12) than for low-betrayal trauma group (zero-order r = .38, semi-partial r = .02). In comparison with traumatic events not involving betrayal, betrayal trauma was associated with higher levels of post-traumatic stress and poorer physical and mental health (Freyd et al., 2005).

In the context of this chapter, case studies 9-12 all involved some level of betrayal trauma because of the previously close relationships which had developed between the supervisors, the faculty, and the program administrators at the universities with the disabled or neurodivergent individual. In addition to the initial betrayal trauma of disability discrimination, the outright refusal of the institutions to support the trainee, intern, or student and instead to back the perpetrator, was an additional source of betrayal trauma, compounding the harm done to the victim. The Freyd et al. (2005) study quantifies the impact of consequences of such the initial betrayal trauma and the subsequent institutional betrayal that these disabled and neurodivergent individuals in the cases above.

Institutional Betrayal in Academia

In case study 12, the university willfully ignored the violations of federal law at the internship site, and dissuaded Heather from legal redress by way of a false promise. The institution masqueraded as an ally while removing the legal leverage that the intern could have used to force the agency to provide the accommodations to which she was entitled, so she could complete her internship successfully. Their deceit and subsequent actions as an educational institution imposed unbearable trauma upon this disabled trainee, with devastating consequences that were life-altering. Without a doubt the institution was acting on its own best interest while ignoring what was in the student's welfare.

The disconnect between "what 'should be' (e.g., people do not intentionally hurt one another) and what is (you have been harmed by another person)" (Freyd et al., 2005, p. 84). This is clear in case 11. This example is betrayal trauma writ large by this institution, as well as by Dr. Tradescantia's unlawful discrimination toward Abelia, the disabled student.

Weaponization of Student Expectations and Codes of Conduct

In general, most graduate schools of psychology have expectations of students' ability to do four things to determine their suitability for the profession: 1) Demonstrate sufficient interpersonal and professional competence; 2) Exhibit self-awareness, self-reflection, and self-evaluation; 3) Be open to feedback and supervision; and 4) Address and resolve issues that interfere with professional development or functioning (adapted from California Southern University's statement on Suitability and Fitness for the Profession, 2026).

In case 11, the faculty and administration were complicit in Dr. Tradescantia's discrimination. The university repeatedly ignored his clear violations of the school's Anti-Discrimination Policy. Moreover, his retaliation after Abelia reporting him contravened the ADA, in addition to his initial prejudicial acts.

Thus, the educational institution weaponized the student codes of conduct, holding Abelia accountable for Dr. Tradescantia's unlawful behavior. The student disciplinary committee was a complete farce, as reporting discrimination is a right afforded by the university itself, as well as the nation's laws. Both he and the university abused this disabled woman, with its vilification of her and besmirching her name and professional reputation. Therefore, the unconscionable consequences delivered by this university and its institutional betrayal are far greater than the initial discrimination Abelia experienced.

Use of DARVO Tactics

Harsey and Freyd (2020) identified a pattern of behaviors often employed by perpetrators of intimate partner violence, in which abusers would deny allegations, employ personal attacks, and take on a persona of victimhood in order to deflect blame from their own abusive behavior. This set of behavioral responses to allegations of wrongdoing have been abbreviated to an acronym, (DARVO), meaning Deny, Attack, Reverse Victim and Offender (Harsey & Freyd, 2020).

When speaking to a mentor outside her educational institution about the aberrant actions taken by her university's clinical psychology program in retaliation for her filing a complaint against Dr. Tradescantia (case study 11), Abelia was stunned to learn that her program was employing DARVO tactics against her.

First, in their refusal to consider Dr. Tradescantia's disability discrimination toward Abelia as a violation of their university's own Anti-Discrimination Policy, the institution was Denying that the faculty's behavior was inappropriate as well as unlawful. In case study 11, both Dr. Tradescantia and the disciplinary committee engaged in personal Attacks against Abelia, twisting the language of the student code of conduct to make it appear that she was unwilling to receive feedback, instead of respectfully pushing back against illegal discrimination.

The disciplinary committee essentially Reversed the role of Victim and Offender by implying that the student was the one in error, rather than the aggrieved party. All of the DARVO tactics were employed by this university against Abelia, the disabled student. Then they further victimized her by placing her on an unnecessary course of corrective action that she clearly could not fulfill due to the nature of her disability. Whether this was intentional or not is speculative; however, since Abelia informed them on multiple occasions that she could not physically comply with its onerous expectations due to her disability, it is a *prima facie* conclusion.

Institutional Betrayal in Clinical Training

In case study 9, the prejudicial actions were taken by the individual supervisor, Dr. Ledebouria, whose discrimination against Jade was based solely upon the trainee's neurodivergence. Yet it was not only the supervisor who harmed the trainee—instead, the collective failure of the entire psychological corporation to hold Dr. Ledebouria accountable for his clearly unlawful behavior compounded the problem. Additionally, the corporation's attorneys intentionally delayed the court proceedings as a calculated strategy to exhaust the financial resources of Jade and his family. Thus, the psychological corporation as an institution further aggravated the matter by employing their David-versus-Goliath tactics against Jade. The harm to this trainee as a result was incalculable.

In case study 10, Dr. Gasteria's prejudicial and unfair treatment of this disabled intern was exacerbated by the large agency. Failing a trainee at their internship should be reserved for the most extreme of cases, only when the intern is impaired permanently, presents a harm to patients, or whose clinical judgment is so inadequate as to make them ineligible to provide necessary services. The large network of clinics inflicted extreme damage upon Zinnia and was likely in breach of contract by their intention to fail her because her disability precluded their preferred method for documentation.

Misuse of the Gatekeeping Function of Psychology

Without question, there are some individuals who should never be allowed into the profession, either as clinical psychologists or as clinical mental health counselors. Such individuals might include those who are predatory or are prone to violence, have inappropriate sexual attraction to clients or colleagues, lack boundaries and have no ability to protect patient confidentiality, lack interpersonal skills or emotional intelligence, or cannot separate their own issues from those of clients. Such people may be more appropriate for other fields of psychology that do not hold the responsibilities of a patient-doctor relationship, and might perhaps be better suited to experimental psychology, social psychology, organizational/industrial psychology—or, to a different discipline altogether.

However, the simple fact that a student or trainee has a disability in one form or another is not acceptable grounds to prevent that otherwise-qualified individual from becoming a clinical psychologist or clinical mental health counselor. And yet, some have been misusing the gatekeeping function of their profession for exactly this reason, as seen in case study 11. Such actions are both illegal and unethical, and yet they are—sadly—not rare.

To do so to otherwise-qualified PWDN does violence to not only the student or trainee, but to the profession of psychology itself.

Politics Behind Institutional Betrayal

Character assassination of those who report discrimination is often employed, as it was in case 11, because the institution—in this case, the university—seeks to maintain its own reputation at the expense of the student. Taking a discrimination complaint seriously, on the other hand, requires a level of humility and openness to scrutiny that is often lacking in educational institutions.

Moreover, some level of an "us and them" mentality may be at play here, as well, in that those in positions of power (e.g., the faculty and administrators) become protective of the accused party. The aggrieved party (e.g., the student) becomes victim to fundamental attribution bias, where internal personality traits are presumed devoid of the context (e.g., external situational factors, such as acts of discrimination).

Because the actors on the part of the university felt threatened by the complaint against the faculty member in case 11, the student disciplinary committee also violated their own Anti-Discrimination Policy in their acts toward the student. Their bizarre and unethical actions were in the service of protecting the institution at all costs, sacrificing their integrity in the process. These same principles were also in effect in cases 9,10, and 12, although in a much less obvious manner.

Potential Involvement of the Dark Triad in Disability Discrimination

The politics behind some of the unconventional behaviors of the institutions involved in cases 9-12 are understandable to a certain degree on an organizational level when analyzed from the perspective of those within the institution, as elucidated above.

However, when viewed on an individual level, in the actions of Dr. Gasteria's refusal of accommodations (case study 10), Dr. Tradescantia's disability discrimination (case study 11), and Dr. Ledebouria's neurodivergence discrimination (case study 9), there may be darker elements at play.

The outright refusal to provide accommodations by clinical supervisors and site directors (Fern, case study 6; and Dr. Gasteria, case study 10), is unlikely to be an element of simply being unaware of disabled individuals' needs and legal rights.

This is a very different thing than the inability of an organization to provide accommodations (Aster, case study 5, Marigold, case study 7). Moreover, the disparate impact of these actions by clinical supervisors and site directors (Fern, case study 6; and Dr. Gasteria, case study 10) had consequential and detrimental effects upon the disabled trainees involved.

Is it possible that some of the individuals involved in the above cases might have personality traits aligning with the "dark triad" concept, as reviewed by Furnham et al. (2013)? The concept of the "dark triad" brings together Machiavellianism, narcissism, and subclinical sociopathy (Furnham et al., 2013), and Dr. Gasteria's intention to fail Zinnia at her internship (case study 10) despite the trainee successfully performing her essential duties in a disability-friendly way implies the cold detachment often seen in sociopathy. In case study 11, Dr. Tradescantia's retaliation against Abelia for filing a complaint based on his disability discrimination and the subsequent actions by the student disciplinary committee smack of Machiavellianism, certainly. And Dr. Ledebouria's neurodivergence discrimination (case study 9) clearly indicates his narcissism. Now, whether all three of these traits were present in each of these clinical supervisors and site directors is unknowable, but certainly all of these elements were present in these cases of trauma induced by training.

However, in case study 8, Dr. Calathea's actions provide abundant evidence to point to the presence of all three: Machiavellianism, narcissism, and sociopathy. This discussion may appear to be hyperbolic, but it is not: his repeated denial of accommodations for Dahlia; falsely claiming that she had not requested them (even after they had been approved by the clinic director, Dr. Alocasia); grading her down for "late" documentation though her notes were completed within the timeline agreed to by Dr. Alocasia, the trainee, and her school; and lying about her on her practicum evaluation. This pattern reflects the "dark triad" traits in action.

One might presume these types of behaviors are innocent mistakes, assuming that it is simply not possible, and that psychologists are immune to sociopathy. But as several of these cases indicate, sociopathy does indeed exist in this field, much as we might prefer to believe the opposite.

Martha Stout (2005) writes that 1 in 25 people (4% of the U. S. population) are sociopaths, and they are found in all professions, especially ones in which they can wield power and manipulate others. Thus, it is not impossible to consider that some would be in the psychology professions, as well.

Lack of Awareness of Disability Laws

Noncompliance Due to Ignorance

While colleges and universities may struggle with exactly how to provide reasonable accommodations for disabled students in certain individual circumstances, in these larger institutions there is more of a fundamental understanding of the Americans with Disabilities Act and Section 504 of the Rehabilitation Act, and the mandate to operate in accordance with these federal laws. In contrast, within free-standing graduate academic programs or professional schools of psychology that are not part of large educational institutions, there appears to be a widespread lack of knowledge of not only these laws, but also of the rights of disabled students, as well as overall ignorance of both the individual and institutional responsibility to comply.

A recent conversation with a colleague who has been a faculty member in psychology for 40 years at an Ivy-league institution recently confirmed this: she was wholly unaware that the ADA was, in fact, a federal law. Therefore, reasonable accommodations are assumed by such individuals to be optional, and noncompliance with these federal laws is not salient for these systems of advanced education in psychology. Moreover, because these federal laws have not been enforced, these egregious violations against PWDN occur with impunity, for the most part. So then, how can we expect schools to comply when their own faculty are ignorant of the protections afforded to disabled and neurodivergent graduate students?

Uneven Power Dynamics

Most such schools are insulated from accountability and responsibility because the aggrieved party (the student) generally does not file a lawsuit against the school, knowing that the educational institution has access to a cadre of lawyers that can tie the case up on litigation for years (as seen in case study 9). Moreover, opposing counsel will likely defame the reputation of the claimant, thus having a further adverse effect on the student and limiting their chances of graduating successfully.

As part of their professional training, graduate students in clinical psychology learn to be sensitive in therapeutic settings to the power differential between themselves as clinicians and their patients. Yet the power differential between a lowly student (who often has limited financial resources) and an institution with an entire legal team is analogous to a David-versus-Goliath scenario.

Furthermore, this unfair advantage is leveraged by faculty and staff accused of wrongdoing, many of whom cover over the misdeeds of institutional employees regardless of the facts of the case, in an us-versus-them tribalistic mentality if a student does indeed have the temerity to file a complaint of discrimination on the basis of disability prejudice. In case study 11, for example, despite numerous witnesses and documented evidence, the university ruled against the student who had filed a formal complaint against the faculty member for violating the anti-discrimination policy. Both the professor and the school had the institutional power, and misused their authority, essentially granting *carte blanche* to other faculty members to do the same to other students.

VI. HOW THE PSYCHOLOGY TRAINING-TO-WORKFORCE PIPELINE CAN IMPROVE

The ABCs of Disability Inclusion

Strides to success for PWDN in the field of psychology include: (a) universal design and accommodations; (b) supervisors initiating discussions about accommodations; (c) transformative teaching (e.g., to include disability and neurodivergent conditions examples in coursework, data examples, planning of exercises, alternative formats for assignments, etc.); (d) proactively addressing systemic barriers; (e) recognizing visible as well as invisible disabilities; (f) using real-world applications of marginalized disability knowledge; (g) calling out ableist behavior (and not excusing or covering for it); (h) honoring the lived experiences of PWDN; (i) enabling students and trainees to feel safe to disclose without fear of stigma or retaliation; (j) challenging discriminatory practices; (k) promoting allyship and mentorship opportunities; (l) ongoing training and assessment for faculty as well as clinical supervisors about issues on disability and neurodivergence; and (m) equitable and inclusive employment, resulting in (n) an empowered workforce (Baughman et al., 2005).

Dissemination of Disability Research

Disability and Neurodiversity are virtual unknowns within the field of psychology (Lund, 2018). These topics rarely are included in any psychology curricula at all (Bogart et al., 2026), though there is a robust literature base in Rehabilitation Psychology, Division 22 of the APA. which is rarely read by those in clinical psychology. Most published research on disability has been "ghettoized" in this way, had has not been widely disseminated throughout other areas of psychology (Olkin & Pledger, 2003). While social psychology has contributed greatly to research on disability prejudice, stigma, and identity development, this critically important contribution to the knowledge base has been unacknowledged and clinical psychology and mental health counseling are largely unaware of its existence.

Adopting a Trauma-Informed and Disability Inclusive Approach Within the Educational Setting

The lack of knowledge about disability and neurodiversity presents a glaring omission within the training structures of educational institutions and clinical training sites, ignoring the largest minority group globally. As we have seen by the case studies above, these recurrent practices in both academia and clinical training impose trauma upon a vulnerable population by those in power, exercising unjust privilege by erecting barriers to degree completion and graduation for no reason other than disability prejudice.

Cultural Humility Regarding Disability and Neurodiversity

Clinical supervision and psychologists in leadership should adopt practices that are both trauma-informed and are reflective of differences in physical ability and appearance, neurodivergence, as well as the reality of invisible disabilities and how their presence impacts the disabled student or trainee.

Just as we are trained to do in a multicultural orientation to BIPOC or LGBTQI+ populations, whether graduate students or trainees, we must adopt a posture of cultural humility toward PWDN, and learn to challenge the able-bodied privilege upon which the infrastructure for psychology education and training have been built.

This is a disability-related social justice issue, situated within the very heart of the helping professions. As a field we must advocate for implementable changes to deconstruct existing structures which are harmful, discriminatory, and exclusionary, while upholding rigorous standards that are equitable, accountable, and ethical.

We Must Deconstruct Institutional Resistance to Inclusion of PWDN

Structural and systemic barriers to inclusion for disabled and neurodivergent students and trainees include ableism, not being represented in curriculum, lack of accommodations in training, lack of continuing education requirements on the topics of neurodiversity and disability. Moreover, the competency in working with disability and neurodivergence is completely ignored in both clinical training and licensing requirements (Baughman et al., 2005).

This systemic exclusion leads to false assumptions about PWDN, bureaucratic burdens, institutional biases, burnout and attrition (Baughman et al., 2005). By adopting a cultural humility approach to inclusion, we can promote a more inclusive and equitable reality for PWDN.

Recommendations to Address the Structural Issues in Academia

It is clear that academic institutions have a great deal of work to do in order to correct the structural inequities that routinely disadvantage PWDN enrolled in their graduate psychology programs. If another minority group, say LGBTQI+ or BIPOC, were demonstrably discriminated against as regularly, and in as spectacular a fashion as those conveyed by the case studies presented in this chapter, it would be front-page news. Many of the prominent Ivy League institutions were recently called to account for their systemic refusals to protect Jewish students from antisemitism on its campuses, and multiple university presidents were forced to step down in the wake of these failures. Some institutions were also sued by the Department of Justice for their refusal to protect Jewish students, faculty, and staff.

Yet there is no corresponding outrage to the illegal actions by graduate schools who are training future mental health professionals. The disability prejudice in these institutions goes far beyond microaggressions, into unnecessary impediments to degree completion for graduate students, with resulting trauma to these trainees, as the anecdotal evidence presented in this chapter demonstrates convincingly. Many former students who are disabled or neurodivergent are left with compromised health, the burden of substantial student loan debt, and the dashed dreams of those who had devoted years to their education for a career they were kept from realizing, as a consequence of the actions of ableist faculty, staff, and administrators.

Sadly, it is not only a student issue: ableism affects the employees of these educational institutions as well (Lindsay & Fuentes, 2022; Gil-Goméz, 2017). Just as the BIPOC community has been asking for years for "people who look like them" to be considered in professorial staff and management positions, so too should educational institutions actively recruit, hire, and promote qualified faculty, staff members, administrators, and executive leadership who are disabled or neurodivergent themselves.

Staffing and Hiring Issues

Smaller colleges and universities that do not have a complete Disability Services Office must at the very least have a dedicated staff member who is either a person with a disability, perhaps has disabled spouse or family member, or has some experiential base from which to understand the challenges faced by PWDN within their student body. It is ludicrous to expect that an able-bodied or neurotypical individual whose duties entail the gathering of medical documentation justifying accommodations, advocating on behalf of PWDN, and educating faculty and staff on the unique needs, strengths, and legal rights of disabled and neurodivergence of students would not at least have some lived experience of their struggles.

Particularly when a disabled or neurodivergent student makes a report of discrimination, a nondisabled staff member should not be making the determination of whether such disability prejudice was or was not in play (as occurred in case 11), as these nondisabled or neurotypical individuals may not even recognize their own able-bodied or neurotypical privilege, thus making their judgment more open to the influence of implicit bias.

The Crucial Role of Directors of Clinical Training

Directors of Clinical Training (DCTs) should be trained on the types of accommodations that might need to be put in place for disabled or neurodivergent trainees to be successful in their clinical placements. Moreover, if students at their practicum or internship placements are not getting the accommodations to which they are legally entitled, DCTs should advocate on the behalf of the disabled trainees with the sites to ensure that accommodations are implemented. The current hands-off approach of most DCTs, who only get involved if there is a problem, is a recipe for failure. These changes will improve not only the graduation rates of their institution, but also would likely strengthen their university's relationships with APPIC, while enhancing the reputation of their respective programs.

Additionally, prior to starting any clinical placements, all disabled and neurodivergent students seeking practicum or internship should be provided by the DCT with a copy of the *APA Resource Guide for Psychology Graduate Students with Disabilities, second edition* (APA, n. d.), to be discussed more fully in a subsequent section. DCTs should work collaboratively with the Office of Disability Services within their programs or universities to ensure that all students registered with the clinical program who are eligible to clinical training have been given a copy of this resource. Moreover, every DCT should not only read it, but be very familiar with it in order to best serve disabled and neurodivergent students. In some cases, the DCTs might need to advocate on behalf of PWDN in clinical placements to enable clinical sites to understand that reasonable accommodations are not optional and are required by federal law. Sites that refuse to provide reasonable accommodations should be excluded from the list of sites approved for that academic training program.

There are far too many changes needed for educational institutions to create learning environments that are truly inclusive and welcoming for disabled graduate students and trainees with neurodivergence, than can be adequately addressed in this chapter. An entire special issue of the *Society for Teaching of Psychology* on this topic was recently released to enable psychology programs to develop a psychology curriculum and teaching environment that comes against ableism and promotes a universal design that can be accessible to all graduate students (Bogart et al., 2026).

Recommendations to Address the Structural Issues in Clinical Training

Likewise, for clinical training sites, an abundant number of changes need to be put in place to ensure that PWDN are not unlawfully discriminated against in practicum, internship, and post-doc placements. Kuemmel and Wilbur (2020) have advanced the concept of a Disability-Affirming Training Environment (DATE), to develop environments within clinical training that are inclusive to PWDN.

The goals of a DATE are to have "attitudinal awareness of disability culture and identity development and taking a strengths-based stance towards disability, willingness to advocate for disability rights, such as universal access, and dedication to establishing accommodations" (Kuemmel & Wilbur, 2020).

Furthermore, Wilbur et al. (2019) outline the responsibility as clinical supervisors to become advocates for PWDN in practicum and internship placements to overcome the structural barriers put in place by the current paradigm of psychology training. Implementation of the DATE concept would go a long way toward addressing the leaks in the training-to-workforce pipeline for future psychology practitioners, to prevent PWDN from falling through the cracks (Lund, 2023).

Clinical placement sites must obtain training on issues of disability and diversity not only with respect to serving *patients* with disabilities, but for how to provide competent supervision to disabled or neurodivergent *trainees and interns*. The *APA Guidelines for Clinical Supervision in Health Service Psychology* (2026b) address competency-based supervision, suggesting a multicultural orientation for supervisors working with diverse trainees. But simply including disability into a multicultural umbrella means that disability once again gets lost and ignored. While some PWDN would endorse being a member of a disability culture, many (if not most), would not.

The APA has current *Guidelines for Assessment and Intervention with Persons with Disabilities* (APA, 2022), which addresses PWDN in the client population, but the APA has yet to develop guidelines for faculty, staff, and clinical supervisors who are providing instruction and training to PWDN as students and trainees. This must be rectified.

Recommendations to Address the Structural Issues Within the Profession Overall

Enhancing Inclusion by Providing Timeline Exemptions for PWDN

APA's Commission on Accreditation Standards of Accreditation (APA CoA) must begin to allow and accredit half-time internship positions to accommodate trainees with disabilities needing this accommodation, though many PWDN can do full-time internships, some cannot due to the nature of their disability. APPIC should also allow half-time, two-year internships into their match system for this same reason. Furthermore, if this adaptation is adopted, it would not only benefit disabled trainees, but would reduce some of the elitism in the profession, as there are a number of students who cannot work full-time due to family obligations, or the need to work to support their families. This will help promote economic diversity in the field, as well.

Likewise, for PWDN, state boards of psychology should consider allowing an exemption or an extension to the period of time in which disabled and neurodivergent trainees can accumulate clinical hours to be eligible for the licensing exam. Given that some disabled people may not have the physical capacity to work full-time, the designated time periods again put an ableist restriction that might fit well for the large body of applicants overall, while penalizing those whose conditions are not amenable to these timelines. In addition, APA also have an as-needed reasonable exemptions for time-limited graduate programs to allow PWDN to complete doctoral programs if necessitated by restrictions from their disability.

Mandating Competency in the PWDN Population on Licensing Exam

Furthermore, the Association of State and Provincial Psychology Boards (ASPBB) should consider adopting a statement of support for the education, training, and competency of psychologists on issues of disability and neurodivergence. There is currently very little teaching on issues of disability in standard curricula in psychology (Bogart et al., 2026), and this will only be remedied by the universities if it becomes a content area covered in the licensing exam. Just as social and cultural bases of behavior is tested in the EPPP, covering social psychology theories, cultural diversity, group dynamics and human behavior in social contexts (Siotia, 2024, June 25), so it should likewise incorporate in questions on the licensing examination regarding the basics of disability, neurodiversity, and issues related to the PWDN in order to ensure basic competency with this population.

Improvements at the Accreditation Level

The American Psychological Association (APA) Council on Accreditation certifies many academic programs for clinical psychology, as well as clinical training sites. The Association of Psychology Postdoctoral and Internship Centers (APPIC) also operates a consortium of advanced clinical training sites for graduate students in clinical, counseling, and educational psychology.

Both APA-accredited and APPIC-affiliated programs and clinical training sites are highly regarded—and, in many states, graduates of other programs without these certifications are not eligible for licensure. Presumably states have adopted these affiliations as proxy certifications of quality education and clinical proficiency. Indeed, several institutions such as the Veterans Administration and its affiliated hospitals and clinics will not hire anyone who has not graduated from both an APA-accredited graduate program and an APA-accredited internship.

Enforcing Compliance with Disability Laws

APPIC requires its member clinical training sites to ensure that trainees are afforded respect and courtesy, stating that practices therein which are dehumanizing towards them by staff are unacceptable (APPIC, 2020). Moreover, it restates that all protected classes including disability not be subjected to discrimination (APPIC, 2020). The membership agreement mandates adherence to all laws and regulations (APPIC, 2020), which would apply to the ADA and Section 504 of the Rehabilitation Act, as well.

But because neither APA's Council on Accreditation nor APPIC explicitly require compliance with legal mandates disallowing discrimination against students on the basis of disability, staff of many accredited programs do engage in discriminatory practices as described in the twelve case studies presented above. Nor do APA and APPIC gather any data whatsoever on programmatic compliance (or lack thereof) with ADA and Section 504 when they accredit either academic programs or clinical training sites.

APPIC's policy for membership requires compliance with APA's ethical code, and makes mention that member sites do not discriminate against individuals with disabilities (APIC, 2020). Yet in case study 11, though the discrimination at the APA-accredited internship site was brought to the attention of the ombudsman at APPIC, no action was taken to hold the agency accountable.

APA's ethical code states that discrimination against any protected class is unethical, and explicitly cites disability as among the categories. Yet again, there is no enforcement of this rule, and no consequences for institutions, programs, or individuals who violate it. Therefore, sites and programs violating the ethical code must be sanctioned accordingly with probation in cases of proven discrimination and loss of accreditation status if a pattern of discriminatory and unlawful actions persist at APPIC-accredited training sites.

APA's Public Policies Regarding Disability

Disability Inclusion

The APA governing Council of Representatives recently issued a policy statement on disability and inclusion to combat stigma and ableist discrimination toward PWDN (Lodi-Smith, 2025). It also honors the lived experience of disabled individuals and promotes inclusivity, by a shift from the deficit-based model of disability (Lodi-Smith, 2025). Finally, it calls for the inclusion of PWDN in research as well as public educational campaigns addressing ableism (Lodi-Smith, 2025).

Full Participation of Psychologists with Disabilities

The United Nations' Convention on the Rights of Persons with Disabilities (CRPD) was supported in a policy statement by the APA governing Council of Representatives (APA, 2014). This document acknowledges that prejudicial attitudes about disability are the primary barrier to PWDN reaching their potential, and establishes that psychological research demonstrates the pervasiveness of stigmatization toward them APA. (2014). It also reaffirmed its 1997 Policy Statement of the Full Participation for Psychologists with Disabilities and addressed the intersection of disability into other minority status, calling for enhanced inclusion within the field of psychology, as well as the elimination of oppression of PWDN (APA, 2014).

A related policy statement adopted by the APA governing Council of Representatives stated: "it is essential for psychologists to understand how stereotypical and stigmatizing language, attitudes, and behaviors can demean and devalue people with disabilities and have an adverse impact on self-concept, self-esteem, self-efficacy, and relationships with others" (APA, 2008). This policy statement in support of the Americans with Disabilities Act recognized the historical maltreatment, discrimination, and stigmatization that PWD have been subjected to, specifically acknowledging both visible and invisible disabilities (APA, 2008).

APA Addresses the Unique Concerns for Disabled and Neurodivergent Interns and Applicants

The APA produced a Resource guide for disabled graduate students regarding the unique difficulties PWDN face when navigating psychology practicum and internship placements (APA Office on Disability Issues in Psychology, n.d.). In it, Arnold Abels advocates that disabled students contact APPIC if they have negative experiences in the selection process when seeking internships (APA Office on Disability Issues in Psychology, n.d.). Williams et al. in this same document outline the biased attitudes toward disabled applicants, involving fear, negative experiences, lack of knowledge and skill regarding disability, overemphasis on limitations (i.e., the deficit-based view of disability), and the tendency to look for information to confirm presumed incompetency on the part of PWDN (APA Office on Disability Issues in Psychology, n.d.). It acknowledges that "psychologists often have received [minimal to no training] on job accommodations, the Americans with Disabilities Act (ADA), and ADA considerations as related to employment interviews" (APA Office on Disability Issues in Psychology, n.d., p. 9). Moreover, it suggests that disabled internship applicants not become defensive when feeling threatened during the interview, by to instead utilize self-presentation/impression management tactics (APA Office on Disability Issues in Psychology, n.d.).

This helpful resource guide explores the complexities regarding whether or not to disclose one's disability, and distinguishes that the accommodations process for PWDN differs at the internship site when compared with that of the educational institutions (APA Office on Disability Issues in Psychology, n.d.). It outlines multiple elements to include in a formal accommodations request, and specifies that the request should be made in writing (APA Office on Disability Issues in Psychology, n.d.). Employer fears about cost of accommodations for qualified workers is often overestimated, when in fact most accommodations costs are less than $500, and half of disabled workers, accommodations are unnecessary (APA Office on Disability Issues in Psychology, n.d.).

While internship is often challenging for all psychology trainees, PWDN have additional sources of stress, including daily demands of living with a disability and its potential complications, health concerns, ableist bias and disability prejudice, as well as issues at the worksite (APA Office on Disability Issues in Psychology, n.d.). Many practicum students or interns choose not to disclose, but concealing their disability imposes additional stress, such as fearing the discovery of disability by others at the internship, and the overall reduction in well-being in terms of affect, cognition, and behavior (APA Office on Disability Issues in Psychology, n.d.). Clinical supervisors often lack understanding of their ability to authorize accommodations or to identify when they are necessary; some may presume accommodations to be unreasonable because they lack training in this area (APA Office on Disability Issues in Psychology, n.d.).

Interns with invisible disabilities in particular are often hesitant to disclose or seek accommodations, taking upon themselves unnecessary and onerous burdens, such as working late in the evening or extra time to complete their job assignments, using personal funds to purchase assistive technology or ergonomic equipment, and neglecting their own needs for self-care (APA Office on Disability Issues in Psychology, n.d.). Many internship sites are located in non-accessible facilities: in one study cited found 20% of sites without any disabled parking spaces; 25% lacked ramps; and most had appropriate ingress to the building wide enough to accommodate a wheelchair, but inner doorways were not ADA-compliant (APA Office on Disability Issues in Psychology, n.d.).

Psychology Leadership: Future Directions for the Profession

Clearly, both APA and APPIC affirm the rights of trainees with disabilities, as evidenced by the foregoing policy statements. Yet these multiple public statements of policy have been issued and ignored repeatedly. The only thing lacking is enforcement.

If APPIC member sites agree to not discriminate and yet engage in disability prejudice and refusal to implement reasonable accommodations, then the clinical placements are not only in violation of federal law, but should face consequences accordingly. Once APPIC becomes aware of a site that is discriminating against a disabled trainee, potentially APPIC could either compel compliance of the member agency as a condition of continued accreditation, or APPIC could immediately revoke the member agency for material breach of its agreement.

The onus should not be placed upon the intern or trainee who has faced discrimination to hold clinical sites or universities accountable. Doing so entails continued stress of a lawsuit by those who already are victims of discrimination; as well as the financial costs, which are excessive to the budget of most trainees. Likewise, graduate students lack the political clout to compel educational institutions to provide academic accommodations or to cease and desist from attitudes and actions that are ablest in nature and prejudicial.

It is time for APA, the leading leadership organization of the profession to now mandate protections for graduate students and psychology trainees who are disabled and neurodivergent. Moreover, the APA must enforce compliance by implementing consequences when educational institutions and clinical sites do not uphold the enforceable standards of the Ethics Code due to discriminatory and unethical practices. In addition, the APA Council on Accreditation should rescind the accreditation status of academic programs that misuse the gatekeeping functions of the profession because of disability prejudice or ableist expectations, which provide barriers to otherwise-qualified PWDN entering the field.

The APA Policy Statement of the Full Participation for Psychologists with Disabilities expressed its commitment to disabled psychologists in terms of physical, social, communicative, and attitudinal access (APA,1997). These policy statements should not just be aspirational goals but must be accompanied by decisive action. Providing policy direction is insufficient to address the systemic inequities laid out in this chapter which prove beyond doubt that the training-to-workforce pipeline in psychology is broken.

By its earlier policy statement, the APA recognizes that lack of access and inclusion of PWD within our profession is indeed a civil rights issue (APA,1997). APA must take steps to address and eradicate the oppression currently placed upon disabled and neurodivergent graduate students and psychology trainees.

CONCLUSION

The current training-to-workforce model in psychology was designed with only abled bodied and neurotypical graduate students and trainees in mind. Thus, it is fundamentally unfair to PWDN, and while some are able to mask their disability or force their disabled bodies and neurodivergent minds to conform to the round hole into which all graduate students and trainees must fit in order to earn their degrees and become licensed.

Earlier in the development of psychology as a discipline, it has historically undermined and excluded women and persons of color, disallowing their entry into educational institutions or prestigious laboratories. From these ignominious origins, the field has grown and expanded in many ways. Among its most recent improvements is the explosion of research on multiculturalism and mandates to ensure that future clinicians would be adequately prepared to sensitively and competently provide therapeutic services to patients of any culture or ethnicity. Understanding of sexual minorities and the gender nonconforming population is slowly being diffused into the field. Psychology is breaking out of its white, heteronormative, and male-dominated history, and has committed itself to the understanding of the complexity of diversity.

And yet, PWDN as both a patient and student population remain lagging behind. Disabled and neurodivergent graduate students and trainees are rarely given a thought in our educational programs, are wholly unrepresented in curricula, and generally are absent from all multicultural research. Despite being the largest minority of all, their absence in psychology renders them virtually invisible (Hagion-Rzepka, 2023).

The clinical training-to-workforce paradigm for aspiring psychologists is ableist in nature and excludes some who slip through the cracks because of the systemic inequities built into it by design. Many of these students and trainees are grievously harmed by their experiences in noninclusive educational and clinical settings because of disability prejudice, unlawful discrimination, and non-inclusive practices that have been perpetuated by fiat. Able-bodied privilege underscores the exclusionary requirements and expectations that are uniformly imposed upon all, without respect for the differences in disabled bodies or neurodivergent minds. As this chapter demonstrates, some disabled or neurodivergent graduate students and trainees are traumatized by their experiences in educational programs and clinical training by uninformed or adversarial persons in positions of power, who wield their authority in an unfair exercise that makes the success of PWDN improbable—and, at times, impossible.

The current situation is untenable, and just as psychology as a field adopted the initiative to become more multiculturally competent, it must now take concrete steps to ensure that PWDN are welcomed, included, valued, and supported as they prepare to enter the field. Their disability status should not preclude them from doing so, as it often does now.

Trauma-informed psychology training with a view to the disabled and neurodivergent community would consider the lasting impact of ableist microaggressions and disability discrimination from a trauma-informed lens, and would not perpetuate these in either its educational or training environments, as it does currently. It would examine the fact that the vast majority of clinical training sites are inaccessible to PWDN. It would honor the intent of and comply with federal law which recognizes disability as a protected class. An educational system that intentionally included PWDN in training would keep in mind issues of accessibility not only in terms of the physical infrastructure, but also would infuse topics of disability and neurodivergence into its curriculum, as well as its clinical training requirements. Moreover, it provide accommodations in both the classroom and clinical placements, and ensure that they are implanted to give the disabled or neurodivergent student the best chance of success.

It would fundamentally restructure the clinical training expectations and apparatus to ensure participation as well as legal compliance.

As Bogart (2014) discussed, rather than trying to "normalize" trainees with disabilities or neurodivergence, instead academics and clinical training staff should enhance the disability self-concept of their practicum students or interns. Improving the visibility of the disability community in both educational institutions and within the profession will help to promote disability pride (Bogart, 2014) while expanding the diversity of our clinician providers, which will better serve our clients. Faculty as well as directors of clinical training and supervisors must study, develop clinical judgment and skill to sensitively and compassionately provide equitable educational and clinical opportunities for PWDN, and their educational and professional organizations must hold them accountable for developing these competencies.

The one-size-fits-all approach to professional training for future psychologists does not adequately serve disabled and neurodivergent student and trainees, and in fact causes substantial harm to them. Thus, our current training paradigm for professional psychology violates our ethical code, which demands that we "first do no harm."

By viewing disability discrimination and exclusion of PWDN within the existing framework for professional training from a trauma-informed lens, we can conclude that the infrastructure of educational and training programs as they stand are outdated and in serious need of restructuring to uphold the social justice values of the profession.

It is, in fact, a cookie-cutter method that does not work because disabled and neurodivergent students, interns, and trainees are not cookie dough to be cut and formed into nondisabled or neurotypical clinicians. They are human beings with minds that think differently and bodies that have less freedom of movement than able-bodied persons. But they are still individuals that can, if we allow them to, contribute meaningfully to our field and make contributions to our understanding of human complexities in terms of meaning and experience.

Enacting these proposed changes would strengthen the field by rendering a more equal opportunity to a large minority which has been historically excluded by design. Doing so would promote a more just, culturally responsive, and welcoming environment for education and training to develop the disabled and neurodivergent clinical providers of tomorrow.

REFERENCES

Americans with Disabilities Act of 1990, Pub. L. No. 101-336, 104 Stat. 327 (1990). congress.gov.

Americans with Disabilities Amendments Act of 2008, Pub. L. No. 110-325. (2008). ADA Amendments Act of 2008, Pub. L. No. 325, Stat. 122 (2008), 3553-3559. congress.gov.

Andrews, E. E., Forber-Pratt, A. J., Mona, L. R., Lund, E. M., Pilarski, C. R., & Balter, R. (2019). # SaytheWord: A disability culture commentary on the erasure of "disability". *Rehabilitation Psychology, 64*(2), 111–118. DOI: 10.1037/rep0000258 PMID: 30762412

APA. (2017). *Ethical principles of psychologists and code of conduct.* American Psychological Association.

APA. (2022). *Guidelines for Assessment and Intervention with Persons with Disabilities.* American Psychological Association. https://www.apa.org/pi/disability/resources/assessment-disabilities

APA. (2026a). *Standards of Accreditation for Health Service Psychology.* APA's Commission on Accreditation Standards of Accreditation. American Psychological Association. https://www.apa.org/ed/accreditation/standards-of-accreditation.pdf

APA. (2026b). *APA Guidelines for clinical supervision in Health Service Psychology.* APA Task Force on Clinical Supervision in Health Service Psychology, American Psychological Association. https://www.apa.org/about/policy/guidelines-supervision.pdf

APA. (2014). *Resolution in support of the U.N. Convention on the Rights of Persons with Disabilities.* American Psychological Association. https://www.apa.org/about/policy/support-un-convention?shem=rimspwouoe,

APA. (2008). *Resolution on the Americans with Disabilities Act.* American Psychological Association. https://www.apa.org/about/policy/disabilities-act?shem=rimspwouoe,

APA. (1997). *Policy statement of the full participation for psychologists with disabilities.* American Psychological Association. https://www.apa.org/about/policy/participation.pdf

APA Office on Disability Issues in Psychology. (n.d.) *APA Resource guide for psychology graduate students with disabilities* (2nd ed.). American Psychological Association. https://www.apa.org/pi/disability/resources/publications/resource-guide ?shem=rimspwouoe,

APPIC (2020). *APPIC member policy for legal and ethical conduct.* Association of Psychology Post-doctoral and Internship Centers. https://www.appic.org/About -APPIC/APPIC-Policies/Member-Policy?shem=rimspwouoe,

ASPPB. (n.d.). *Current examination for professional practice in psychology (EPPP)®content areas*. https://asppb.net/exams/asppb-examination-for-professional -psychology-eppp/eppp-exam-topics/

Banaji, M. R., & Greenwald, A. G. (2013). *Blind spot: Hidden biases of good people*. Delacorte Press.

Bargiela, S., Steward, R., & Mandy, W. (2016). The experiences of late-diagnosed women with autism spectrum conditions: An investigation of the female autism phenotype. *Journal of Autism and Developmental Disorders*, *46*(10), 3281–3294. DOI: 10.1007/s10803-016-2872-8 PMID: 27457364

Baughman, K., Leventhal, L., Black, S., & Friedheim, R. E. (2005). The missing link: Disability inclusion in psychology education, training, and employment. [Poster]. *APA Annual Conference*, Los Angeles.

Bogart, K. R., Heydarian, N. M., Hughes, A. S., Lund, E. M., & Rosa, N. M. (2026). Special issue introduction: Creating an anti-ableist psychology curriculum and teaching environment. *Teaching of Psychology*, *1-4*(2), 115–118. Advance online publication. DOI: 10.1177/00986283251412268

Bogart, K. R., Lund, E. M., Rottenstein, A., & Bouchard, L. (2017). Who self-identifies as disabled? An examination of impairment and contextual predictors. *Rehabilitation Psychology*, *62*(4), 553–562. DOI: 10.1037/rep0000132 PMID: 28581320

Bogart, L. R. (2014). The role of disability self-concept in adaptation to congenital or acquired disability. *Rehabilitation Psychology*, *59*(1), 107–115. DOI: 10.1037/ a0035800 PMID: 24611927

Bolton, M. J. (2023). De-centering neuronormativity is an imperative in humanistic psychotherapy: Towards a neurodiversity-informed, person-centered approach. *The Person-Centered Journal*, 1-39. DOI: 10.31234/osf.io/q2t8h

Bumgardner, K. (2023). Ableism in education: Professor perpetuation of disability discrimination through accommodation non-compliance. *Scripps Senior Theses*. 2184. https://scholarship.claremont.eduScripps_theses/2184

California Southern University. (2026). *Statement on suitability and fitness for the profession.* https://calsouthern.smartcatalogiq.com/en/2025-2026/general-catalog/school-of-behavioral-sciences/doctor-of-psychology-clinical-specialization)

Conover, K. J., Israel, T., & Nylund-Gibson, K. (2017). Development and validation of the Ableist Microaggressions Scale. *The Counseling Psychologist*, *45*(4), 570–599. DOI: 10.1177/0011000017715317

Dunn, D. S., & Burkaw, S. (2013). Disability identity: Exploring narrative accounts of disability. *Rehabilitation Psychology*, *58*(2), 148–157. DOI: 10.1037/a0031691 PMID: 23437994

Family Educational Rights and Privacy Act of 1974, 20 U.S.C. §232g. govinfo.gov

Freyd, J. J., Kles, B., & Allard, C. B. (2005). Betrayal trauma: Relationship to physical health, psychological distress, and a written intervention. *Journal of Trauma & Dissociation*, *6*(3), 83–104. DOI: 10.1300/J229v06n03_04 PMID: 16172083

Fung, L. K. (2021). *Neurodiversity: From phenomenology to neurobiology and enhancing technologies*. American Psychiatric Association. DOI: 10.1176/appi.books.9781615379514

Furnham, A., Richards, S. C., & Palhus, D. L. (2013). The dark triad of personality: A 10-year review. *Social and Personality Psychology Compass*, *7*(3), 199–216. DOI: 10.1111/spc3.12018

Galiana-Simal, A., Vela-Romero, M., Romero-Vela, V. M., Oliver-Tercero, N., García-Olmo, V., Benito-Castellanos, P. J., Muñoz-Martinez, V., & Beato-Fernandez, L. (2020). Sensory processing disorder: Key points of a frequent alteration in neurodevelopmental disorders. *Cogent Medicine*, *7*(1), 1736829. DOI: 10.1080/2331205X.2020.1736829

Gil-Goméz, E. N. (2017). (In)visibilities: A woman faculty of color search for a disabled identity that fits. In Massé, M. A., & Bauer-Maglin, N. (Eds.), *Staging women's lives in academia: Gendered life stages in language and literature workplaces*. SUNY Press.

Hagion-Rzepka, C. (2023). The invisible minority: Addressing disability in graduate psychology training programs. In Jesus, Â. (Ed.), *Instructional Approaches for Health Professions Education.* IGI Global Scientific.

Harsey, S., & Freyd, J. J. (2020). Deny, attack, reverse victim and offender (DARVO): What is the influence on perceived perpetrator and victim credibility? *Journal of Aggression, Maltreatment & Trauma*, *29*(8), 897–916. DOI: 10.1080/10926771.2020.1774695

Kuemmel, A., & Wilbur, R. (2020). Thirty-one years after the ADA: The perplexity of disability. *APPIC 2020 Conference*.

Leedham, A., Thompson, A. R., Smith, R., & Freeth, M. (2020). 'I was exhausted trying to figure it out': The experiences of females receiving an autism diagnosis in middle to late adulthood. *Autism, 24*(1), 135–146. DOI: 10.1177/1362361319853442 PMID: 31144507

Lett, K. (2018). *Impact of ableist microaggressions on university students with self-identified disabilities*. University of Regina.

Liasidou, A., & Gregoriou, A. (2024). A systematic literature review of intersectionality and disability in education. *British Journal of Sociology of Education, 45*(4), 584–608. DOI: 10.1080/01425692.2024.2340562

Lindsay, S., & Fuentes, K. (2022, April 07). It is time to address ableism in academia: A systematic review of the experiences and impact of ableism among faculty and staff. *Disabilities*, *2*(2), 178–203. DOI: 10.3390/disabilities2020014

Lodi-Smith, J. (Sep 4, 2025). From the Board: APA council approves major policy changes—Master's-level practice, disability inclusion, and traditional wisdom integration. Society for Personality and Social Psychology. *SPSP News Blog*. https://spsp.org/news/spsp-news/board-apa-council-approves-6-major-policy-changes?shem=rimspwouoe,

Lund, E. M. (2023). Addressing the leaking pipeline: Supporting disabled graduate student teachers in psychology. *Teaching of Psychology, 50*(2), 99-104. DOI: 10.1177/00986283211103642

Lund, E. M. (2018). Disability as diversity in professional psychology: A continued call for research and action. *Training and Education in Professional Psychology*, *12*(4), 295–296. DOI: 10.1037/tep0000218

Lund, E. M., Khazeem, L. R., & DeJesus, C. R. (2023). Addressing intersectional identities and experiences professional psychology trainees with disabilities. A call for action. *Training and Education in Professional Psychology*, *17*(2), 185–190. DOI: 10.1037/tep0000403

McDonald, K. E., Keys, C. B., & Balcazar, F. E. (2007). Disability, race/ethnicity and gender: Themes of cultural oppression, acts of individual resistance. *American Journal of Community Psychology*, *39*(1-2), 145–161. DOI: 10.1007/s10464-007-9094-3 PMID: 17294120

Nario-Redmond, M. (2024). Ableism: The many manifestations of disability prejudice. In Bennett, G., & Goodall, E. (Eds.), *The Palgrave Encyclopedia of Disability*., DOI: 10.1007/978-3-031-40858-8_8-1

Nerenberg, J. (2020). *Divergent mind: Thriving in a world that wasn't designed for you*. Harper One.

Olkin, R. (1999). *What psychotherapists should know about disability*. Guilford Press.

Olkin, R., Hayward, H., Abbene, M. S., & VanHeel, G. (2019). The experiences of microaggressions against women with visible and invisible disabilities. *The Journal of Social Issues*, *75*(3), 757–785. https://doi.org/. DOI: 10.1111/josi.12342

Rehabilitation Act of 1973, 29 U.S.C. § 794. 28 CFR 35.104.

Siotia, S. (2024, June 25). AP-LS Student Committee Preparing for the EPPP: Essential Tips and Tricks. [blog post]. American-Psychology Law Society. http://www.apls-students.org/the-intersection-a-blog/preparing-for-the-eppp-essential-tips-and-tricks

Smith, C. P., & Freyd, J. J. (2014). Institutional betrayal. *The American Psychologist*, *69*(6), 575–587. DOI: 10.1037/a0037564 PMID: 25197837

Stout, M. (2005). *The sociopath next door*. Broadway Books.

Tran, S., Krauter, M., & Bogart, K. R. (2025). Ableism: The time has come to understand bias against people with disabilities. In Nelson, T. D. (Ed.), *Handbook of prejudice, stereotyping, and discrimination* (3rd ed., pp. 276–299). Routledge.

Watson, N. (2002). Well, I know this is going to sound very strange to you, but I don't see myself as a disabled person: Identity and disability. *Disability & Society*, *17*(5), 509–527. DOI: 10.1080/09687590220148496

Wilbur, R. C., Kuemmel, A., & Lackner, R. J. (2019). Who's on first? Supervising psychology trainees with disabilities and establishing accommodations. *Training and Education in Professional Psychology*, *13*(2), 111–118. DOI: 10.1037/tep0000231

Williams, M. T. (2020). Psychology cannot afford to ignore the many harms caused by microaggressions. *Perspectives on Psychological Science*, *15*(1), 38–43. DOI: 10.1177/1745691619893362 PMID: 31801042

Wolbring, G., & Nasir, L. (2024). Intersectionality of disabled people through a Disability Studies, Ability-based studies, and intersectional pedagogy lens: A survey and a scoping review. *Societies (Basel, Switzerland)*, *14*(9), 176. DOI: 10.3390/soc14090176

World Health Organization. (2019). *International statistical classification of diseases and related health problems* (11th ed.). (ICD-11). https://icd.who.int/

Chapter 6
A Resilience-Integrated Framework for Trauma Treatment to Enhance Adaptive Capacity

Sarah E. Stewart-Spencer
http://orcid.org/0009-0009-7952-4213
Stewart-Spencer Consulting, LLC, USA

ABSTRACT

This chapter examines limitations in traditional trauma treatment approaches that emphasize reactive symptom reduction and assume traumatic exposure has ended. Such models are insufficient for individuals in high-demand professions who experience ongoing and cumulative trauma. This chapter proposes that integrating resilience skill development directly into trauma treatment is essential for promoting long-term psychological stability and adaptive functioning. Resilience is conceptualized as a teachable, dynamic clinical process rather than an innate trait or supplementary self-care strategy. This chapter introduces the PEACE Resilience Model, a structured framework aligned with phase-oriented trauma treatment that embeds resilience development across stabilization, reprocessing, and reintegration. The model emphasizes psychoeducation, self-awareness, foundational health practices, acute stress coping, and personalized resilience planning. This chapter provides an evidence-informed roadmap for ethical and effective practice

DOI: 10.4018/979-8-3373-8597-6.ch006

INTRODUCTION. A RESILIENCE-INTEGRATED FRAMEWORK FOR TRAUMA TREATMENT TO ENHANCE ADAPTIVE CAPACITY

Trauma treatment has traditionally been implemented as a reactive approach with a primary focus on symptom reduction following adverse exposure. Clients typically present to therapy with traumatic stress symptoms requiring stabilization and relief from distress. Prevailing treatment models conceptualize trauma as discrete or time-limited, with minimal attention to anticipated future exposure or sustained vulnerability (Billings & Nicholls, 2025; Sonu et al., 2024). Symptom-focused interventions reduce trauma-related stress, such as hyperarousal, hypervigilance, and intrusive or flooding memories, providing an opportunity for stabilization. Recent advances in treating Complex Post-Traumatic Stress Disorder (CPTSD) have demonstrated meaningful and hopeful progress in symptom reduction and stabilization (Karatzias et al., 2023). At the same time, adaptive capability may receive less attention in symptom-focused treatment, which can suggest that treatment ends when symptoms subside. Within these approaches, recovery is often framed as the absence of pathology rather than the presence of adaptive functioning to navigate future exposure (Leitch & McCaw, 2024). Disruptions in identity, purpose, moral frameworks, and worldview commonly accompany trauma (Condon et al., 2023), suggesting that treatment may benefit from extending beyond symptom-reduction or stabilization. Providers may reinforce passive recovery with repair-oriented approaches instead of models grounded in readiness, durability, and long-term adaptation.

Limitations of Reactive Trauma Treatment

Although advances in trauma treatment represent meaningful progress, their effectiveness may be influenced by the assumption that clients will not experience or anticipate another traumatic exposure. For some individuals, symptom-focused treatment can be sufficient to sustain recovery. However, this assumption may be less applicable for populations where trauma exposure is part of their vocational culture. For populations whose responsibilities or duties place them in harm's way, such as high-demand professionals (HDPs), trauma exposure is an accepted reality. HDPs include first responders, military members, healthcare professionals, in-field journalists, crisis workers, and legal and social service providers, among other public-service roles in which the work itself entails repeated proximity to crisis, suffering, or threat. HDPs are individuals whose roles require sustained performance under pressure, rapid decision-making in complex situations, and an unwavering commitment to the well-being, safety, or success of others. These roles often come with elevated expectations, long hours, emotional strain, ethical dilemmas, and high visibility. While each field presents unique challenges, the shared thread is continuous exposure to trauma and/or chronic stress that accumulates over time. HDPs function under stress that impacts mental, emotional, and relational health.

Cumulative Trauma and High-Demand Professionals

Repeated trauma exposure is an inherent characteristic of populations that serve in crucial, essential roles. Cumulative and anticipatory trauma require unique assessment and treatment considerations. For example, the neurobiological and psychological impacts of ongoing threat and stress change the recovery landscape (Kalisch et al., 2015; McEwen & Akil, 2020) and extend beyond traditional PTSD symptom clusters. For HDPs, trauma is not confined to isolated incidents; it is woven into the fabric of their vocation. With repeated exposure, entrenched symptom patterns develop that reduce recovery efficiency (Karatzias et al., 2023) leaving the individual vulnerable to complicated recovery trajectories. This unique characteristic necessitates adjustments to adequately meet their treatment needs.

High-demand professionals face more challenges than traumatic-stress related symptoms alone. Protective mechanisms, such as sleep, physical activity, relational connection, and embodied regulation practice, are often overlooked or minimized as self-care strategies rather than essential self-sustaining mechanisms to mitigate repeated trauma exposure. Wang et al. (2023) identified physical activity as a protective mechanism. Emerging evidence indicates that individuals exposed to ongoing career-related trauma demonstrate elevated dropout rates for trauma therapies compared to their civilian counterparts (Emerson, 2026). HDPs are more likely to view their lived reality of trauma exposure as part of what they signed up for. A system-level inefficiency exists in high-demand professions characterized by repeated cycles of intervention and symptom reduction, without the development of protective mechanisms. This creates revolving-door care and burnout within care systems due to greater service stabilization needs. Viewing these limitations collectively suggests that treatment for HDPs may benefit from intentional cultivation of adaptive capacity and a shift beyond episodic repair.

Reframing Resilience as a Core Competency

These limitations underscore the need for a more developmentally oriented approach to trauma care. Resilience training can fill this gap. Resilience is a dynamic process of adaptation and recovery in response to adverse experiences or challenges. It is often conflated with stoicism or the ability to bounce back quickly, reinforcing the misconception that resilience means an individual has less distress or does not need support in challenging moments. There are various definitions of resilience in the literature, which may have contributed to divergent views (Vella & Pai, 2019). Leitch and McCaw (2024) proposed a new definition of resilience:

The responsive capacity to adapt or bounce back after adverse or traumatic experiences; to anticipate and mitigate stressors; and to be generative during times of relative stability. (p. 189)

Previously held notions of resilience viewed it as a given personality or innate genetic trait. However, prevailing views position resilience as an accessible skill cultivated by intentional practice and skill-based learning (Bergeman & Nelson, 2024; Vella & Pai, 2019). It reflects the capacity to mobilize internal and external resources in response to stress. Resilience is now understood as situationally expressed, influenced by developmental history, relational supports, cultural context, and ongoing environmental demands. Connor and Davidson (2003) noted that internal and external stressors are ever-present and that an individual's ability to cope with these events is influenced by both successful and unsuccessful adaptations to previous disruptions (p. 76). Rutter (2006) suggested that ongoing exposure to risk or adversity is a key factor in resilience development. This viewpoint lends itself to therapeutic integration as resilience can be strengthened, weakened, or reshaped by accumulated experiences, including therapeutic intervention. When resilience is conceptualized as a developmental process, rather than a required trait, the opportunity opens for clinical cultivation instead of passive expectation.

The unique proactive stance of resilience cannot be equated with self-care that seeks to replenish deficits. Seshadri et al. (2025) suggested that resilience cannot be relegated to self-care homework, and Connor and Davidson (2003) implied that resilience can be a meaningful treatment target. Positioning resilience primarily as self-care inadvertently equates it to supplementary treatment rather than a learnable capacity with therapeutic importance. Resilience-named interventions are being tested in rigorous designs to learn more about how to intertwine with current approaches (Ekbäck et al., 2021). Resilience training can reduce symptoms post-intervention at three months (Seshadri et al., 2025). Purposeful expansion of internal reserves and preparation for life's challenges serve as the central mission of resilience building. Because HDPs anticipate ongoing trauma exposure as part of their career, resilience may serve as a mitigating factor for weathering these challenges. For organizations and service systems serving HDPs, resilience-integrated trauma treatment also represents a workforce sustainability strategy, supporting retention, performance stability, and ethical service delivery.

Resilience deserves equal clinical focus with trauma treatment, not as an adjunct intervention. Sinkler et al. (2023) suggested that trauma recovery is positively influenced by clients' levels of resilience. If resilience represents adaptive capacity, then developing resilience becomes a legitimate clinical aim rather than an ancillary wellness recommendation. Resilience encompasses regulation skills, physiological care, self-awareness, cognitive agility, and self-mastery. Elevating it to a clinical competency positions clinicians for building future-oriented protection and making it integral to treatment. Equipping high-demand professionals beyond repair toward preparation for re-exposure demonstrates ethical care, indicating that resilience is not merely an enhancement but a clinical responsibility.

Resilience skill-building integrated into trauma work is the next evolution of mental health approaches (Leitch & McCaw, 2024; Sonu et al., 2024), especially for high-demand professionals such as first responders (Rimon & Shelef, 2025). Leitch and McCaw (2024) stated:

This framework [resilience with trauma-informed care] includes attention to adversity and its sequelae, in addition to actively incorporating strengths, protective factors, and an expanded definition of resilience. The shift beyond the pathology-focused traditional biomedical model also aligns with the movement toward whole-person care and its emphasis on health promotion, well-being, and a lifelong capacity for growth and learning. (p. 188)

Rimon and Shelef (2025) highlighted that cultivating resilience reduces stress and burnout and lowers risk for moral injury. Emerging models increasingly centralize skills training, positioning it as a focal component of treatment rather than a separate or supplemental intervention (Karatzias et al., 2023). Resilience building to minimize future trauma exposure has empirical support regarding PTSD development (Ptak et al., 2025), providing protective durability against ongoing exposure.

Treatment providers may benefit from additional direction or training on integrating trauma treatment with resilience strategies. Several lines of evidence suggest this area remains underdeveloped. Systematic reviews of resilience-focused interventions in healthcare settings describe a heterogeneous literature in which structured, manualized models integrated with trauma treatment are relatively uncommon (Unjai et al., 2024). Cook et al. (2017) surveyed doctoral programs and reported that many graduates enter the field without structured coursework in trauma, and Sadusky et al. (2021) reported that fewer than one-third of counselor education programs explicitly mentioned trauma-related content. While doctoral programs in counselor education primarily emphasize research, teaching, and supervision rather than advanced clinical practice (Council for Accreditation of Counseling and Related Educational Programs [CACREP], 2024), the available literature suggests that trauma-specific preparation is not consistently embedded at the master's level either (Cook et al., 2017; Sadusky et al., 2021). Resilience-integrated trauma training appears even more limited across training levels.

Counselor education programs do not hold explicit standards or competencies on resilience-based skill building. For example, the 2024 CACREP Standards reference resilience under the Foundational Counseling Curriculum within the counselor identity role, in which counselors are expected to promote resilience and optimum development across the lifespan (CACREP, 2024). However, the absence of a detailed or standalone competency domain leaves room for variation in how programs operationalize resilience and designate clinical practice or skill acquisition for counselors embracing resilience strategies as a discrete clinical competency. Leitch and McCaw (2024) emphasized that healthcare professionals generally need more training on both trauma and resilience.

Intersectional and Structural Considerations

A clinical model for high-demand professionals cannot be deployed apart from the structural conditions that produce both the work and the trauma. High-demand professionals are not a homogenous category, and the lived experience of repeated occupational trauma is shaped by intersecting identities including race, gender, sexuality, class, disability, and immigration status (Crenshaw, 1991; Sonu et al., 2024). Female first responders, BIPOC clinicians and crisis workers, immigrant healthcare professionals, and queer service members may carry not only the cumulative trauma inherent to their roles but also the additional weight of workplace discrimination, tokenization, and minority stress, all of which shape help-seeking, dropout, and treatment response (Carter, 2007; Meyer, 2003). Resilience-integrated trauma care that ignores these intersections risks framing adaptive capacity as a uniform clinical target, when in practice the resources available to cultivate it are unevenly distributed by structural factors well outside the therapy room.

Equally important is the ethical complexity that some high-demand roles occupy in relation to the communities they serve. Law enforcement, detention, military, and certain healthcare and child welfare roles can be sources of trauma for the very populations they encounter, particularly communities of color, immigrant communities, and other historically marginalized groups (Alang et al., 2017; Bor et al., 2018). Trauma-informed care for HDPs must therefore hold two truths simultaneously: that occupational trauma exposure is real and warrants competent clinical response, and that resilience-building should not function simply to return workers to systems that may themselves perpetuate harm. Within the PEACE Resilience Model, this awareness invites clinicians to use psychoeducation and expanding awareness as opportunities for moral reflection rather than only symptom recognition, to ground activating healthy habits in cultural and community context rather than universal prescription, and to support resilience plans that include space for ethical questioning of professional roles when warranted. Resilience-integrated trauma treatment is most consistent with trauma-informed values when it is also informed by intersectional and structural critique. This positions providers to deliver care that is clinically rigorous, culturally responsive, and ethically accountable to the broader systems in which their clients work.

Integrating Resilience Within Phase-Oriented Trauma Treatment

Existing phase-oriented frameworks have long served as the organizing backbone of trauma treatment. Cutting across theoretical orientations, phase-oriented trauma treatment frameworks tend to converge on three primary stages: stabilization, trauma reprocessing, and reintegration (Herman, 1992, 2015). While four-phase models also exist, differences tend to take one of these three primary objectives and divide it into another phase at the beginning or end of treatment. These phases are not linear but represent a fluid process in which the client demonstrates readiness for progression. Stabilization focuses on regulation, psychoeducation, rapport-building, and creating internal safety. This phase is not completed or finished; rather, it continues as the foundation that parallels subsequent phases. The reprocessing phase is the intervention phase of trauma treatment, employing approaches such as Eye Movement Desensitization and Reprocessing (EMDR), prolonged exposure, hypnotherapy, and narrative exposure therapy, among others. The final phase, reintegration, focuses on restoring connections for the client, both internally, to parts of self, meaning, and self-narrative, and externally, with personal, professional, and community-oriented relationships. The triphasic framework provides a robust foundation for treatment but largely developed within the assumption that trauma exposure has ceased. Past trauma is addressed, while future adversity is not explicitly addressed. Phases do not consistently account for ongoing exposure.

Clinicians often introduce resilience-related content in the reintegration phase (e.g., relapse prevention, wellness planning, and maintaining self-care practices), following trauma reprocessing. There are multiple reasons resilience content may be positioned later in treatment, including an intentional sequencing decision to prioritize stabilization and symptom reduction before asking clients to engage in future-oriented skill building. However, positioning resilience exclusively at the end of treatment may also risk framing it as an adjunct to recovery rather than a mechanism of recovery. Because trauma directly compromises regulatory capacity, there may be value in introducing resilience-related skills earlier in treatment to support stabilization. Delaying resilience building until after trauma reprocessing may miss opportunities presented during stabilization. Early integration of resilience content may also have the potential to decrease therapeutic dropout, dysregulation, and avoidance, although this is presented here as a proposed outcome warranting empirical investigation rather than an established finding. Related literature suggests that strengthening regulation and engagement skills early in treatment is associated with retention and reduced avoidance in trauma-focused care (Imel et al., 2013; Najavits, 2015), offering preliminary conceptual support. Early introduction of resilience training may create a developmental process in which adaptive capacity is cultivated alongside trauma resolution.

A structured resilience model designed to operate in parallel with established triphasic trauma treatment may address this gap with several potential benefits for high-exposure trauma populations. It elevates resilience to a core clinical competency with equal attention during trauma resolution. Trauma and resilience share a clinical focus to restore psychological and physiological systems. For example, trauma disrupts regulation, self-perception, relational trust, and meaning-making, while resilience reflects the restoration and strengthening of the same systems. Resilience training moves beyond supplementary or add-on status to hold a central place in treatment planning. Additionally, an integrated or parallel approach may enhance adaptive capacity, thereby increasing potential for trauma reprocessing. Clients build skills that advance their readiness for trauma reprocessing through self-observation of physiological shifts, mobilizing regulation tools, and reorientation to agency. Early integration also organizes resilience into a sequence of teachable domains that correspond with evolving treatment needs over time. Because the triphasic model is not linear, skills can be revisited throughout the triphasic model or experientially re-encountered at later stages. Skill application is cultivated within the context of lived reality.

The PEACE Resilience Model

The PEACE Resilience Model is a practical, skills-based approach designed to mitigate ongoing trauma exposure and enhance self-mastery, originally developed for first responders and subsequently adapted for high-demand professionals (Agliata & Stewart-Spencer, 2026). The model conceptualizes resilience as a structured, teachable process with intentional cultivation. It functions as a translational framework, supporting the transfer of resilience research into sustainable clinical practice. As illustrated in Figure 1, this model is designed to integrate with phase-oriented trauma treatment frameworks rather than function as a secondary or post-treatment approach.

PEACE is an acronym for five interrelated domains: Psychoeducation on trauma, Expanding awareness, Activating healthy habits, Coping with acute stress, and Establishing a resilience plan. The five domains are best understood as the ingredients of resilience rather than as five separate stages with resilience added at the end. Each domain is itself a resilience-building practice. Psychoeducation builds resilience by reducing stigma, normalizing trauma responses, and equipping clients with the cognitive frame to recognize what they are experiencing. Expanding awareness builds resilience by training the metacognitive and interoceptive capacities that allow regulation to occur. Activating healthy habits builds resilience by cultivating the physiological, relational, and motivational conditions on which adaptive capacity depends. Coping with acute stress builds resilience by rehearsing applied regulation under realistic future-exposure conditions. Establishing a resilience plan builds resilience by consolidating these capacities into a personalized, evolving practice that the client owns. Resilience is therefore present from the first domain forward; the final domain does not introduce resilience but personalizes and sustains it. In this sense, the PEACE Resilience Model does not house resilience under a single stage of treatment but distributes it across every interaction.

Conceptualizing the domains as ingredients of resilience also clarifies how the model integrates with the triphasic frame. Resilience-building is not delayed until reintegration; it is woven into stabilization, into reprocessing readiness, and into reintegration alike. Resilience functions as a practical scaffold for embedding adaptive capacity across the triphasic model of trauma care, couched in the therapeutic process.

Figure 1. Integration of the PEACE resilience model across triphasic trauma treatment

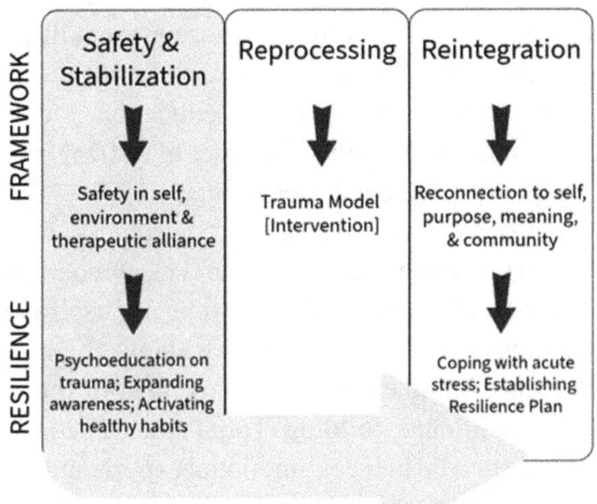

[Figure 1 depicts resilience development as a continuous horizontal through-line across all five PEACE domains and all three triphasic phases (stabilization, trauma reprocessing, reintegration). Each domain intersects with one or more phases, but resilience is shown as active from the first session rather than introduced only at the final domain.]

Operationalizing Resilience Across Five Domains

The first domain of the PEACE Resilience Model centers on psychoeducation on trauma. In the PEACE framework, psychoeducation is itself a resilience-building practice rather than an introductory preface to resilience work. Psychoeducation is a core component of treating trauma-exposed populations (Lanza et al., 2018; Rubinstein et al., 2025) and is often included in resilience workshops, interventions, and resiliency models (Unjai et al., 2024). A variety of topics for psychoeducation are noted in the literature, such as resilience enhancement (Babanataj et al., 2019; Henshall et al., 2020) and emotional intelligence (Mao et al., 2021). Psychoeducation is also considered an active ingredient in trauma work for stabilization (Dubi et al., 2017). In the PEACE Resilience Model, psychoeducation builds knowledge about types of trauma, mechanisms, and characteristics to reduce stigma. From the first session, clients are also introduced to resilience itself, its definition, its evidence base as a learnable capacity, and its role across the full course of treatment, so that the resilience frame is established before any subsequent skill is taught. Reducing self-blame reframes trauma responses as normative reactions to abnormal stress, enhancing cognitive reappraisal. While psychoeducation is commonly delivered through workshops or didactic learning (Unjai et al., 2024), embedding it into a therapeutic space offers individualized processing.

The second domain of PEACE is expanding awareness, which increases self-observation and monitoring of the stress response (i.e., sympathetic nervous system response). Like psychoeducation, expanding awareness is itself a resilience capacity: the metacognitive and interoceptive sensitivity that allows clients to detect activation early enough to intervene. Regulation and management of the stress response are frequently addressed in resilience building (Unjai et al., 2024). This domain illustrates how physiological state influences emotional experience, cognitive appraisal, and behavioral reactivity (Langer et al., 2025). Expanding awareness around the autonomic nervous system enables early detection of dysregulation and fosters intentional engagement with regulation. Avoidance, emotional numbing, isolation, and distraction are commonly reported coping strategies in high-demand professionals, such as first responders (Dautovich et al., 2023). Expanding capacity for detecting stress response activation invites opportunities for intentional intervention. This domain, aligning with stabilization (Herman, 1992, 2015), cultivates confidence in containing stress responses while building readiness for internal safety for trauma reprocessing.

The third and most expansive domain of the PEACE Resilience Model focuses on activating healthy habits through intentional practice of foundational health. Activating healthy habits is the most concrete expression of resilience as a daily, embodied practice; the cumulative effect of these habits is itself the buildup of resilience capacity

(Agliata & Stewart-Spencer, 2026). Trauma disrupts core aspects of physiological and relational systems of health, such as sleep, autonomic balance, and relational engagement (Porges, 2022). This domain addresses systemic vulnerabilities and deepens stabilization to elicit greater recovery ownership. This domain is conceptually grounded in Maslow's (1943, 1954) hierarchy of needs, emphasizing physiological stability, safety, relational connection, self-esteem or agency, and self-actualization. This humanistic perspective aligns with third-wave resilience research that views adverse experiences as internal motivational fuel toward self-actualization (Vella & Pai, 2019). It may also serve as an operationalized approach to building reserve capacity, which Bergeman and Nelson (2024) described as reserve capabilities that individuals can draw upon to effectively respond to adversity.

Reframing basic human needs as resilience building blocks, rather than lifestyle recommendations, centralizes the client's role in restoring and expanding capacity for adaptation through adversity. Constructing resilience on physiological health, consistent with the foundation of Maslow's (1943, 1954) hierarchy, creates a compassionate developmental lens for clients. For example, without proper sleep or nutrition, expectations for performance in higher-level skills may need to be adjusted, such as self-appraisal or cognitive agility. Limitations in higher-level skills are reframed as unmet needs rather than lack of motivation or resistance. Recalibrated expectations also foster realistic, context-specific routines for high-demand professionals to maintain or reimplement during times of occupational stress or trauma exposure. Resilience skills that are intentionally practiced increase the protective nature of resilience (Vella & Pai, 2019). These skills are practiced within the therapeutic relationship, giving clients the opportunity to evaluate and adapt their approach, addressing what Connor and Davidson (2003) described as a pathway to successful coping. This progression fosters confidence and reinforces self-efficacy. Clients observe tangible evidence of their capacity to influence internal states, which aids readiness for trauma reprocessing or transition to reintegration. The client's role in resilience skill building during the third domain becomes a sustainable and transferable practice for future stress contexts.

The fourth domain of the PEACE Resilience Model is coping with acute stress. This domain is a resilience-building practice in its own right, in that it rehearses the applied use of regulation skills under the realistic anticipation of future exposure. This domain embraces realistic expectations that trauma exposure will occur again and that clients have a prepared plan to manage future crises. Approximately 70% of the general population worldwide will experience at least one lifetime traumatic event (Kessler et al., 2017), while first responders may encounter 400 to 600 traumatic events over the course of their careers (Avon and Somerset Police Federation, 2021). Traditional trauma treatment addresses reactions to acute stress retroactively. This domain emphasizes proactive response through regulation and grounding techniques as well as structured recovery rituals. This domain reiterates psychoeducation learned earlier by reminding clients of emotional and physiological manifestations of trauma. Critical incidents create high-stakes environments where impaired judgment opens potential consequences impacting professional, personal, or relational livelihoods (Arnsten, 2015). Creating metacognitive awareness of distress markers empowers clients in early intervention, potentially limiting consequences during or after critical incidents. This domain aims to restore normalcy through empowered preparation and client agency.

The fifth domain of the PEACE Resilience Model focuses on establishing a resilience plan. This domain does not introduce resilience for the first time; rather, it consolidates the resilience capacities that have been built across the preceding four domains into a personalized, sustainable practice. Clients consolidate their therapeutic gains, evaluate adaptations, and translate skills into real-world practice. Protocols for PTSD suggest that trauma recovery benefits from strategies that reinforce gains, explicitly address prevention, and consider long-term maintenance planning (Rubinstein et al., 2025). Treatment termination becomes more than symptom-reduction. Clients have authorship over resilience with explicit framing of its dynamic and evolving nature. Resilience is not static (Bergeman & Nelson, 2024). Plans to maintain it must shift across developmental stages, occupational transitions, health changes, and broader life circumstances. Recalibration in the face of change or growth elicits ownership over the process. Nestled within reintegration in the trauma treatment phase, the fifth domain of PEACE supports reconnection to a restored sense of self and a reconnected sense of purpose through reclaimed autonomy (Condon et al., 2023).

Implementation and Future Directions

Implementation of the PEACE Resilience Model requires attention to clinician training, organizational support, and contextual adaptation. Because formal curricula dedicate minimal resources to integrating resilience skill building (CACREP, 2024; Cook et al., 2017; Sadusky et al., 2021), providers may benefit from supervision and guidance in how to practically deploy these strategies. Providers benefit from structured supervision and ongoing professional development to maintain fidelity to resilience-integrated practices. Organizational leadership plays a critical role in allocating time, resources, and policy support to further integration. Advocating for resilience models at a systemic level may further enhance cultural relevance within counselor education programs.

Trauma treatment has made substantial advances in symptom-reduction and supporting recovery from adverse experiences. However, for populations encountering ongoing trauma exposure, current approaches may remain insufficient. High-demand professionals, such as first responders and emergency healthcare providers, may benefit from treatments that go beyond episodic stabilization. Enhancing adaptive capabilities through integrated resilience skill training in triphasic treatment frameworks creates a pathway for sustained psychological durability. Resilience skill-building, established as a core clinical competency, positions providers to empower clients with teachable, dynamic, adaptive capacities. The PEACE Resilience Model operationalizes this integration by treating each of its five domains as an ingredient of resilience, so that resilience is built across the full arc of trauma care rather than added as a supplementary or post-process intervention. The PEACE Resilience Model is designed to offer seamless entry into phase-oriented trauma treatment. There is value in resilience-integrated trauma treatments with long-term adaptation over professional careers. Continued research, training, and model refinement are needed, including empirical evaluation of the proposed benefits of early resilience integration on client engagement, dropout, and outcomes. Future work also needs to examine how the model functions across intersecting identities and within structurally complex occupational systems, ensuring that resilience-integrated care strengthens individual adaptive capacity without becoming a tool that returns workers to harmful systems unchanged. Incorporating resilience into trauma treatment does not diminish healing past wounds; rather, it equips individuals not only to survive adversity but to engage in meaningful self-protection to fulfill the vocations to which they are called.

REFERENCES

Agliata, A. K., & Stewart-Spencer, S. (2026). *Mastering resilience: Strategies for high-demand professionals*. C3: Connect. Communicate. Collaborate. https://a.co/d/03xpmiAU

Alang, S., McAlpine, D., McCreedy, E., & Hardeman, R. (2017). Police brutality and Black health: Setting the agenda for public health scholars. *American Journal of Public Health, 107*(5), 662–665. DOI: 10.2105/AJPH.2017.303691 PMID: 28323470

Arnsten, A. F. T. (2015). Stress weakens prefrontal networks: Molecular insults to higher cognition. *Nature Neuroscience, 18*(10), 1376–1385. DOI: 10.1038/nn.4087 PMID: 26404712

Avon and Somerset Police Federation. (2021, September 15). *Capture data on traumatic incidents*. Police Federation of England and Wales. https://www.polfed.org/avonsom/news/news-articles/capture-data-on-traumatic-incidents/

Babanataj, R., Mazdarani, S., Hesamzadeh, A., Gorji, M. H., & Cherati, J. Y. (2019). Resilience training: Effects on occupational stress and resilience of critical care nurses. *International Journal of Nursing Practice, 25*(1), e12697. Advance online publication. DOI: 10.1111/ijn.12697 PMID: 30338603

Bergeman, C. S., & Nelson, N. A. (2024). Building a dynamic adaptational process theory of resilience (ADAPTOR): Stress exposure, reserve capacity, adaptation, and consequence. *The American Psychologist, 79*(8), 1063–1075. DOI: 10.1037/amp0001280 PMID: 39531707

Billings, J., & Nicholls, H. (2025). PTSD and complex PTSD, current treatments and debates: A review of reviews. *British Medical Bulletin, 156*(1), ldaf015. Advance online publication. DOI: 10.1093/bmb/ldaf015 PMID: 41004137

Bor, J., Venkataramani, A. S., Williams, D. R., & Tsai, A. C. (2018). Police killings and their spillover effects on the mental health of Black Americans: A population-based, quasi-experimental study. *Lancet, 392*(10144), 302–310. DOI: 10.1016/S0140-6736(18)31130-9 PMID: 29937193

Carter, R. T. (2007). Racism and psychological and emotional injury: Recognizing and assessing race-based traumatic stress. *The Counseling Psychologist, 35*(1), 13–105. DOI: 10.1177/0011000006292033

Condon, M., Bloomfield, M. A. P., Nicholls, H., & Billings, J. (2023). Expert international trauma clinicians' views on the definition, composition and delivery of reintegration interventions for complex PTSD. *European Journal of Psychotraumatology*, *14*(1), 2165024. Advance online publication. DOI: 10.1080/20008066.2023.2165024 PMID: 37052098

Connor, K. M., & Davidson, J. R. T. (2003). Development of a new resilience scale: The Connor-Davidson Resilience Scale (CD-RISC). *Depression and Anxiety*, *18*(2), 76–82. DOI: 10.1002/da.10113 PMID: 12964174

Cook, J. M., Simiola, V., Ellis, A. E., & Thompson, R. (2017). Training in trauma psychology: A national survey of doctoral graduate programs. *Training and Education in Professional Psychology*, *11*(2), 108–114. DOI: 10.1037/tep0000150

Council for Accreditation of Counseling and Related Educational Programs. (2024). *2024 CACREP standards*. https://www.cacrep.org/for-programs/2024-cacrep-standards/

Crenshaw, K. (1991). Mapping the margins: Intersectionality, identity politics, and violence against women of color. *Stanford Law Review*, *43*(6), 1241–1299. DOI: 10.2307/1229039

Dautovich, N. D., Katjijova, M., Cyrus, J. W., & Kliewer, W. (2023). Duty-related stressors, adjustment, and the role of coping processes in first responders: A systematic review. *Psychological Trauma: Theory, Research, Practice, and Policy*, *15*(Suppl. 2), S286–S296. DOI: 10.1037/tra0001258 PMID: 35653742

Dubi, M., Powell, P. W., & Gentry, E. (2017). *Trauma, PTSD, grief & loss: The 10 core competencies for evidence-based treatment*. PESI Publishing & Media.

Ekbäck, E., Granåsen, G., Svärling, R., Blomqvist, I., & Henje, E. (2021). Clinical effectiveness of training for awareness resilience and action online compared to standard treatment for adolescents and young adults with depression: Study protocol and analysis plan for a pragmatic, multi-center randomized controlled superiority trial. *Frontiers in Psychiatry*, *12*, 674583. Advance online publication. DOI: 10.3389/fpsyt.2021.674583 PMID: 34707516

Emerson, L. (2026, January 15). *Servicemembers, veterans are quitting psychotherapy treatment for post-traumatic stress disorder*. U.S. Medicine. https://www.usmedicine.com/clinical-topics/ptsd/servicemembers-veterans-are-quitting-psychotherapy-treatment-for-post-traumatic-stress-disorder/

Henshall, C., Davey, Z., & Jackson, D. (2020). The implementation and evaluation of a resilience enhancement programme for nurses working in the forensic setting. *International Journal of Mental Health Nursing*, *29*(3), 508–520. DOI: 10.1111/inm.12689 PMID: 31930654

Herman, J. L. (1992). *Trauma and recovery: The aftermath of violence—From domestic abuse to political terror*. Basic Books.

Herman, J. L. (2015). *Trauma and recovery: The aftermath of violence—From domestic abuse to political terror* (2nd ed.). Basic Books.

Imel, Z. E., Laska, K., Jakupcak, M., & Simpson, T. L. (2013). Meta-analysis of dropout in treatments for posttraumatic stress disorder. *Journal of Consulting and Clinical Psychology*, *81*(3), 394–404. DOI: 10.1037/a0031474 PMID: 23339535

Kalisch, R., Müller, M. B., & Tüscher, O. (2015). A conceptual framework for the neurobiological study of resilience. *Behavioral and Brain Sciences*, *38*, e92. Advance online publication. DOI: 10.1017/S0140525X1400082X PMID: 25158686

Karatzias, T., McGlanaghy, E., & Cloitre, M. (2023). Enhanced Skills Training in Affective and Interpersonal Regulation (ESTAIR): A new modular treatment for International Classification of Diseases, 11th revision, complex posttraumatic stress disorder (CPTSD). *Brain Sciences*, *13*(9), 1300. Advance online publication. DOI: 10.3390/brainsci13091300 PMID: 37759901

Kessler, R. C., Aguilar-Gaxiola, S., Alonso, J., Benjet, C., Bromet, E. J., Cardoso, G., Degenhardt, L., de Girolamo, G., Dinolova, R. V., Ferry, F., Florescu, S., Gureje, O., Haro, J. M., Huang, Y., Karam, E. G., Kawakami, N., Lee, S., Lepine, J. P., Levinson, D., & Koenen, K. C. (2017). Trauma and PTSD in the WHO World Mental Health Surveys. *European Journal of Psychotraumatology*, *8*(sup5, Suppl. 5), 1353383. Advance online publication. DOI: 10.1080/20008198.2017.1353383 PMID: 29075426

Langer, K., Wolf, O. T., Merz, C. J., & Jentsch, V. L. (2025). The effects of stress hormones on cognitive emotion regulation: A systematic review and integrative model. *Neuroscience and Biobehavioral Reviews*, *170*, 106040. Advance online publication. DOI: 10.1016/j.neubiorev.2025.106040 PMID: 39909150

Lanza, A., Roysircar, G., & Rodgers, S. (2018). First responder mental healthcare: Evidence-based prevention, postvention, and treatment. *Professional Psychology, Research and Practice*, *49*(3), 193–204. DOI: 10.1037/pro0000192

Leitch, L., & McCaw, B. (2024). Time to move forward: Resilience and trauma-informed care. *The Permanente Journal*, *28*(1), 188–192. DOI: 10.7812/TPP/23.076 PMID: 37862407

Mao, L., Huang, L., & Chen, Q. (2021). Promoting resilience and lower stress in nurses and improving inpatient experience through emotional intelligence training in China: A randomized controlled trial. *Nurse Education Today*, *107*, 105130. Advance online publication. DOI: 10.1016/j.nedt.2021.105130 PMID: 34543939

Maslow, A. H. (1943). A theory of human motivation. *Psychological Review*, *50*(4), 370–396. DOI: 10.1037/h0054346

Maslow, A. H. (1954). *Motivation and personality*. Harper & Row.

McEwen, B. S., & Akil, H. (2020). Revisiting the stress concept: Implications for affective disorders. *The Journal of Neuroscience : The Official Journal of the Society for Neuroscience*, *40*(1), 12–21. DOI: 10.1523/JNEUROSCI.0733-19.2019 PMID: 31896560

Meyer, I. H. (2003). Prejudice, social stress, and mental health in lesbian, gay, and bisexual populations: Conceptual issues and research evidence. *Psychological Bulletin*, *129*(5), 674–697. DOI: 10.1037/0033-2909.129.5.674 PMID: 12956539

Najavits, L. M. (2015). The problem of dropout from "gold standard" PTSD therapies. *F1000prime Reports*, *7*, 43. Advance online publication. DOI: 10.12703/P7-43 PMID: 26097716

Porges, S. W. (2022). Polyvagal theory: A science of safety. *Frontiers in Integrative Neuroscience*, *16*, 871227. Advance online publication. DOI: 10.3389/fnint.2022.871227 PMID: 35645742

Ptak, M. K., Smith, D., Pridgen, S., & Held, P. (2025). Pre-treatment resilience as a predictor of veterans' post-traumatic stress disorder symptom outcomes immediately and up to 12-months following intensive cognitive processing therapy. *Journal of Clinical Psychology*, *81*(12), 1213–1220. DOI: 10.1002/jclp.70029 PMID: 41074762

Rimon, A., & Shelef, L. (2025). Moral injury among medical personnel and first responders across different healthcare and emergency response settings: A narrative review. *International Journal of Environmental Research and Public Health*, *22*(7), 1055. Advance online publication. DOI: 10.3390/ijerph22071055 PMID: 40724122

Rubinstein, D., Abargil, M., Duek, O., & Harpaz-Rotem, I. (2025). RESET post-traumatic stress disorder: Clinical protocol integrating reconsolidation, exposure, and short-term emotional transformation. *European Journal of Psychotraumatology*, *16*(1), 2540141. Advance online publication. DOI: 10.1080/20008066.2025.2540141 PMID: 40815290

Rutter, M. (2006). Implications of resilience concepts for scientific understanding. *Annals of the New York Academy of Sciences*, *1094*(1), 1–12. DOI: 10.1196/annals.1376.002 PMID: 17347337

Sadusky, A., Berger, E. P., & Toporkova, L. (2021). Examination of trauma training for postgraduate psychology students. *Clinical Psychologist*, *25*(3), 306–315. DOI: 10.1080/13284207.2021.1913047

Seshadri, A., Fuller-Tyszkiewicz, M., Harper, L., Clark, M. M., Singh, B., Chesak, S., Kung, S., Bobo, W. V., & Wieneke, K. (2025). Randomized controlled trial of stress management and resiliency training for depression (SMART-D)—Pilot study. *PLoS One*, *20*(8), e0328539. Advance online publication. DOI: 10.1371/journal.pone.0328539 PMID: 40828809

Sinkler, M. A., Alejo, A., Agel, J., Hendrickson, S., Breslin, M. A., & Vallier, H. A. (2023). The development of a Trauma Resiliency Scale (tRS-18). *Journal of Orthopaedic Research*, *41*(9), 2040–2045. DOI: 10.1002/jor.25550 PMID: 36919222

Sonu, S., Mann, K., Potter, J., Rush, P., & Stillerman, A. (2024). Toward integration of trauma, resilience, and equity theory and practice: A narrative review and call for consilience. *The Permanente Journal*, *28*(1), 151–168. DOI: 10.7812/TPP/23.105 PMID: 38206776

Unjai, S., Forster, E. M., Mitchell, A. E., & Creedy, D. K. (2024). Interventions to promote resilience and passion for work in health settings: A mixed-methods systematic review. *International Journal of Nursing Studies Advances*, *7*, 100242. Advance online publication. DOI: 10.1016/j.ijnsa.2024.100242 PMID: 39380624

Vella, S. C., & Pai, N. B. (2019). A theoretical review of psychological resilience: Defining resilience and resilience research over the decades. *Archives of Medicine and Health Sciences*, *7*(2), 233–239. DOI: 10.4103/amhs.amhs_119_19

Wang, Y., Ashokan, A., & Mitra, R. (2023). Physical exercise as a resilience factor in depression and anxiety: A systematic review and meta-analysis. *Neuroscience and Biobehavioral Reviews*, *146*, 105071. Advance online publication. DOI: 10.1016/j.neubiorev.2023.105071

Chapter 7
Narrative Ownership, Storytelling, and the Politics of Voice

Wednesdae Reim Ifrach
http://orcid.org/0000-0002-3567-6778
Moravian University, USA

ABSTRACT

This chapter examines storytelling in trauma contexts as a political practice shaped by power, history, and social location rather than an inherently therapeutic act. Challenging dominant assumptions that healing requires disclosure, it shows how compelled or premature storytelling can reproduce harm, particularly for marginalized survivors. Drawing on trauma studies, decolonial theory, and epistemic justice, the chapter introduces narrative sovereignty as an ethical framework that affirms survivors' rights to author, withhold, revise, or reclaim their stories on their own terms, including through silence, art, ritual, or collective action. It distinguishes between internal trauma integration and external narration, emphasizing consent, autonomy, and harm reduction as core principles of ethical story work. Beyond individual therapy, the chapter centers collective storytelling practices such as art activism, zines, and community archives- as sites of resistance and healing that situate trauma within structural and historical contexts.

INTRODUCTION: STORY AS POWER, STORY AS SURVIVAL

Storytelling is a fundamental human practice that shapes how individuals make meaning of experience, including trauma. Long before writing, people shared stories to pass down history and imagine futures (Asakura et al., 2023; Mattingly,

DOI: 10.4018/979-8-3373-8597-6.ch007

1998). Through stories, communities transmit wisdom, negotiate norms, and ground themselves in a sense of belonging. Narratives weave together emotion, memory, and meaning, shaping how individuals understand themselves and each other. In this context, "narrative" refers to the ways individuals organize and interpret their experiences through story, whether spoken, written, embodied, or symbolic. In the aftermath of violence or catastrophe, telling one's story can help survivors find coherence in chaos and have their suffering acknowledged. The urge to speak is often tied to the need for recognition of pain, yet storytelling always unfolds within cultural and power structures that influence survivor agency and narrative control.

In the discourse of trauma recovery, storytelling is often hailed as inherently healing. Research indicates that narrating trauma can integrate memories and reduce distress (Brison, 1999; Herman, 1992), and many survivors do find relief when sharing their narrative in supportive contexts. However, disclosure is not universally beneficial. For some, retelling a traumatic event triggers re-experiencing rather than relief (Herman, 2015; Perry & Szalavitz, 2017). Others may stay silent because sharing feels unsafe; their stories could be misunderstood, exploited, or even weaponized against them. Marginalized survivors face even greater risks: their accounts often clash with dominant cultural narratives or are dismissed as not credible (Fricker, 2007; Rosen, 2021). Recognizing survivors as experts of their own experiences fosters respect and affirms that choosing to speak or remain silent is both a personal and political act. This chapter frames trauma narratives and storytelling as a site of power, politics, and possibility. Stories of harm are not simply personal expressions; they are embedded within broader histories of colonialism, racism, sexism, and ableism (Farmer, 2004; Spivak, 1988). These power dynamics determine which narratives are allowed to be heard, whose voices resonate, and whose are suppressed. Trauma-informed care committed to social justice must therefore uphold narrative sovereignty. Narrative sovereignty refers to the right of individuals and communities to control how their stories are created, shared, interpreted, and circulated. This entails recognizing survivors' right to author, withhold, revise, or reclaim their stories on their own terms. This perspective also challenges the assumption that healing always requires verbal disclosure. Self-determination means acknowledging that silence, art, ritual, and collective action are equally valid ways of making meaning from pain, fostering trust and cultural respect in the process.

This chapter proceeds in four parts. First, it examines how power shapes who can speak and be heard. Second, it explores the harms of narrative exploitation, erasure, and weaponization. Third, it introduces narrative sovereignty as an ethical framework for trauma-informed practice. Finally, it considers how collective storytelling functions as a site of resistance and healing within marginalized communities.

Storytelling has long been a survival strategy for communities facing oppression. Enslaved people preserved culture through songs and folktales; Indigenous nations passed down oral histories that teach cosmology and values; queer elders shared coming-out stories and queer history to guide younger generations. In each case, stories function as anchors that hold communities together when other structures fail them. Survival narratives, however, are vulnerable to co-optation. When dominant institutions, researchers, or media appropriate these stories, the storytelling that once sustained the community can become a spectacle (McKenzie-Mohr & Lafrance, 2014; Smith, 2021; Spivak, 1988). A trauma-informed framework must therefore be critical of how stories are solicited, edited, and consumed. It must critically examine who benefits when a story is told and who profits from the circulation of trauma, fostering awareness of potential harm and encouraging ethical practices.

The core argument of this chapter is that trauma-informed care must move beyond the simplistic exhortation to "share your story" and toward protecting narrative self-determination. Healing does not flow automatically from disclosure. It emerges when people reclaim the authority to name their experiences and define their meanings (Asakura et al., 2023; Elliott et al., 2005; Perry & Winfrey, 2021). Clinicians, researchers, and advocates can support this by creating safe spaces, respecting pacing, and honoring individual choices to speak or remain silent. Recognizing these possibilities requires relinquishing control over the narratives they hope to elicit and being attentive to how professional practices might perpetuate narrative oppression. This chapter traces the politics of voice across history and institutions, illuminates harms associated with narrative exploitation, outlines principles of narrative sovereignty, and offers guidance for ethical story work in clinical and community settings. Throughout the chapter, survivors, particularly those from marginalized communities, are centered as experts of their own experiences. The goal is to foster conditions in which their stories, silences, and alternative expressions are respected.

WHO GETS TO TELL THE STORY?

This section examines how structural power determines whose stories are recognized as credible and whose are dismissed or silenced. Historically, structural power has dictated whose stories are heard and whose are silenced. Colonial authorities collected Indigenous and enslaved people's narratives but filtered them through their own interpretations to justify the empire. Later, medical and legal institutions often pathologized or dismissed the testimonies of women, queer people, and people of color. Survivors from marginalized groups still confront a "credibility discount" in courts and public discourse; trauma that deviates from expected norms is too often disbelieved or sanitized. Reclaiming narrative voice means recognizing survivors and communities as the experts of their own experiences and challenging the hierarchies that deem only certain voices credible. It requires creating space for trauma narratives in whatever form they emerge, whether through words, art, or silence, without imposing outside interpretations.

EXPLOITED, ERASED, WEAPONIZED: NARRATIVE HARM IN TRAUMA CONTEXTS

This section outlines the primary forms of narrative harm that emerge when trauma stories are controlled or used by institutions. Historical patterns underscore how those in power have exploited trauma narratives. For example, 19th-century "salvage anthropology" saw Western researchers collect Indigenous stories under the pretense of preservation, while ignoring their own role in colonial violence. Contemporary calls for survivors to "share your story" can unwittingly replicate this dynamic by placing the onus on the oppressed to explain their suffering rather than on oppressors to change harmful systems.

Modern social movements demonstrate that increased narrative visibility can both empower survivors and reproduce existing inequalities. The #MeToo movement, for instance, empowered many survivors to break long-held silences. However, public attention often centered on celebrities and familiar villains, sidelining women of color, trans and undocumented survivors, and even commodifying survivors' stories for profit. Similarly, humanitarian campaigns may feature refugees' trauma narratives to evoke pity while reinforcing "savior" tropes that position Western audiences as rescuers.

Narrative exploitation occurs when institutions solicit trauma narratives for their own agendas rather than the storyteller's well-being. In research, for example, survivors may be asked to recount painful experiences as data, only to see interviews archived and papers published with little benefit to those who shared their experiences. In therapy, some approaches implicitly require detailed trauma disclosure as a condition of healing. However, forcing survivors to tell their story before they feel ready can be re-traumatizing, echoing the loss of control at the heart of trauma. Trauma-informed practice recognizes that not everyone benefits from narrating their trauma on the same timeline; survivors must be free to decide if, when, and how much to share.

Narrative erasure is another harm. Institutions often minimize or hide stories that expose wrongdoing or threaten their image. Whistleblowers and survivors who speak out about abuse by influential figures frequently find their accounts discredited or buried. Some are even legally silenced through non-disclosure agreements or pressured to stay quiet "for the good of the community." By erasing inconvenient stories, institutions maintain the status quo and signal that their reputation matters more than survivors' pain.

Weaponization refers to using a survivor's story against them. In legal contexts, survivors' narratives are often twisted to discredit or punish them. Asylum seekers, for example, may be denied protection because typical trauma symptoms, fragmented memories, or visible distress are misread as lies. Domestic violence survivors can find their trauma responses, such as anger or anxiety, used against them in custody disputes, casting them as "unstable" rather than focusing on the abuser's actions. In child welfare cases, parents who disclose past struggles while seeking help risk having those admissions turned against them as evidence of unfitness. In these ways, stories shared in good faith can boomerang into tools of judgment and control (Espiritu Gandhi & Nguyen, 2023). This underscores that storytelling is not inherently safe; without protective conditions, it can reproduce harm.

Our broader culture often commodifies trauma narratives in depoliticizing ways. Media and entertainment frequently package individual stories of suffering as sensational content, focusing on personal tragedies while obscuring systemic causes. This constant consumption of decontextualized trauma can numb the public and reinforce the idea that violence is an individual misfortune rather than a product of structural inequities. To resist this pattern, there must be a shift from passively consuming trauma stories to actively witnessing them as calls to action and solidarity.

NARRATIVE SOVEREIGNTY: CONSENT, AUTONOMY, AND SELF-DETERMINED STORYTELLING

This section introduces narrative sovereignty as a guiding ethical principle and explores how to operationalize it in practice. At the heart of ethical storytelling lies narrative sovereignty, the principle that individuals and communities have the power to control their own stories, deciding if and how those stories are told, to whom, and for what purposes. Stories are more than information; they are part of one's identity and culture. When a story is taken without consent, misrepresented, or shared out of context, it violates not only personal boundaries but also communal integrity. Misappropriating a narrative can wound a community's psyche as profoundly as a physical injury.

Practicing narrative sovereignty starts with reframing how stories are invited. Too often, survivors feel expected to disclose trauma to get help or be believed. This expectation can replicate coercion by implying that remaining silent will result in negative consequences. Instead, storytelling should be a voluntary invitation, never a requirement. No survivor should be penalized for declining to share. Practitioners and researchers must make it clear that speaking out is optional and that silence will be respected. Moreover, when someone does choose to tell their story, they deserve transparency and control at every step. Survivors should know why they are being asked to share, how their narrative will be used, who will hear it, and how long it will circulate. Consent in narrative work is an ongoing process, not a one-time form; it must be specific, revisited over time, and non-coerced.

Narrative sovereignty also recognizes that processing trauma and narrating trauma are not the same. A survivor can work through pain emotionally, physically, and spiritually without ever constructing a public story about it. Many healing practices, such as somatic therapy, mindfulness, ritual, art, and community ceremony, allow people to process trauma internally or within a trusted group without turning it into a verbal account for others. Sharing one's story with an outside audience is a separate step: it involves translating private experiences into a form that others can receive. Some survivors may ultimately find it empowering to do so, but others may not, and both choices are valid. Recognizing this distinction helps practitioners support healing without automatically pushing for storytelling. It also respects cultural differences: in some communities, trauma is handled through collective rituals, song, or purposeful silence rather than individual talk. Honoring narrative sovereignty means accepting that there is no single "right" way to heal; telling a public trauma narrative is one path, not the only path.

Supporting narrative self-determination in practice means helping survivors make informed choices about if and how to share. Survivors can reflect on several considerations when deciding whether to tell their stories: Which parts of their experience they want to share, and which they prefer to keep private, when they feel ready to talk about it, with whom they feel safe sharing (only in confidence, or in a larger forum), why they want to tell it (for personal catharsis, to educate others, to seek justice), and in what form they wish to express their story.

By reflecting on these factors (ideally with a supportive advocate or therapist), survivors retain agency over their narratives. This process can prevent unintended harms, such as sharing too much, too soon, or in an unsafe setting, by ensuring that any storytelling aligns with the survivor's readiness and goals.

Narrative sovereignty operates not only at the individual level but also at the collective level. Communities have shared narratives, origin myths, migration histories, and collective traumas that are part of their cultural heritage and should not be appropriated or commodified without communal consent. Indigenous data sovereignty movements, for example, assert community control over how information about Indigenous peoples is stored and used, providing a model for collective narrative stewardship. Similarly, community-led archives and cultural centers allow communities to curate their own histories and decide how and when to share them with outsiders. Honoring collective narrative sovereignty challenges Western notions of individual authorship and instead respects communal ownership of stories and communal decision-making about their use.

Affirming narrative sovereignty does not mean hiding the truth or avoiding complex stories; it means those truths should be told by those who lived them, on their own terms. There is a crucial difference between silencing a survivor and respecting a survivor's choice not to share with a particular audience or at a specific time. Sometimes survivors choose public storytelling as an act of witness to demand change; other times, they decide that keeping their story within a trusted circle, or only within themselves, is the safer and more healing option. Allies and professionals must relinquish any sense of entitlement to someone else's story. They should carefully consider whether the urge to encourage a survivor to "share" truly serves that survivor, or instead repeats an extractive pattern that benefits the listener or the institution. Situating narrative sovereignty within broader movements for decolonization and self-determination highlights that storytelling is deeply political, tied to struggles for land, resources, and cultural survival as much as to individual healing.

In clinical and community practice, embracing narrative sovereignty means shifting from clinician-led interpretation to collaborative meaning-making. Instead of viewing the professional as the expert who analyzes a client's story, ethical story work treats the survivor as the expert of their own life. For example, narrative therapy approaches people as the authors of their stories and helps them "re-author" the meaning of their experiences (Mohatt et al., 2014). A survivor might separate themselves from a problem-saturated trauma narrative and identify themes of strength or resilience that had been overshadowed. This process counteracts epistemic injustice by validating the survivor's perspective as essential to understanding their trauma and recovery.

Ethical story work also means continually negotiating consent and boundaries in therapeutic settings. A client's comfort with sharing can change over time, so practitioners should regularly check in about what feels safe to discuss and what feels off-limits. Consent initially given to discuss a specific event should not be assumed to cover all future sessions or broader uses, such as case presentations or research. Practitioners must remain mindful of how they document and handle stories. For instance, clinical notes should be written with the assumption that the client might read them, using respectful and context-rich language rather than stigmatizing labels. Whenever possible, inviting clients to review or even co-write notes can foster transparency and shared ownership of their narrative.

Avoiding narrative colonization is another key principle. Professionals must be careful not to impose their own interpretations or cultural biases onto a survivor's story. Instead of assuming what an experience means, the practitioner should ask the survivor for their interpretation of that experience. It is important to acknowledge that healing and storytelling can take many forms. If a survivor is more comfortable expressing themselves through poetry, art, or even through pauses and silence, that choice should be honored. No one form of storytelling should be privileged as more "real" or "intelligent" than another. Validating nonverbal and creative expression reduces the risk of re-traumatization that can occur when survivors are forced into a narrow mode of disclosure that does not fit them.

In fact, incorporating cultural traditions and creative modalities can greatly enrich trauma work. Expressive arts therapies allow survivors to externalize feelings that might be impossible to articulate verbally. Painting, music, dance, or drama can engage the senses and create a safe distance from overwhelming memories. Movement-based practices (like dance or yoga) help survivors reconnect with their bodies and regain a sense of agency and pleasure in bodily experience, countering trauma's tendency to make the body feel like an unsafe place. Likewise, community rituals, such as healing circles drawing on Indigenous traditions, provide nonhierarchical spaces for collective storytelling and listening, reinforcing social bonds and shared resilience. These approaches serve as a reminder that storytelling is not always about a literal spoken narrative; it can also be embedded in actions, gestures, and collective experiences.

Harm-reduction principles also inform ethical story work. A harm-reduction lens meets survivors where they are, without judgment, and focuses on safety and choice. For instance, if a survivor is using a risky coping strategy to deal with trauma symptoms, a harm-reduction approach would not begin by demanding abstinence or complete disclosure of the trauma. Instead, it might involve acknowledging that the survivor's existing coping strategies are adaptive under the circumstances. The practitioner and survivor can then collaboratively explore safer alternatives and work on building stability. With greater stability, if and when the survivor chooses to confront the trauma narrative, they can do so with support. This approach aligns with transformative justice, which seeks to address harm without relying on punitive systems that often re-traumatize survivors or further marginalize them. For clinicians, this could mean supporting a survivor's pursuit of accountability and healing outside of the criminal justice system (if involving police or courts would cause more harm). Instead, the focus can be on community-based or restorative options that prioritize the survivor's sense of safety and justice.

Practitioners must also reflect on their own narrative power. Holding someone's story is a privilege that carries responsibility. Therapists, researchers, and advocates act as gatekeepers when they decide how a story is stored, interpreted, or shared with others. Professionals should continually reflect on their intentions and practices in handling survivors' stories. They need to ensure that the use of a survivor's story genuinely benefits the survivor, rather than advancing the professional's own agenda. They must obtain the survivor's informed consent for each specific use of the story and anticipate how sharing it (even anonymously) might impact the survivor. Importantly, practitioners should involve the survivor in decisions about how their story will be used. By maintaining this kind of ethical reflexivity and accountability, professionals can move from being owners of others' stories to guardians of them, protecting the dignity and intent of those narratives.

COMMUNITY NARRATIVES, COLLECTIVE STORYWORK, AND RESISTANCE

This section shifts from individual to collective storytelling, highlighting how communities use narrative as a tool of resistance and survival. Individual therapy is one way to heal narratives, but marginalized communities have long used collective storytelling as a vital practice of survival, resilience, and resistance. Even before formal mental health systems existed, communities shared stories through oral traditions, rituals, performances, and mutual aid to find meaning in suffering and maintain identity amid violence and dispossession. In grassroots organizing, art activism, and social movements, storytelling is not just a form of expression but also a strategic tool for building solidarity, mobilizing resistance, and envisioning alternative futures. When people share personal struggles in community spaces, private pain becomes public knowledge, helping individuals realize that their experiences are not isolated problems but connected to larger historical and structural forces like racism, colonialism, patriarchy, ableism, and economic exploitation. Through this process, collective storywork creates counter-narratives. These stories actively challenge dominant myths, oppose medicalized or criminalized portrayals, and affirm identities and histories that have been systematically erased or distorted.

Art activism provides one of the most potent avenues for marginalized communities to reclaim narrative authority through creative media. Across global contexts, artists employ music, visual art, dance, theater, spoken word, and digital production to render visible experiences of trauma, resistance, grief, and survival that are often unspeakable within dominant discourse. These creative practices frequently draw on ancestral traditions while simultaneously responding to present political conditions, producing hybrid forms that carry both memory and critique. Importantly, the emphasis in community-based art activism is rarely on producing a polished artifact for institutional validation. Instead, the focus rests on the relational process of creation itself: the shared labor, witnessing, experimentation, and mutual recognition that occur as people tell their stories together. Within these spaces, participants not only reclaim narrative control but also strengthen collective bonds, interrupt isolation, and cultivate cultural continuity as a source of healing.

Zines, small, self-published booklets, offer another vital grassroots platform for narrative sovereignty. By allowing marginalized creators to bypass mainstream publishing gatekeepers, zines enable people to circulate stories in their own voices, using their own aesthetics, language, and values. Their low cost and accessibility make them a profoundly democratic form of media production; with minimal resources, anyone can author, reproduce, and distribute their work. Historically, zines have played a central role within feminist, queer, disabled, and punk communities as vehicles for sharing personal testimony, political analysis, poetry, artwork, and survival strategies that were excluded from or actively censored by dominant media. Circulated through community centers, independent bookstores, mail networks, and now digital archives, zines form decentralized webs of relation and recognition. As counter-narratives, they disrupt imposed silences, validate experiences rarely represented in mass culture, and allow communities to speak to one another outside of institutional surveillance.

Community archives similarly enable marginalized groups to preserve and curate their own histories in ways that resist erasure and misrepresentation. Often organized through grassroots collectives, mutual aid networks, or local cultural centers, these archives gather photographs, letters, oral histories, zines, ephemera, and everyday objects that institutional archives have traditionally deemed unworthy of preservation. What distinguishes community archives is not only what they collect, but how they collect it. Operating through participatory and relational ethics, contributors retain decision-making power over what is preserved, how materials are described, and who is granted access. This practice challenges extractive research methods and relocates authority within the community itself. The act of archiving becomes a form of political work: by deciding which stories matter and how they are framed, communities assert ownership over their collective memory, protect themselves against historical revisionism, and sustain intergenerational continuity.

Collective storywork functions as an act of resistance precisely because it refuses the privatization of trauma. Rather than locating suffering solely within individual psyches, community storytelling recognizes harm as the outcome of interlocking systems of oppression. When survivors share their stories in communal settings, they encounter validation that disrupts shame. They also cultivate mutual support and generate shared strategies for survival and transformation. These practices give rise to what might be called narrative infrastructure: community-run platforms, publications, rituals, performances, and traditions. Such infrastructure ensures that voices remain audible even when dominant institutions ignore, distort, or commodify them. Through this sustained circulation of stories, communities enact narrative sovereignty collectively, claiming the right to be custodians of their own meanings, memories, and futures.

Looking forward, digital technology will continue to reshape the terrain of collective storytelling in complex and contradictory ways. Online platforms allow marginalized storytellers to connect across geographic boundaries and build transnational networks of solidarity with unprecedented speed. Podcasts, social media, live streams, and virtual gatherings can dramatically expand access to stories, particularly for those who face barriers to physical participation due to disability, surveillance, poverty, or migration status. At the same time, corporate-controlled platforms introduce significant risks. Personal narratives are frequently monetized as data, algorithmic systems reward spectacle over nuance, and public visibility can expose vulnerable storytellers to harassment, doxing, and state surveillance. In response, many communities are developing independent digital infrastructures that prioritize care, consent, and security. These include community-run servers, encrypted group communication tools, cooperative media platforms, and digital literacy initiatives that teach participants how to protect privacy, retain ownership of their content, and resist algorithmic distortion. Through such efforts, communities work to ensure that digital media strengthen rather than undermine narrative sovereignty.

Cultivating a rich ecosystem of storytelling spaces, artistic, archival, digital, and ritual, enables communities to build resilience amid ongoing conditions of structural violence. These spaces affirm that recovery from trauma is not solely an intrapsychic process but a fundamentally relational and political one. They also model alternatives to the top-down approaches characteristic of state and market institutions. These community-driven approaches demonstrate that care, accountability, and meaning-making can be created collectively from the ground up. For clinicians and researchers, engaging with community narratives demands humility, reflexivity, and an ethic of solidarity rather than expertise-driven authority. It requires showing up with resources that are offered without extraction. Clinicians and researchers must recognize that community knowledge often exceeds academic theory in depth, nuance, and applicability. To effectively support these spaces, practitioners should explore ways to integrate community-led storytelling into existing clinical and policy structures, addressing systemic barriers and fostering genuine collaboration. It also entails advocating for funding structures and public policies that sustain community-led narrative spaces rather than subordinating them to institutional agendas.

Ultimately, those who enter these storytelling spaces from outside must understand themselves as guests. Their role is to witness, support, and protect, not to define, manage, or redirect. When institutions genuinely honor community narrative autonomy and provide material support while stepping aside from control, they help foster conditions in which healing is co-created, histories are safeguarded, and liberation becomes collectively imaginable and actionable. It is essential to establish clear boundaries and ongoing dialogue to ensure external support enhances, rather than undermines, community sovereignty, preventing paternalism or tokenism from taking root.

CONCLUSION: TOWARD A FUTURE OF SOVEREIGN STORYTELLING

Reclaiming narrative sovereignty is essential to justice-oriented trauma care because it redistributes power over meaning-making back to survivors. Throughout this chapter, it has been demonstrated that stories of suffering are never neutral; they are always entangled with power, shaping whose pain is considered legible, whose testimony is doubted, who is rendered visible, and who is erased. This chapter traced how colonialism, racial capitalism, patriarchy, heteronormativity, cisnormativity, and ableism have systematically stripped Indigenous, Black, queer, disabled, and otherwise marginalized people of authorship over their own experiences. It also examined the profound harms that occur when trauma narratives are exploited for institutional legitimacy, consumed as spectacle, erased from historical memory, or weaponized for carceral, medical, and bureaucratic control. In response, the chapter advocates for consent-based, autonomy-centered narrative practices that restore survivors' agency. Healing emerges from environments where people define their experiences and choose when, how, and whether to share their stories, fostering hope and empowerment.

This chapter emphasizes that ethical trauma care requires practitioners and allies to decenter their own interpretive authority and instead adopt practices that actively safeguard survivor agency. This includes slowing down dominant clinical timelines, cultivating deep listening rather than information extraction, and practicing cultural humility that treats lived experience as primary knowledge rather than supplementary data. It also requires honoring nonverbal, somatic, artistic, spiritual, and fragmented modes of expression as fully valid narrative forms, rather than privileging linear, verbally articulated stories that conform to Western therapeutic norms. Harm-reduction principles offer an essential ethical anchor here, emphasizing choice, pacing, and the minimization of secondary harm. Ongoing, contextual consent must be understood not as a one-time procedural step but as a dynamic, relational practice that is revisited repeatedly across time, settings, and power differentials. Within this framework, silence itself becomes intelligible not as resistance or pathology, but as a meaningful, protective, and sometimes necessary narrative choice.

Equally central is the recognition that narrative sovereignty is not only an individual right but also a collective and political project. Community storytelling, art-making, archiving, and activism generate counter-narratives that resist dominant scripts of deficit, deviance, and disposability. These practices contest the historical positioning of marginalized people as objects of knowledge and instead reclaim them as producers of meaning, theory, and culture. Through these collective forms, trauma is re-situated within social, historical, and structural contexts, rather than collapsed into individualized pathology. In doing so, communities nurture resilience and mutual care. They also generate frameworks for accountability, repair, and transformation that go beyond the limits of individualized therapeutic intervention.

Moving toward a future of sovereign storytelling requires sustained commitment at both individual and structural levels. At the personal level, professionals, researchers, advocates, and allies must learn to function as guardians rather than gatekeepers of stories. This means listening more than speaking, refusing voyeurism, obtaining consent at every stage of engagement, and honoring boundaries without coercion or retaliation when survivors choose not to disclose. By doing so, conditions for relational safety are fostered, allowing trust to grow organically. In such environments, survivors can share their stories, if and when they choose, in ways that feel self-directed and meaningful. It is also crucial to cultivate spaces that welcome diverse forms of expression, including art, movement, ritual, digital media, and collective testimony, so that survivors are not forced into a single, clinically sanctioned narrative mode. Crucially, justice-oriented practice requires advocating for policies that decouple access to care, housing, legal protections, and material resources from mandatory disclosure of trauma. Survivors should never have to relive or expose their pain to be deemed deserving of support.

This work also demands rigorous and ongoing political education. Professionals must actively engage intersectional, decolonial, disability justice, mad studies, and queer-of-color frameworks to understand how power shapes both whose stories are heard and how those stories are interpreted. Without such analysis, even well-intentioned practitioners risk reproducing narrative violence through misrecognition, over-interpretation, cultural flattening, or epistemic dismissal. Reflexivity must therefore be treated not as an optional add-on, but as a core clinical and scholarly competency. Embracing reflexivity empowers practitioners to act ethically and confidently in their work with trauma survivors.

At the structural level, institutions must confront and dismantle the conditions that sustain narrative oppression. Doing so will disrupt entrenched hierarchies and financial interests. Media institutions need to move beyond commodifying and sensationalizing trauma. Instead, they must commit to practices that elevate survivors' voices on their own terms, providing fair compensation, editorial control, and protections from harm. Research bodies must shift from extractive models to genuinely participatory, community-led methodologies in which communities retain ownership of data, interpretation, and dissemination. Legal, medical, educational, and social service systems must ensure that disclosing trauma does not trigger punishment, surveillance, family separation, criminalization, immigration consequences, or loss of benefits. These risks currently deter many survivors, especially those from marginalized communities, from seeking support. Funders, likewise, must prioritize long-term investment in community-based storytelling, archiving, and arts initiatives that preserve suppressed histories and cultivate liberatory counter-narratives. They should not privilege short-term, outcome-driven metrics that prioritize institutional reputations over community needs.

None of these transformations will unfold without resistance. Institutional inertia, professional defensiveness, and deeply embedded ideologies of control, risk management, and "objectivity" will continue to obstruct meaningful reform. Nevertheless, narrative sovereignty is not a peripheral concern; it is a cornerstone of self-determination, dignity, and collective survival. Genuine healing begins to emerge when individuals are free to choose how, when, and whether to narrate their lives. Healing is further enabled when communities possess the resources and authority to protect, interpret, and transmit those narratives across generations. In such a future, storytelling no longer functions as a technology of extraction, discipline, or proof, but as a practice of solidarity, memory, and world-making. Justice, then, is not only argued for in policy or pursued through institutions; it is enacted in the everyday practices through which people reclaim authorship over their lives and speak themselves into liberation. In this way, narrative sovereignty becomes not only a clinical ethic but a broader practice of justice, through which individuals and communities reclaim authorship over their lives.

REFERENCES

Asakura, K., Miller, J., Nakash, O., & O'Neill, P. (2023). Toward "Decolonizing" Clinical Social Work Practice and Education. *Smith College Studies in Social Work, 93*(2–4), 73–82. DOI: 10.1080/00377317.2023.2279389

Brison, S. J. (1999). Trauma narratives and the remaking of the self. In Bal, M., Crewe, J., & Spitzer, L. (Eds.), *Acts of Memory: Cultural Recall in the Present* (pp. 39–54). University Press of New England.

Elliott, D. E., Bjelajac, P., Fallot, R. D., Markoff, L. S., & Reed, B. G. (2005). Trauma-informed Or trauma-denied: Principles and implementation of trauma-informed services for women. *Journal of Community Psychology, 33*(4), 461–477. DOI: 10.1002/jcop.20063

Espiritu Gandhi, E. L., & Nguyen, V. (2023). *The Routledge Handbook of Refugee Narratives*. Routledge. DOI: 10.4324/9781003131458

Farmer, P. (2004). An anthropology of structural violence. *Current Anthropology, 45*(3), 305–325. DOI: 10.1086/382250

Fricker, M. (2007). *Epistemic Injustice: Power and the Ethics of Knowing*. Oxford University Press., DOI: 10.1093/acprof:oso/9780198237907.001.0001

Herman, J. L. (1992). *Trauma and Recovery: The Aftermath of Violence, from Domestic Abuse To Political Terror*. Basic Books.

Herman, J. L. (2015). Justice from the victim's perspective. *Violence Against Women, 21*(6), 638–658. DOI: 10.1177/1077801205274450 PMID: 16043563

Mattingly, C. (1998). *Healing Dramas and Clinical Plots: The Narrative Structure of Experience*. Cambridge University Press. DOI: 10.1017/CBO9781139167017

McKenzie-Mohr, S., & Lafrance, M. (Eds.). (2014). *Women Voicing Resistance: Discursive and Narrative Explorations*. Routledge. DOI: 10.4324/9780203094365

Mohatt, N. V., Thompson, A. B., Thai, N. D., & Tebes, J. K. (2014). Historical trauma as public Narrative: A conceptual review. *Social Science & Medicine, 106*, 128–136. DOI: 10.1016/j.socscimed.2014.01.043 PMID: 24561774

Perry, B. D., & Szalavitz, M. (2017). *The Boy Who Was Raised as a Dog: And Other Stories From a Child Psychiatrist's Notebook* (3rd ed.). Basic Books.

Perry, B. D., & Winfrey, O. (2021). *What Happened to You? Conversations on Trauma, Resilience and Healing*. Flatiron Books.

Rosen, L. T. (2021). Mapping out epistemic justice in the clinical space. *Philosophy, Ethics, and Humanities in Medicine; PEHM, 16*(1), 9. Advance online publication. DOI: 10.1186/s13010-021-00110-0 PMID: 34696799

Smith, L. T. (2021). *Decolonizing Methodologies: Research and Indigenous Peoples* (3rd ed.). Zed Books., DOI: 10.5040/9781350225282

Spivak, G. C. (1988). Can the subaltern speak? In C. Nelson & L. Grossberg (Eds.), *Marxism And the Interpretation of Culture* (pp. 271–313). Macmillan.

Chapter 8
Community-Based and Collective Healing Models:
Evaluation and Measurement of Trauma-Informed System Implementation

Deepak Gupta
http://orcid.org/0000-0003-3929-1362
Institute of Technology and Management, Gwalior, India

Saodat Musaeva
Termez University of Economics and Service, Termez, Uzbekistan

Nasiba Jumaniyazova
Mamun University, Khiva, Uzbekistan

Mukhayya Djumaniyazova
Urgench State University, Urgench, Uzbekistan

Asqar Ismailov
Tashkent State University of Economy, Tashkent, Uzbekistan

Narzulloeva Salomatbonu Sunatulloevna
Bukhara State Pedagogical Institute, Bukhara, Uzbekistan

ABSTRACT

This chapter examines community-based and collective healing approaches within trauma-informed care frameworks, focusing on evaluation methodologies and measurement strategies for systemic implementation. Drawing from intersectional perspectives and evidence-based research, the chapter explores how collective trauma responses—including historical, racial, and community-level adversities—require healing models that extend beyond individual clinical interventions. The discussion integrates cultural considerations, community-driven practices, and systems-level

DOI: 10.4018/979-8-3373-8597-6.ch008

accountability measures. Through critical analysis of existing evaluation frameworks, the chapter proposes comprehensive assessment tools that capture both process and outcome measures across multiple ecological levels.

1. INTRODUCTION

The recognition of trauma as a fundamental public health concern has catalyzed a paradigm shift in how systems of care conceptualize and respond to adversity. Traditional approaches to trauma treatment have predominantly focused on individual pathology and clinical interventions, often overlooking the collective, historical, and structural dimensions of traumatic experiences. This individualistic framework proves insufficient when addressing traumas that are inherently collective in nature—those stemming from systemic oppression, community violence, forced displacement, historical injustices, and structural inequities that affect entire populations across generations.

Community-based and collective healing models emerge from this critical gap, offering frameworks that honor the social ecology of trauma while centering community wisdom, cultural practices, and collective resilience. These approaches recognize that healing from collective trauma requires interventions that occur at multiple levels simultaneously—individual, relational, organizational, community, and systemic. As Forkey et al. (2021) emphasize in their comprehensive framework for trauma-informed care in pediatric settings, effective trauma response must address not only individual symptoms but also the environmental contexts that perpetuate or ameliorate traumatic stress.

The implementation of trauma-informed systems represents a fundamental organizational transformation that extends beyond protocol changes or staff training. It requires deep cultural shifts in how institutions understand power, engage with communities, and measure success. Yet, as Purtle (2021) documents in a systematic review of trauma-informed organizational interventions, the field lacks standardized, validated approaches to evaluating these complex system-level changes. This evaluation gap poses significant challenges: without robust measurement frameworks, organizations struggle to assess fidelity to trauma-informed principles, demonstrate effectiveness, identify areas for improvement, and justify continued investment in systemic transformation.

This chapter addresses these critical needs by examining community-based and collective healing models within the context of trauma-informed system implementation. We explore evaluation methodologies that honor the complexity of collective healing while providing actionable data for continuous quality improvement. The discussion integrates insights from implementation science, community psychology, cultural psychology, and health equity frameworks to propose comprehensive measurement approaches that are both rigorous and culturally responsive.

1.1. Purpose and Scope

This chapter serves multiple interconnected purposes. First, it provides a comprehensive overview of community-based and collective healing approaches, situating these models within broader trauma-informed care frameworks. Second, it critically examines existing evaluation methodologies for trauma-informed system implementation, identifying strengths, limitations, and gaps in current measurement practices. Third, it proposes an integrated evaluation framework that addresses multiple dimensions of system transformation while centering equity, cultural responsiveness, and community partnership.

The scope encompasses diverse settings where trauma-informed approaches are being implemented—including healthcare systems, child welfare agencies, educational institutions, juvenile justice programs, mental health services, and community-based organizations. While recognizing the unique considerations within each setting, the chapter emphasizes cross-cutting principles and measurement strategies applicable across contexts. Special attention is given to systems serving populations that have experienced collective and historical traumas, including communities of color, immigrant and refugee populations, Indigenous communities, and other marginalized groups where trauma-informed approaches must be fundamentally grounded in cultural safety and structural competence.

1.2. Theoretical Foundations

The theoretical foundation of this chapter draws from multiple disciplinary perspectives. Ecological systems theory provides a framework for understanding how trauma impacts and healing occurs across nested environmental levels. Implementation science offers methodological guidance for studying complex organizational change processes. Critical race theory and intersectionality frameworks illuminate how systems of oppression create and maintain collective trauma while shaping differential access to healing resources. Community psychology principles emphasize participatory approaches, empowerment, and the importance of context in intervention design and evaluation.

Bailey, Feldman, and Bassett (2021) articulate how structural racism operates as a root cause of racial health inequities through racist policies embedded in systems and institutions. Their framework demonstrates that addressing health disparities requires examining and transforming the structural and policy-level determinants that create differential exposure to trauma and differential access to healing resources. This structural lens is essential for understanding why community-based and collective healing approaches must include explicit attention to power, equity, and systemic transformation rather than focusing solely on individual or interpersonal interventions.

2. CONCEPTUALIZING COLLECTIVE TRAUMA AND COMMUNITY HEALING

Understanding collective trauma and community healing requires expanding beyond diagnostic frameworks focused on individual symptomatology. Collective trauma refers to traumatic experiences that affect entire groups, communities, or populations simultaneously or across generations. These traumas are often rooted in systemic oppression, mass violence, forced displacement, environmental catastrophes, or historical injustices that target specific populations based on race, ethnicity, religion, nationality, or other group identities.

2.1. Forms of Collective Trauma

Collective trauma manifests in multiple forms, each requiring nuanced understanding and culturally grounded responses. Historical trauma encompasses traumatic experiences that occurred in the past but continue to impact communities through intergenerational transmission of both biological and psychosocial effects. Conching and Thayer (2021) present a comprehensive conceptual model for understanding biological pathways through which historical trauma affects health, with particular emphasis on epigenetic modifications that may transmit traumatic stress responses across generations. Their framework illustrates how historical experiences of genocide, slavery, forced relocation, and cultural suppression can have enduring biological impacts that intersect with ongoing social and economic marginalization.

Racial trauma represents another critical form of collective trauma, stemming from experiences of racism, discrimination, and race-based violence. Williams, Metzger, Leins, and DeLapp (2021) developed the UConn Racial/Ethnic Stress and Trauma Survey to assess racial trauma within a DSM-5 framework, recognizing that experiences of racism can meet criteria for traumatic stressors while also producing unique patterns of psychological distress not fully captured by standard PTSD criteria. Their work demonstrates the importance of culturally specific assessment tools that acknowledge the particular phenomenology of race-based trauma.

Community violence and collective victimization affect neighborhoods and communities through chronic exposure to violence, crime, and social disorder. Negi, Cepeda, and Valdez (2021) documented crime victimization patterns among immigrant Latino day laborers following Hurricane Katrina, illustrating how disaster contexts can exacerbate vulnerability to violence while highlighting the intersection of immigration status, economic marginalization, and community-level trauma. Migration-related trauma affects refugee and immigrant populations who experience forced displacement, persecution, family separation, dangerous migration journeys, and resettlement challenges. These experiences often compound across individual, family, and community levels while intersecting with acculturative stress and discrimination in host countries.

2.2. Mechanisms of Collective Healing

Community-based healing approaches operate through multiple interconnected mechanisms that address the multilevel nature of collective trauma. Social support and collective efficacy provide protective buffers against traumatic stress while facilitating recovery. When communities come together in shared healing practices, they activate social support networks, reduce isolation, and create opportunities for collective meaning-making. Cultural practices and traditional healing ceremonies offer pathways for processing trauma that honor community values, spiritual beliefs, and ancestral wisdom.

Goodkind, LaNoue, Lee, Freeland, and Freund (2021) examined a community-based cultural mental health intervention for American Indian youth and their families, demonstrating the feasibility and acceptability of interventions grounded in Indigenous cultural practices and community partnership. Their findings illustrate how culturally rooted healing practices can address historical trauma while strengthening cultural identity and community connections. The intervention integrated traditional healing ceremonies, cultural activities, and community gatherings with evidence-based mental health strategies, creating a synergistic approach that honored both cultural wisdom and scientific evidence.

Collective narrative and storytelling enable communities to construct shared understandings of traumatic experiences, resist silencing and erasure, and reclaim agency in defining their own experiences. When trauma survivors come together to share stories, they often discover commonalities that reduce shame, validate experiences, and build solidarity. These narrative practices can occur through formal testimony projects, community dialogues, artistic expression, or informal sharing within trusted relationships. The process of collective meaning-making helps communities integrate traumatic experiences into broader narratives of resistance, resilience, and survival.

2.3. Community-Based Intervention Models

Several evidence-informed models have emerged for addressing collective trauma through community-based approaches. These models share common features including emphasis on cultural grounding, community partnership, attention to social determinants, and integration of multiple intervention levels. Ellis et al. (2021) examined psychosocial factors influencing diverse behaviors and attitudes among Somali refugee youth in the United States, highlighting the complex interplay between pre-migration trauma, resettlement stress, cultural identity, and community support. Their research underscores the necessity of interventions that address multiple levels of influence while being deeply grounded in cultural understanding and community engagement.

Miller, Brown, Shramko, and Svetaz (2021) articulated ten clinical pearls for applying trauma-informed practices to the care of refugee and immigrant youth. Their framework emphasizes understanding migration experiences holistically, recognizing family separation as a significant trauma, attending to legal and documentation status as ongoing stressors, building trust through cultural humility, and connecting families to community resources. These principles extend beyond clinical settings to inform system-level trauma-informed approaches that recognize the unique needs of immigrant and refugee populations.

Community-based participatory research (CBPR) approaches offer methodological frameworks for developing and evaluating community healing interventions in partnership with affected communities. CBPR emphasizes shared power, mutual respect, co-learning, capacity building, and long-term commitment to community well-being. In trauma-focused work, participatory approaches ensure that interventions are culturally appropriate, address community-identified priorities, and build on existing community strengths and resources. Moreover, the participatory process itself can be healing, as community members exercise agency in defining problems and solutions rather than being positioned as passive recipients of expert-driven interventions.

Figure 1. Multi-level trauma-informed implementation framework

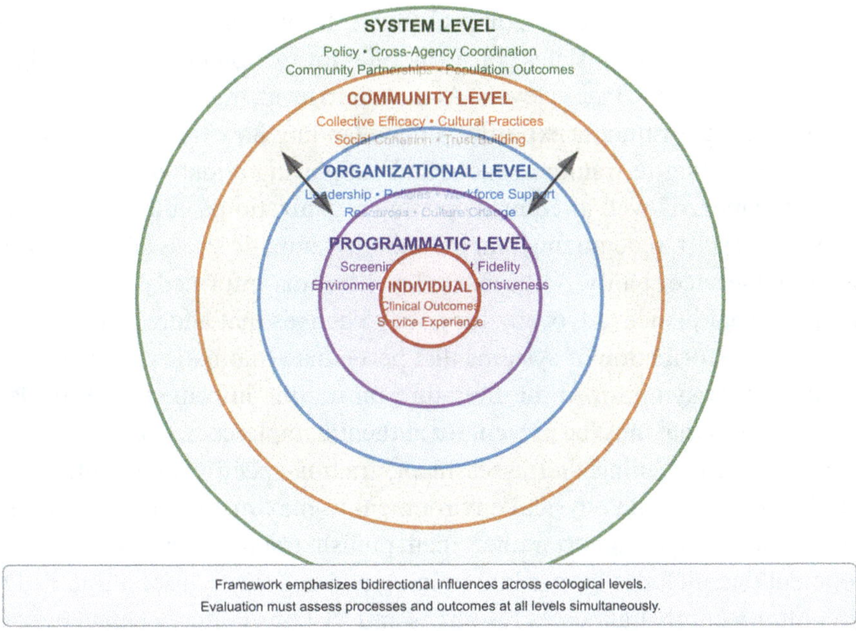

Figure 1 illustrates the ecological nature of trauma-informed implementation, showing how change must occur simultaneously across five nested levels: individual, programmatic, organizational, community, and system. The bidirectional arrows emphasize that influences flow in both directions—individual experiences shape organizational culture, just as organizational policies affect individual wellbeing. Comprehensive evaluation requires assessing both processes and outcomes at all levels, as success at one level depends on alignment with others.

3. TRAUMA-INFORMED SYSTEM IMPLEMENTATION

Implementing trauma-informed approaches at the system level requires comprehensive organizational change that extends far beyond individual staff training or program modifications. System implementation involves transforming organizational culture, policies, practices, and physical environments to create contexts that promote safety, trustworthiness, peer support, collaboration, empowerment, and attention to cultural and gender issues—the six key principles identified by the Substance Abuse and Mental Health Services Administration (SAMHSA) as foundational to trauma-informed care.

3.1. Core Principles and Framework

Levenson (2021) provides a comprehensive framework for trauma-informed social work practice that translates core principles into actionable practice behaviors across micro, mezzo, and macro levels. At the micro level, trauma-informed practice involves screening for trauma exposure, understanding how trauma affects current functioning, avoiding re-traumatization, and supporting client empowerment and choice. At the mezzo level, it requires creating organizational cultures that support both clients and staff, recognizing that secondary traumatic stress affects workforce wellbeing and service quality. At the macro level, trauma-informed practice demands attention to social justice, advocacy for policy changes that address root causes of trauma, and transformation of systems that perpetuate traumatic experiences.

Reeves (2021) synthesized the literature on trauma-informed care to identify essential elements that must be present for authentic implementation. These include universal trauma screening and assessment, trauma-specific interventions when indicated, attention to the physical environment to maximize safety and minimize triggers, policies that support rather than punish trauma responses, workforce development that includes both initial training and ongoing consultation, and leadership commitment that allocates resources and sustains culture change over time. The synthesis reveals that partial implementation—adopting some elements while neglecting others—compromises effectiveness and may even cause harm by raising expectations for safety that the system cannot fulfill.

3.2. Implementation Challenges and Barriers

Despite growing consensus about the importance of trauma-informed approaches, implementation faces numerous challenges. Hanson and Lang (2021) offer a critical examination of trauma-informed care among agencies serving maltreated youth and their families, identifying significant gaps between stated commitment and actual practice. They document how agencies often adopt trauma-informed language without making substantive changes to policies and practices that may be inherently traumatizing, such as frequent placement moves, restrictive behavior management strategies, or punitive responses to trauma-driven behaviors.

Resource constraints present persistent challenges, as trauma-informed implementation requires sustained investment in training, consultation, environmental modifications, and additional staffing to reduce caseloads and allow time for relationship-building. Organizations serving vulnerable populations often operate with limited budgets, creating tensions between ideal practices and fiscal realities. Moreover, funding structures may incentivize quantity over quality, rewarding high throughput rather than the slower, more relational work that trauma-informed practice requires.

Workforce issues compound implementation challenges. Hatcher, Bride, Oh, King, and Catrett (2021) assessed secondary traumatic stress among juvenile justice education workers, finding significant levels of compassion fatigue and burnout that affect both staff wellbeing and their capacity to provide trauma-informed services. Organizations must attend to workforce trauma and implement strategies to prevent secondary traumatic stress, including reasonable caseloads, regular supervision and peer support, clear boundaries between work and personal life, and organizational cultures that normalize self-care and help-seeking. Without addressing workforce wellness, trauma-informed implementation cannot be sustained.

3.3. Implementation Strategies

Successful implementation requires strategic approaches grounded in implementation science frameworks. Marsac et al. (2021) documented the process of implementing a trauma-informed approach across pediatric health care networks, identifying critical success factors. These include strong leadership commitment demonstrated through resource allocation and policy changes, creation of implementation teams with representatives from all organizational levels and departments, use of champions who advocate for trauma-informed practices and support peer learning, staged implementation that begins with assessment and planning rather than immediate practice changes, and integration with existing quality improvement initiatives rather than positioning trauma-informed care as a separate add-on.

Palfrey et al. (2021) described achieving service change through implementation of a trauma-informed care training program within a mental health service. Their approach emphasized creating a training curriculum tailored to organizational context, using train-the-trainer models to build internal capacity, providing ongoing coaching and consultation beyond initial training, and establishing feedback loops that allowed staff to voice concerns and shape implementation processes. Importantly, they found that training alone was insufficient—organizational policies, supervision structures, and performance evaluation systems needed to align with trauma-informed principles to support practice change.

Phased implementation approaches allow organizations to build capacity gradually while learning from early experiences. Initial phases typically focus on awareness-building and assessment, helping staff understand trauma prevalence and impact while assessing organizational readiness and identifying areas for change. Middle phases involve policy development, environmental modifications, and practice changes in pilot areas. Later phases expand successful practices across the organization while establishing systems for ongoing quality monitoring and continuous improvement.

This staged approach prevents overwhelming staff and allows for adaptation based on emerging data and feedback.

Figure 2. Implementation phases and outcome trajectories over time

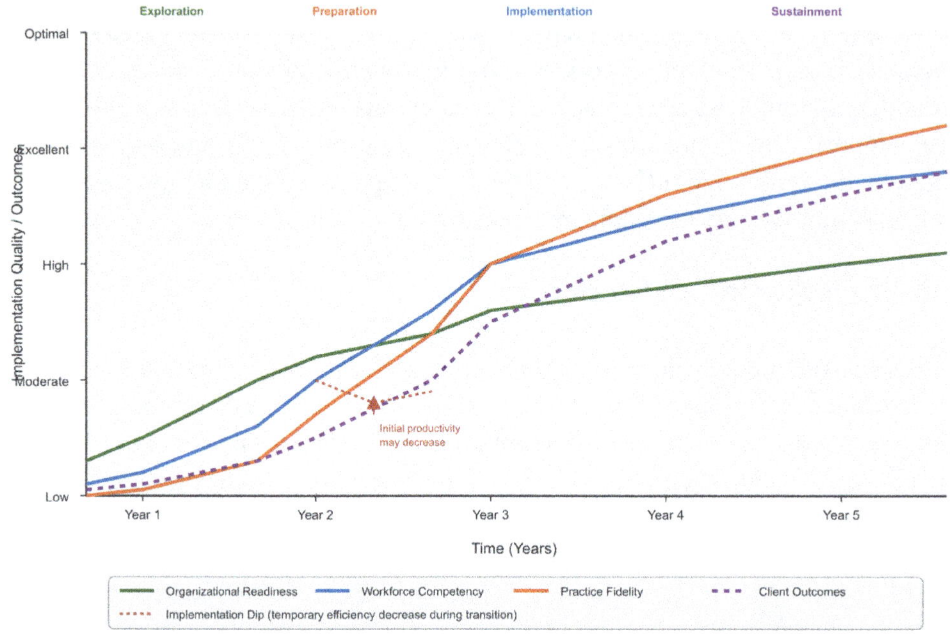

Figure 2 reveals a critical implementation reality: various indicators change at different paces across the five-year timeline. Organizational readiness and workforce competency begin improving during exploration and preparation phases, while practice fidelity and client outcomes lag behind. Note the "implementation dip"—the temporary decrease in efficiency during transition to new practices. This phenomenon is normal but often triggers premature abandonment of trauma-informed approaches. The graph demonstrates why longitudinal measurement is essential; snapshots at any single point miss the full trajectory. Patience and sustained commitment are required for meaningful transformation.

4. EXPANDING CONCEPTUALIZATIONS OF ADVERSITY

Traditional trauma frameworks have relied heavily on Adverse Childhood Experiences (ACE) measures that focus primarily on household dysfunction and individual maltreatment. While ACE research has been instrumental in establishing links between early adversity and later health outcomes, the original ACE framework has significant limitations. It emphasizes individual and family-level adversities while neglecting community and structural factors that profoundly shape health and wellbeing. Moreover, the original ACE items were developed with predominantly white, middle-class populations and may not capture adversities most relevant to marginalized communities.

4.1. Expanded ACE Frameworks

Cronholm et al. (2021) pioneered efforts to expand the concept of adversity by developing an expanded ACE framework that includes community-level adversities alongside traditional household items. Their expanded measure adds items assessing community violence exposure, discrimination, foster care placement, and economic hardship. Research using this expanded framework demonstrates that community-level adversities contribute independently to health outcomes beyond traditional ACEs, and that the expanded measure better captures adversity experiences among urban, diverse populations. This expansion represents an important step toward more comprehensive adversity assessment that recognizes social and structural determinants of trauma exposure.

Liu, Kia-Keating, and Nylund-Gibson (2021) examined patterns of adversities and pathways to health among White, Black, and Latinx youth, identifying distinct adversity profiles that vary by race and ethnicity. Their findings reveal that youth of color experience higher rates of both traditional and community-level adversities, and that different adversity patterns have varying health impacts across racial groups. These results underscore the necessity of culturally responsive approaches to adversity assessment and intervention that account for differential exposure to various forms of adversity and differential impacts of those exposures across sociocultural contexts.

The Philadelphia ACE Survey expanded the original framework even further, adding items about witnessing violence, experiencing racism, living in unsafe neighborhoods, experiencing bullying, and living in foster care. Research using this expanded survey found that among a diverse urban sample, these additional items were highly prevalent and significantly associated with poor health outcomes. Notably, many youth who scored zero on traditional ACEs scored positive on expanded items, suggesting that traditional measures miss substantial adversity among certain populations. These findings have important implications for trauma-informed practice—systems that screen only for traditional ACEs may fail to identify many youth who have experienced significant trauma.

4.2. Intersectionality and Compounding Adversities

Intersectionality frameworks illuminate how multiple marginalized identities interact to shape trauma exposure and access to resources. Individuals who hold multiple marginalized identities—such as being a woman of color, an immigrant with a disability, or a transgender youth of color—often experience compounding adversities that cannot be understood by simply adding together separate identity-based oppressions. Instead, these identities intersect to create unique patterns of marginalization and distinct forms of trauma.

For example, the experiences of racism faced by Black women cannot be fully understood by examining racism and sexism separately—instead, they experience gendered racism that reflects the intersection of these identities. Similarly, undocumented immigrant youth of color face intersecting vulnerabilities related to immigration status, race, age, and often economic marginalization. Trauma-informed systems must develop capacity to recognize and respond to these intersecting identities and compounding adversities rather than treating identity dimensions in isolation.

Measurement approaches must also reflect intersectional thinking. This means moving beyond additive models that simply count the number of marginalized identities to examining how specific identity intersections shape experiences. It requires disaggregating data by multiple identity dimensions simultaneously rather than examining each dimension separately. It demands qualitative and mixed-methods approaches that capture the lived experiences of individuals at various identity intersections. And it necessitates involving community members with intersecting marginalized identities in all phases of research and evaluation to ensure that measurement approaches accurately reflect their experiences and priorities.

5. EVALUATION FRAMEWORKS FOR TRAUMA-INFORMED SYSTEMS

Evaluating trauma-informed system implementation presents unique methodological challenges. Unlike discrete interventions with defined start and end points, system transformation is an ongoing, iterative process involving multiple components implemented at different levels across extended timeframes. Traditional outcome evaluation approaches prove insufficient, as they cannot capture the complexity of organizational change processes or attribute outcomes to specific intervention components within dynamic systems contexts.

5.1. Multi-Level Evaluation Models

Comprehensive evaluation of trauma-informed system implementation requires multi-level frameworks that assess changes across individual, program, organizational, and system levels. At the individual level, evaluation examines whether trauma-informed practices improve outcomes for people receiving services—including symptom reduction, functional improvement, service satisfaction, and reduction in re-traumatization experiences. Individual-level measures should include both standardized clinical assessments and patient-reported outcome measures that capture service users' perspectives on care quality and helpfulness.

Cloitre, Hyland, Prins, and Shevlin (2021) validated the International Trauma Questionnaire (ITQ) as a measure for assessing treatment-related change in PTSD and complex PTSD. Their research demonstrates the importance of measures specifically designed to detect change over time, with strong psychometric properties including sensitivity to treatment effects. For evaluation of trauma-informed systems, such measures can assess whether implementation efforts translate into meaningful clinical improvement for service users experiencing trauma-related symptoms.

Program-level evaluation examines fidelity to trauma-informed principles within specific programs or services. This includes assessing whether programs conduct universal trauma screening, provide trauma-specific evidence-based treatments when indicated, create physically and emotionally safe environments, involve service users in treatment planning and decision-making, and connect individuals to peer support and community resources. Program-level measures often employ structured observation protocols, file reviews, and stakeholder interviews to assess alignment between stated trauma-informed principles and actual practices.

Organizational-level evaluation focuses on system-wide factors that enable or constrain trauma-informed practice. This includes assessment of organizational policies, leadership commitment and resource allocation, workforce training and support, physical environment modifications, and cultural change processes. Organizational climate measures can assess staff perceptions of safety, support, and alignment with trauma-informed values. Administrative data can track workforce stability, supervision frequency, training completion, and resource utilization patterns that reflect organizational priorities.

System-level evaluation examines how organizations interact with other entities in the service ecosystem and whether broader system transformations occur. This includes assessing coordination and collaboration across agencies, policy changes that support trauma-informed approaches, community partnerships and engagement, and reduction in system-level practices that cause trauma such as unnecessary foster care placements, school suspensions, or juvenile justice involvement. System-level evaluation often requires examining administrative databases across agencies and conducting community surveys to assess population-level indicators.

5.2. Process and Outcome Measures

Evaluation frameworks must include both process measures that assess implementation activities and outcome measures that assess results. Process measures document what implementation activities occurred, when, for whom, and with what level of fidelity. These measures are essential for understanding whether poor outcomes reflect ineffective interventions or inadequate implementation. Common process measures include training completion rates, policy adoption timelines, practice observation scores, and implementation milestone achievement.

Kassam-Adams et al. (2021) developed a method for assessing content validity in model-based creation and iteration of eHealth interventions, providing guidance applicable to trauma-informed system implementation evaluation. Their approach emphasizes involving multiple stakeholder groups in defining what should be measured and validating that measures capture priority constructs. This participatory approach to measurement development ensures that evaluation frameworks reflect diverse perspectives on what constitutes successful trauma-informed implementation rather than relying solely on researcher or administrator priorities.

Outcome measures should reflect the full range of intended impacts. Proximal outcomes include changes in knowledge, attitudes, and self-efficacy among staff following training. Intermediate outcomes include changes in practices, policies, and organizational culture. Distal outcomes include improved client experiences and clinical outcomes, reduced restraint and seclusion use, decreased staff turnover, and population-level health improvements. Importantly, trauma-informed implementation may also prevent negative outcomes—such as reducing re-traumatization, avoiding unnecessary child removals, or preventing school expulsions. Evaluation frameworks should attend to both improvement in positive outcomes and reduction in negative outcomes.

Longitudinal measurement is essential given that system transformation occurs over extended timeframes and impacts may not be immediately apparent. Initial implementation efforts often require substantial investment before positive outcomes emerge. Early phases may even show temporary decreases in some efficiency measures as staff adjust to new practices and organizations invest resources in training and infrastructure. Evaluation frameworks must include repeated measures over multiple years to capture implementation trajectories and longer-term impacts. This temporal dimension also allows for examination of sustainability—whether trauma-informed changes persist and become embedded in organizational culture or fade over time.

5.3. Implementation Science Frameworks

Implementation science offers frameworks specifically designed for studying complex intervention implementation in real-world settings. The Consolidated Framework for Implementation Research (CFIR) identifies five major domains that influence implementation: intervention characteristics, outer setting (including policies and community context), inner setting (organizational characteristics), characteristics of individuals involved, and implementation process. These domains provide a comprehensive lens for evaluating factors that enable or impede trauma-informed implementation.

The RE-AIM framework guides evaluation by examining five dimensions: Reach (proportion and characteristics of people affected), Effectiveness (impact on outcomes), Adoption (proportion and representativeness of settings that adopt practices), Implementation (consistency and fidelity of delivery), and Maintenance (extent practices are sustained over time). Applying RE-AIM to trauma-informed system implementation helps ensure evaluation addresses both internal validity (effectiveness) and external validity (generalizability and sustainability).

The Exploration, Preparation, Implementation, Sustainment (EPIS) framework describes four phases of implementation, each with distinct activities and evaluation needs. During Exploration, evaluation focuses on assessing readiness, identifying needs, and selecting appropriate approaches. During Preparation, evaluation examines planning processes, capacity-building activities, and barrier identification. During Implementation, evaluation monitors fidelity, documents adaptations, and tracks early outcomes. During Sustainment, evaluation assesses whether practices become routinized and whether outcomes persist. This phased approach to evaluation aligns measurement with implementation stages rather than applying the same measures across all phases.

6. CULTURALLY RESPONSIVE EVALUATION APPROACHES

Culturally responsive evaluation recognizes that conventional evaluation approaches often reflect dominant cultural values and may not adequately capture experiences, outcomes, or processes meaningful to diverse communities. For trauma-informed system evaluation, cultural responsiveness is not optional—it is essential for valid measurement and ethical practice. Evaluation frameworks must be designed in partnership with communities served, employ culturally appropriate methods, and include measures that reflect community-defined indicators of success.

6.1. Principles of Cultural Humility in Evaluation

Cultural humility provides a framework for approaching evaluation with openness to learning from communities rather than assuming evaluator expertise. This stance involves recognizing power differentials inherent in evaluation relationships, committing to ongoing self-reflection about one's own cultural assumptions and biases, and maintaining lifelong learning about diverse cultural perspectives. In trauma-informed system evaluation, cultural humility means acknowledging that communities affected by trauma hold expertise about their own experiences and healing needs that may differ from professional or academic understandings.

Oral et al. (2021) emphasize that trauma-informed care represents the future of healthcare precisely because it requires attention to social context, cultural values, and historical experiences that shape both trauma exposure and healing possibilities. Their vision of trauma-informed care explicitly includes cultural responsiveness as a core element rather than an add-on consideration. This integration means that evaluation frameworks must assess cultural responsiveness as a dimension of implementation quality—examining whether organizations demonstrate cultural humility, employ culturally diverse staff, offer interpretation and translation services, incorporate cultural healing practices, and partner with cultural community organizations.

6.2. Community Partnership in Evaluation Design

Authentic community partnership in evaluation requires involving community members from the earliest stages of planning rather than consulting them only after evaluation frameworks are already developed. Community partners should participate in defining evaluation questions, selecting or developing measures, determining data collection methods, interpreting findings, and deciding how results are disseminated and used. This participatory approach ensures that evaluation addresses questions communities care about and produces actionable information relevant to their priorities.

Partnership also requires attending to power dynamics and ensuring community partners have genuine influence over evaluation processes. This means providing compensation for community members' time and expertise, offering capacity-building opportunities so community partners can develop evaluation skills, using accessible language rather than technical jargon, being transparent about constraints and decision-making processes, and following through on commitments. When power imbalances are not addressed, participatory approaches can become extractive—benefiting researchers or organizations while providing little value to communities and potentially reinforcing experiences of exploitation that mirror historical traumas.

Mixed-methods approaches combining quantitative and qualitative data are particularly valuable for culturally responsive evaluation. Quantitative measures allow for systematic tracking of implementation progress and outcomes across large samples. Qualitative methods provide depth and context, capturing nuances that standardized measures may miss and allowing participants to share experiences in their own words. Community-based participatory approaches often employ photovoice, digital storytelling, community mapping, and other creative methods that honor diverse ways of knowing and communicating. These approaches can be especially meaningful for communities whose experiences have been historically silenced or distorted in dominant narratives.

6.3. Equity-Centered Measurement

Equity-centered measurement explicitly examines whether trauma-informed implementation reduces disparities in service access, quality, and outcomes. This requires disaggregating data by race, ethnicity, language, immigration status, sexual orientation, gender identity, disability status, and other dimensions of identity to identify differential impacts. Evaluation should examine not only average effects but also whether implementation benefits all groups equitably or primarily benefits already-advantaged populations while leaving disparities unchanged or even widening them.

Equity-focused evaluation also assesses organizational practices that may perpetuate disparities. This includes examining whether trauma screening and assessment tools are culturally valid across populations served, whether evidence-based treatments are accessible to people with limited English proficiency or those facing economic barriers, whether staffing reflects the diversity of service users, and whether organizational policies inadvertently disadvantage certain groups. For example, policies requiring extensive documentation may create barriers for undocumented immigrants, while inflexible scheduling may exclude people working multiple jobs or lacking transportation.

Importantly, equity-centered evaluation recognizes that equal outcomes may not represent equity when starting points differ dramatically. Communities that have experienced historical trauma and ongoing marginalization may require additional resources and supports to achieve comparable wellbeing. Evaluation frameworks should assess whether implementation includes explicit efforts to address historical and structural inequities rather than assuming that uniform approaches will produce equitable outcomes. This might include examining whether organizations allocate additional resources to communities facing greatest adversity, whether they employ targeted outreach to underserved populations, and whether they partner with community organizations that have established trust with marginalized groups.

7. COMPREHENSIVE ASSESSMENT FRAMEWORK FOR TRAUMA-INFORMED IMPLEMENTATION

Building on the preceding analysis, this section proposes a comprehensive assessment framework for evaluating trauma-informed system implementation with particular attention to community-based and collective healing approaches. The framework integrates multiple evaluation traditions including implementation science, cultural responsiveness, participatory evaluation, and equity-focused measurement. It addresses process and outcome measures across individual, organizational, and system levels while centering community partnership and cultural grounding.

Figure 3. Comprehensive evaluation cycle for trauma-informed systems

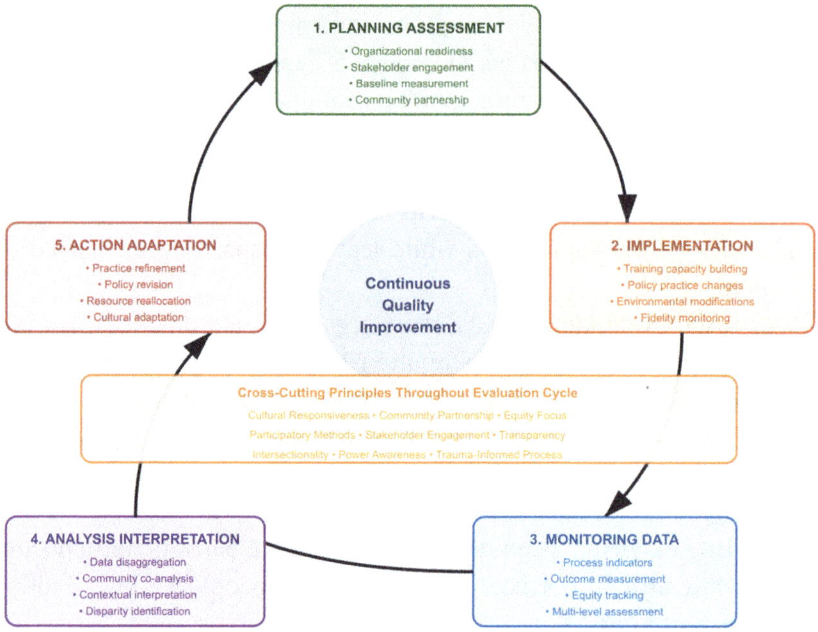

Figure 3 depicts evaluation as a continuous cycle rather than a one-time assessment. The five phases—Planning & Assessment, Implementation, Monitoring & Data Collection, Analysis & Interpretation, and Action & Adaptation—form an ongoing loop of quality improvement. Cross-cutting principles (cultural responsiveness, community partnership, equity focus, participatory methods, stakeholder engagement, transparency, intersectionality, power awareness, and trauma-informed process) must permeate all phases. This cyclical approach ensures that evaluation findings directly inform practice refinement, creating systems that continuously evolve based on evidence and community feedback rather than remaining static after initial implementation.

Table 1. Multi-level assessment domains for trauma-informed system implementation

Assessment Level	Key Domains	Example Measures	Data Sources
Individual	Clinical outcomes, Service experience, Safety perceptions, Empowerment	ITQ, Patient satisfaction surveys, Re-traumatization incidents, Choice and voice measures	Clinical records, Service user surveys, Focus groups, Incident reports
Programmatic	Screening practices, Treatment fidelity, Environment safety, Cultural responsiveness	Screening rates, EBT implementation checklists, Environmental audits, Cultural competency assessments	Administrative data, File reviews, Observation protocols, Staff surveys
Organizational	Policy alignment, Workforce support, Leadership commitment, Resource allocation	Policy audits, Staff wellness measures, Budget analysis, Organizational climate surveys	Document review, HR data, Financial records, Leadership interviews
System	Cross-agency coordination, Policy advocacy, Community partnerships, Population outcomes	Referral networks, Policy tracking, Partnership assessments, Community health indicators	Cross-system databases, Legislative records, Community surveys, Population health data
Community	Collective efficacy, Cultural healing practices, Community trust, Social cohesion	Community surveys, Participatory assessments, Cultural practice documentation, Network analysis	Community forums, Ethnographic methods, Asset mapping, Resident interviews

7.1. Implementation Process Indicators

Process indicators track implementation activities and fidelity across phases. During the exploration phase, indicators include completion of organizational readiness assessments, engagement of diverse stakeholders in planning, identification of implementation champions, and development of logic models or theory of change frameworks. During preparation, indicators include completion of staff training, revision of policies and procedures to align with trauma-informed principles, environmental modifications to enhance safety, and establishment of data collection systems.

During active implementation, process indicators include rates of trauma screening and assessment, utilization of trauma-specific interventions, documentation of service user choice and voice in treatment planning, frequency of case consultation focused on trauma-informed approaches, and monitoring of environmental safety and triggers. Sustainment phase indicators include continued training for new staff, integration of trauma-informed principles into quality improvement processes, ongoing policy review and revision, and maintenance of workforce support systems.

7.2. Outcome Measurement Across Domains

Outcome measures must capture both intended positive changes and reduction in harmful practices. Individual-level outcomes include reduction in trauma symptoms, improved functional status, enhanced quality of life, increased hope and empowerment, and stronger connections to supportive relationships. Service experience outcomes include higher satisfaction ratings, perception of being treated with dignity and respect, involvement in decision-making, and absence of re-traumatizing experiences during service provision.

Organizational outcomes include decreased use of coercive interventions such as restraint, seclusion, or involuntary medication; reduced critical incident rates; improved staff retention and satisfaction; decreased burnout and secondary traumatic stress; and stronger organizational climate characterized by psychological safety and collaborative relationships. System-level outcomes include reduced unnecessary placements in restrictive settings, decreased involvement in juvenile justice or other punitive systems, improved coordination across service sectors, and population-level improvements in wellbeing indicators.

For community-based and collective healing approaches specifically, outcome measures should assess community-level changes including increased collective efficacy, stronger social cohesion, revitalization of cultural healing practices, enhanced community trust in institutions, and improved relationships between service systems and communities. These outcomes require methods beyond individual surveys, including community forums, participatory evaluation approaches, and cultural community indicators co-developed with community partners.

7.3. Equity and Disparities Monitoring

Comprehensive assessment frameworks must include systematic monitoring of equity and disparities. This requires disaggregating all process and outcome measures by relevant demographic and identity variables including race, ethnicity, language, immigration status, gender identity, sexual orientation, disability status, and socioeconomic position. Analyses should examine whether implementation reaches all populations equitably, whether practices are implemented with similar fidelity across groups, and whether outcomes improve comparably for all groups.

Importantly, equity monitoring should not only examine whether disparities narrow but also whether absolute outcomes improve for marginalized groups. An intervention that improves outcomes for everyone equally may reduce relative disparities while maintaining absolute gaps in wellbeing. Conversely, targeted interventions that improve outcomes primarily for marginalized groups can reduce absolute disparities while relative gaps persist due to historical and structural inequities. Both absolute and relative measures of disparity should be tracked to provide comprehensive understanding of equity impacts.

8. CHALLENGES AND FUTURE DIRECTIONS

Despite significant progress in conceptualizing and implementing trauma-informed systems, substantial challenges remain. This section examines persistent challenges while identifying promising directions for advancing the field.

8.1. Methodological Challenges

Purtle (2021) conducted a systematic review of evaluations of trauma-informed organizational interventions that include staff trainings, identifying significant methodological limitations across the literature. Most evaluations employed weak research designs without comparison groups, relied heavily on self-report measures susceptible to social desirability bias, focused on proximal outcomes like knowledge and attitudes rather than practice changes or client outcomes, and lacked sufficient follow-up to assess sustainability. These limitations make it difficult to draw firm conclusions about effectiveness or to identify which implementation strategies produce better outcomes.

Attribution poses particular challenges in system-level evaluation. When implementing comprehensive changes across multiple organizational levels simultaneously, isolating the effects of specific components becomes nearly impossible. Moreover, outcomes are influenced by countless factors beyond implementation efforts—including broader policy changes, economic conditions, community events, and natural variation over time. Sophisticated analytic approaches including quasi-experimental designs with propensity score matching, interrupted time series analyses, and comparative case studies can strengthen causal inference, but perfect experimental control remains elusive in real-world system transformation.

Measurement burden creates tensions between comprehensive assessment and practical feasibility. Organizations implementing trauma-informed approaches often have limited evaluation capacity and must balance measurement needs against service delivery demands. Overly burdensome evaluation can contribute to staff burnout and reduce enthusiasm for implementation. Future work should focus on developing brief, valid measures that provide actionable information without overwhelming systems. Technology-enabled data collection through electronic health records and automated data extraction can reduce burden while improving data quality and timeliness.

8.2. Sustainability and Scalability

Sustaining trauma-informed system transformation over time presents significant challenges. Initial enthusiasm and dedicated resources during implementation phases often wane as organizations face competing priorities, leadership changes, budget constraints, and staff turnover. Without ongoing attention and investment, trauma-informed practices may erode, policies may go unenforced, and organizational culture may revert to previous patterns. Building sustainability requires embedding trauma-informed principles into core organizational structures including hiring practices, performance evaluation, quality improvement processes, and budgeting rather than treating trauma-informed care as a special initiative.

Scaling successful implementation across diverse contexts raises questions about adaptation and fidelity. What works in one organizational or community context may not translate directly to others with different populations, resources, constraints, and cultures. Yet excessive adaptation may compromise core principles and effectiveness. Implementation science frameworks increasingly recognize the importance of planned, principled adaptation that maintains fidelity to core functions while allowing surface structure modifications to fit local contexts. Evaluation frameworks should track adaptations and examine their impacts on outcomes to build knowledge about when and how adaptation supports or undermines effectiveness.

8.3. Addressing Root Causes

A fundamental tension exists between trauma-informed approaches focused on ameliorating trauma impacts versus addressing root causes of trauma exposure. Bailey et al. (2021) argue compellingly that addressing racial health inequities requires confronting structural racism and racist policies that create differential trauma exposure and differential access to resources. While trauma-informed services can help individuals cope with trauma and reduce re-traumatization within service systems, they cannot eliminate trauma if the social conditions producing trauma remain unchanged.

Truly transformative trauma-informed approaches must therefore include explicit attention to prevention and social change alongside response and treatment. This means organizations implementing trauma-informed practices should also engage in advocacy for policies that reduce poverty, discrimination, violence, and other structural sources of trauma. It means building partnerships with community organizing efforts working to transform the social conditions that produce trauma. And it means recognizing that while trauma-informed services are necessary, they are not sufficient—fundamental social transformation is required to prevent trauma at its source.

8.4. Future Research Priorities

Several research priorities emerge from this analysis. First, the field needs rigorous effectiveness studies employing strong research designs to establish whether trauma-informed system implementation actually improves outcomes and to identify which implementation strategies and components are most impactful. Second, research should examine mechanisms of change—how and why trauma-informed approaches work when they do, and what barriers prevent success when they fail. Third, cost-effectiveness studies are needed to make the business case for trauma-informed implementation and guide resource allocation decisions.

Fourth, research should examine long-term sustainability and trajectories of implementation over extended timeframes. Most existing research captures early implementation phases; understanding what happens five or ten years later is essential for guiding efforts to maintain gains. Fifth, comparative effectiveness research should examine different models of trauma-informed implementation to identify optimal approaches for specific contexts. Sixth, research must center equity explicitly, examining whether trauma-informed approaches reduce or exacerbate disparities and identifying strategies that promote equitable implementation and outcomes.

Finally, research should examine community-based and collective healing approaches more thoroughly. The evidence base for these approaches remains limited despite their theoretical importance and community endorsement. Rigorous evaluation of collective healing interventions, using culturally appropriate methodologies and community-defined outcomes, could strengthen the empirical foundation while honoring community wisdom. Such research must be conducted in genuine partnership with communities, ensuring that research processes themselves embody trauma-informed and culturally responsive principles.

Emerging interdisciplinary research also offers instructive parallels for advancing trauma-informed evaluation methodology. Precision medicine approaches in oncology have demonstrated the value of multi-omic biomarker integration for capturing complex biological phenomena that resist reduction to single indicators—a lesson applicable to multi-dimensional trauma measurement. For example, Abuhassan et al. (2026a) showed that aptasensor platforms enable highly sensitive detection in colorectal cancer diagnostics, while Abuhassan et al. (2026b) demonstrated that multi-omic biomarker integration substantially improves diagnostic precision in ovarian cancer; analogously, trauma-informed evaluation would benefit from integrating multiple data streams rather than relying on any single outcome measure. Similarly, Abuhassan et al. (2026c) developed next-generation nano-biosensors for hepatocellular carcinoma that exemplify the precision achievable when detection tools are tailored to specific biological contexts—a principle that resonates with calls for culturally tailored assessment instruments in trauma research. Al-khreisat et al. (2026) highlighted the importance of examining microenvironment crosstalk in cancer stem cell plasticity, underscoring how contextual and relational factors shape outcomes; parallel attention to ecological context is equally essential in trauma-informed systems evaluation. AlRamadneh et al. (2025) examined miR-34-mediated regulation of apoptosis and autophagy in glioblastoma, illustrating how regulatory mechanisms operating at the molecular level can have cascading effects on cell fate—a dynamic that mirrors how policy and organizational changes cascade through service systems to affect individual outcomes. Farah et al. (2026) and Daoud et al. (2025) explored targeted delivery strategies for cancer stem cells using ferroptosis pathways and nanocarrier platforms respectively, reflecting a broader shift toward precision-targeted intervention that holds relevance for tailoring trauma-informed interventions to specific population subgroups. Torshizi et al. (2026) provided mechanistic insights into curcumin's regulation of NF-κB and Nrf2 inflammatory signaling pathways, illustrating how anti-inflammatory mechanisms operate at multiple molecular levels simultaneously—analogous to how trauma-informed interventions must address stress dysregulation at individual, relational, and systemic levels concurrently. Kenjayev et al. (2026) examined pH-sensitive nanoparticles in radiotherapy, demonstrating that responsiveness to environmental conditions can enhance therapeutic efficacy; similarly, trauma-informed interventions that are sensitive and adaptive to community context produce more effective outcomes. Khan et al. (2025) conducted a systematic review and meta-analysis on circulating tumor DNA as a predictive biomarker for postsurgical recurrence, underscoring the value of longitudinal biological monitoring—a design principle that informs recommendations for sustained longitudinal evaluation in trauma-informed implementation research. Finally, advances in artificial intelligence and machine learning offer promising tools for analyzing complex, high-dimensional evaluation datasets. Gupta et al. (2026a) examined digital hoboism within algorithmic culture, raising critical questions about how digital technologies reshape identity and belonging—considerations relevant to understanding how trauma-affected communities navigate digitally mediated service systems. Gupta et al. (2026b) addressed explainability and transparency requirements in AI architectures, issues of paramount importance when deploying algorithmic tools in social service evaluation contexts where accountability and interpretability are ethical imperatives. Taken together, these cross-disciplinary advances underscore the importance of methodological innovation, precision measurement, contextual sensitivity, longitudinal design, and technological transparency—principles that should guide the next generation of trauma-informed evaluation research.

9. CONCLUSION

This chapter has examined community-based and collective healing models within the context of trauma-informed system implementation, with particular attention to evaluation and measurement approaches. Several key themes emerge from this analysis. First, collective trauma requires collective healing—individual clinical interventions, while valuable, are insufficient for addressing traumas rooted in systemic oppression, historical injustice, and community violence. Community-based approaches that honor cultural practices, build collective efficacy, and address social determinants are essential complements to individual treatment.

Second, implementing trauma-informed approaches at the system level requires comprehensive organizational transformation extending far beyond training or program changes. Successful implementation demands attention to policies, practices, physical environments, workforce support, leadership commitment, and organizational culture. Partial implementation risks being ineffective or even harmful by creating expectations that cannot be fulfilled.

Third, evaluation of trauma-informed implementation must be comprehensive, culturally responsive, and equity-focused. Multi-level frameworks assessing process and outcomes across individual, programmatic, organizational, and system levels provide the most complete picture of implementation progress and impacts. Evaluation must move beyond narrow clinical outcomes to examine service experiences, organizational climate, workforce wellbeing, community partnerships, and population-level indicators. Moreover, evaluation must explicitly examine equity—disaggregating data by identity dimensions and assessing whether implementation reduces disparities in access, quality, and outcomes.

Fourth, cultural responsiveness and community partnership are not optional enhancements but essential elements of trauma-informed practice and evaluation. Conventional approaches developed without input from affected communities often fail to capture relevant experiences, outcomes, and healing processes. Participatory approaches that involve community members throughout evaluation—from question formulation through interpretation and use of findings—produce more valid, useful, and ethically sound knowledge while building community capacity and honoring community expertise.

Fifth, while trauma-informed approaches are necessary, they are not sufficient for eliminating trauma. Truly transformative approaches must address root causes—

confronting structural racism, economic inequality, violence, and other social conditions that produce trauma. Organizations implementing trauma-informed practices should simultaneously engage in advocacy and partnership with social change efforts working to transform these underlying conditions.

The field of trauma-informed care has made remarkable progress over the past two decades, moving from a relatively obscure concept to widespread adoption across multiple service sectors. This progress creates both opportunities and responsibilities. The opportunity is to leverage growing awareness and commitment to create systems that truly promote healing, reduce re-traumatization, and address historical and structural traumas. The responsibility is to ensure that trauma-informed becomes more than a buzzword—that implementation is deep and authentic rather than superficial, that evaluation is rigorous and culturally responsive, and that approaches evolve based on evidence and community wisdom.

Moving forward requires sustained commitment from multiple stakeholders. Researchers must conduct rigorous evaluation using strong designs, culturally appropriate methods, and meaningful outcomes while partnering authentically with communities. Practitioners must move beyond rhetoric to substantive practice changes while advocating for organizational and systemic transformation. Administrators must allocate resources, revise policies, and sustain culture change rather than treating trauma-informed care as a temporary initiative. Policymakers must create enabling conditions through funding, regulation, and policy that support trauma-informed approaches while addressing root causes of trauma exposure. And communities must be centered as knowledge holders and partners whose experiences, priorities, and wisdom guide all aspects of implementation and evaluation.

The comprehensive assessment framework proposed in this chapter provides a roadmap for evaluating trauma-informed implementation while centering community-based and collective healing approaches. By attending to multiple levels, employing mixed methods, prioritizing cultural responsiveness, monitoring equity, and partnering with communities, this framework aims to support both accountability and continuous improvement. Yet frameworks are only tools—their value depends on how they are implemented. Used mechanistically without attention to context and relationships, even well-designed frameworks can become instruments of surveillance rather than supports for healing. Used thoughtfully in partnership with affected communities, they can generate knowledge that advances justice and wellbeing.

Ultimately, the vision that should guide trauma-informed system transformation extends beyond reducing symptoms or preventing re-traumatization, important as those goals are. The deeper aspiration is to create systems and societies where all people can thrive—where trauma exposure is minimized through just social conditions, where healing resources are accessible to all who need them, where cultural practices and community wisdom are honored, where institutions operate with humility and accountability, and where collective wellbeing is prioritized alongside individual wellness. Achieving this vision requires not only trauma-informed services but fundamental transformation of the social structures that produce trauma. Community-based and collective healing models point toward this broader transformation, offering pathways for healing that acknowledge social ecology of trauma while honoring community resilience, cultural strength, and collective agency. Through rigorous yet humble evaluation that centers community partnership and equity, we can support this transformation while remaining accountable to those most affected by trauma and most invested in collective healing.

REFERENCES

Abuhassan, Q., Al-Assi, G., Rekha, M. M., Chanania, K., Bavanilatha, M., Arora, V., Sinha, A., & Hayitova, M. (2026b). Multi-omic biomarker detection in ovarian cancer. *Clinica Chimica Acta*, *581*, 120758. Advance online publication. DOI: 10.1016/j.cca.2025.120758 PMID: 41349936

Abuhassan, Q., Atoom, A. M., Roopashree, R., Kanwar, J. B., Sudhakar, T., Sharma, V., Chauhan, A. S., & Ruziyev, O. (2026a). Aptasensors in colorectal cancer: Emerging tools for precision diagnostics. *Clinica Chimica Acta*, *581*, 120751. Advance online publication. DOI: 10.1016/j.cca.2025.120751 PMID: 41352752

Abuhassan, Q., Saleh, K., Roopashree, R., Kanwar, J. B., Sudhakar, T., Sharma, V., Chauhan, A. S., & Khaitova, S. (2026c). Next-generation nano-biosensors for hepatocellular carcinoma. *Clinica Chimica Acta*, *555*, 120805. DOI: 10.1016/j.cca.2025.120805 PMID: 41461225

Al-khreisat, M. J., Abdulsahib, W. K., Jasim, I. K., Malathi, H., Nayak, P. P., Anand, D. A., Mukherjee, G., Sinha, A., & Ruziyev, O. (2026). Targeting cancer stem cell plasticity and tumor microenvironment crosstalk: A comprehensive review. *Discover. Oncology*, *17*(1), 145. DOI: 10.1007/s12672-025-04297-y PMID: 41422192

AlRamadneh, T. N., Abdulsahib, W. K., Ismael, S. H., Roopashree, R., Nayak, P. P., Nandhini, S. U., Arora, V., Chauhan, A. S., & Ruziyev, O. (2025). Crossroads of cell fate: miR-34-mediated regulation of apoptosis and autophagy in glioblastoma. *Discover. Oncology*, *16*(1), 2177. Advance online publication. DOI: 10.1007/s12672-025-04021-w PMID: 41313571

Bailey, Z. D., Feldman, J. M., & Bassett, M. T. (2021). How structural racism works—Racist policies as a root cause of U.S. racial health inequities. *The New England Journal of Medicine*, *384*(8), 768–773. DOI: 10.1056/NEJMms2025396 PMID: 33326717

Cloitre, M., Hyland, P., Prins, A., & Shevlin, M. (2021). The International Trauma Questionnaire (ITQ) measures reliable and clinically significant treatment-related change in PTSD and complex PTSD. *European Journal of Psychotraumatology*, *12*(1), 1930961. DOI: 10.1080/20008198.2021.1930961 PMID: 34211640

Conching, A. K. S., & Thayer, Z. (2021). Biological pathways for historical trauma to affect health: A conceptual model focusing on epigenetic modifications. *Social Science & Medicine*, *230*, 74–82. DOI: 10.1016/j.socscimed.2019.04.001 PMID: 30986608

Cronholm, P. F., Forke, C. M., Wade, R., Bair-Merritt, M. H., Davis, M., Harkins-Schwarz, M., Pachter, L. M., & Fein, J. A. (2021). Adverse childhood experiences: Expanding the concept of adversity. *American Journal of Preventive Medicine, 49*(3), 354–361. DOI: 10.1016/j.amepre.2015.02.001 PMID: 26296440

Daoud, E., Abdulsahib, W. K., Ismael, S. H., Roopashree, R., Ray, S., Nellore, J., Mukherjee, G., Chauhan, A. S., & Kholiyeva, M. (2025). Nanomedicine and nutraceutical-based nanocarriers for specific delivery to cancer stem cells: Targeted drug delivery at the STEM frontier. *Discover. Oncology*, *16*(1), 4057. DOI: 10.1007/s12672-025-04057-y PMID: 41286210

Ellis, B. H., Abdi, S. M., Lazarevic, V., White, M. T., Lincoln, A. K., Stern, J. E., & Horgan, J. G. (2021). Relation of psychosocial factors to diverse behaviors and attitudes among Somali refugee youth in the United States. *The American Journal of Orthopsychiatry*, *86*(4), 393–403. DOI: 10.1037/ort0000121 PMID: 26618939

Farah, H., Abdulsahib, W. K., Ismael, S. H., Roopashree, R., Ray, S., Nandhini, S. U., Arora, V., Chauhan, A. S., & Buriyeva, D. (2026). Emerging small molecule strategies target cancer stem cells through ferroptosis and metabostemness. *Discover. Oncology*, *17*(1), 111. DOI: 10.1007/s12672-025-04259-4 PMID: 41390898

Forkey, H., Szilagyi, M., Kelly, E. T., Duffee, J., Springer, S. H., Fortin, K., Jones, V. F., Vaden Greiner, M. B., Ochs, T. J., Partap, A. N., Davidson Sagor, L., Allen Staat, M., Thackeray, J. D., Waite, D., & Weber Zetley, L. (2021). Trauma-informed care. *Pediatrics*, *148*(2), e2021052580. DOI: 10.1542/peds.2021-052580 PMID: 34312292

Goodkind, J. R., LaNoue, M., Lee, C., Freeland, L., & Freund, R. (2021). Feasibility, acceptability, and initial findings from a community-based cultural mental health intervention for American Indian youth and their families. *Journal of Community Psychology*, *40*(4), 381–405. DOI: 10.1002/jcop.20517 PMID: 25414529

Gupta, D., Azizbek, I., Suxrob, P., & Abdullaeva, I. Ravshan kizi, B. M., Abdukabilovna, T. D., & Jumayev, U. (2026a). Digital hoboism. In E. Kaygisiz (Ed.), *Digital ideologies in the age of algorithmic culture* (pp. 307-338). IGI Global Scientific Publishing. https://doi.org/DOI: 10.4018/979-8-3373-4531-4.ch010

Gupta, D., Nigora, A., Gulkhayo, G., Nuriddin, E., Karimov, S., Otabek, M., & Kuanishbay, S. (2026b). Explainable and transparent AI architectures. In Pakshad, P., & Omar, M. (Eds.), *Examining vulnerabilities and adversarial exploitation of AI and LLMs* (pp. 297–324). IGI Global Scientific Publishing., DOI: 10.4018/979-8-3373-8252-4.ch011

Hanson, R. F., & Lang, J. (2021). A critical look at trauma-informed care among agencies and systems serving maltreated youth and their families. *Child Maltreatment, 21*(2), 95–100. DOI: 10.1177/1077559516635274 PMID: 26951344

Hatcher, S. S., Bride, B. E., Oh, H., King, D. M., & Catrett, J. F. (2021). An assessment of secondary traumatic stress in juvenile justice education workers. *Journal of Correctional Health Care, 17*(3), 208–217. DOI: 10.1177/1078345811401509 PMID: 21571748

Kassam-Adams, N., Marsac, M. L., Kohser, K. L., Kenardy, J., March, S., & Winston, F. K. (2021). A new method for assessing content validity in model-based creation and iteration of eHealth interventions. *Journal of Medical Internet Research, 17*(4), e95. DOI: 10.2196/jmir.3811 PMID: 25881584

Kenjayev, Y., Khalikova, N., Eshqobilov, O., Axmedov, U., Babamuratov, A., & Xursanov, A. (2026). Utilizing pH-sensitive nanoparticles in cancer radiotherapy: Mechanisms and therapeutic potential. *Journal of Nanoparticle Research, 28*(2), 36. DOI: 10.1007/s11051-026-06553-w

Khan, A. U., Jasim, Y. H., Shahid, K., Saidov, J., Atamuratova, Z., & Urazbaeva, D. (2025). Circulating tumor DNA as a predictive biomarker for colorectal cancer postsurgical recurrence: A systematic review and meta-analysis. *Clinical & Translational Oncology, 28*(4), 1348–1362. Advance online publication. DOI: 10.1007/s12094-025-04073-y PMID: 41107654

Levenson, J. (2021). Trauma-informed social work practice. *Social Work, 62*(2), 105–113. DOI: 10.1093/sw/swx001 PMID: 28339563

Liu, S. R., Kia-Keating, M., & Nylund-Gibson, K. (2021). Patterns of adversities and pathways to health among White, Black, and Latinx youth. *Child Abuse & Neglect, 86*, 89–99. DOI: 10.1016/j.chiabu.2018.09.007 PMID: 30273815

Marsac, M. L., Kassam-Adams, N., Hildenbrand, A. K., Nicholls, E., Winston, F. K., Leff, S. S., & Fein, J. (2021). Implementing a trauma-informed approach in pediatric health care networks. *JAMA Pediatrics, 170*(1), 70–77. DOI: 10.1001/jamapediatrics.2015.2206 PMID: 26571032

Miller, K. K., Brown, C. R., Shramko, M., & Svetaz, M. V. (2021). Applying trauma-informed practices to the care of refugee and immigrant youth: 10 clinical pearls. *Children (Basel, Switzerland), 6*(8), 94. DOI: 10.3390/children6080094 PMID: 31434278

Negi, N. J., Cepeda, A., & Valdez, A. (2021). Crime victimization among immigrant Latino day laborers in post-Katrina New Orleans. *Hispanic Journal of Behavioral Sciences*, *35*(3), 354–369. DOI: 10.1177/0739986313488089 PMID: 39371044

Oral, R., Ramirez, M., Coohey, C., Nakada, S., Walz, A., Kuntz, A., Benoit, J., & Peek-Asa, C. (2021). Adverse childhood experiences and trauma informed care: The future of health care. *Pediatric Research*, *79*(1), 227–233. DOI: 10.1038/pr.2015.197 PMID: 26460523

Palfrey, N., Reay, R. E., Aplin, V., Cubis, J. C., McAndrew, V., Riordan, D. M., & Raphael, B. (2021). Achieving service change through the implementation of a trauma-informed care training program within a mental health service. *Community Mental Health Journal*, *55*(3), 467–475. DOI: 10.1007/s10597-018-0272-6 PMID: 29705979

Purtle, J. (2021). Systematic review of evaluations of trauma-informed organizational interventions that include staff trainings. *Trauma, Violence & Abuse*, *21*(4), 725–740. DOI: 10.1177/1524838018791304 PMID: 30079827

Reeves, E. (2021). A synthesis of the literature on trauma-informed care. *Issues in Mental Health Nursing*, *36*(9), 698–709. DOI: 10.3109/01612840.2015.1025319 PMID: 26440873

Torshizi, S. S., Aboqader, R. F., Muhammadov, N., Khujaniyozova, O., Ruzmetova, Z., Hayitova, M., Shahreza, M. S., Girish, M. S., Dehkordi, F. S., & Vahed, S. (2026). Curcumin in redox and inflammatory signaling: Mechanistic insights into NF-κB and Nrf2 pathway regulation. *Journal of Chemical Health Risks*, *16*(1), 1–13. DOI: 10.60829/jchr.2025.1205763

Williams, M. T., Metzger, I. W., Leins, C., & DeLapp, C. (2021). Assessing racial trauma within a DSM-5 framework: The UConn Racial/Ethnic Stress & Trauma Survey. *Practice Innovations (Washington, D.C.)*, *3*(4), 242–260. DOI: 10.1037/pri0000076

Chapter 9
The Role of Advocacy, Policy, and Activism in Trauma Recovery:
The Politics of Recovery

Melissa Galica
http://orcid.org/0009-0001-1851-1998
Grand Canyon University, USA

ABSTRACT

This chapter argues that trauma recovery is inseparable from the systems that shape survivors' lives. Through the lenses of advocacy, policy, and activism, it demonstrates how trauma-informed care must extend beyond individual intervention to address the structural conditions that produce and perpetuate harm. Advocacy offers concrete, immediate support as survivors navigate housing, healthcare, employment, and legal systems. Policy establishes the broader conditions under which safety, stability, and access become possible. Activism mobilizes collective power to challenge inequities, shift narratives, and demand systemic change. Integrating these lenses reveals trauma recovery as both an individual and collective process, requiring coordinated efforts across practitioners, organizations, and communities. The chapter concludes with a call to stewardship, inviting readers to recognize their spheres of influence and to participate in creating conditions where justice, dignity, and healing can take root. Trauma-informed care becomes not only a practice, but a shared responsibility.

DOI: 10.4018/979-8-3373-8597-6.ch009

INTRODUCTION

Trauma research demonstrates that recovery does not unfold solely in therapy rooms or through individual coping strategies. It is shaped by the policies, institutions, and social conditions that structure people's lives. This chapter argues that advocacy, policy, and activism are not peripheral to trauma recovery but central to it; they are essential components of trauma-informed care when practiced through a social justice lens. To understand what recovery truly demands, we must look beyond the intrapsychic and into the environments that constrain or enable healing. The following stories illustrate how systemic forces shape survivors' daily realities and why recovery must be understood as both personal and political, grounded in lived experience as well as in theory.

A young mother in Detroit keeps a folder of hospital bills and denial letters, each one a reminder of how racial bias in maternal health care nearly cost her life. A disabled warehouse worker in El Paso carries human resources notices documenting repeated refusals to provide Americans with Disabilities Act accommodations, reminders that his body is seen as expendable. A refugee family in Minneapolis stores asylum paperwork in a plastic grocery bag as they navigate hearings that will determine whether they can remain together. A formerly incarcerated man in Atlanta keeps eviction notices folded in his pocket, each one a barrier to rebuilding stability after release. None of these folders contains therapy notes or symptom checklists. They contain evidence of institutional decisions that determine who is believed, who is protected, and who is repeatedly exposed to harm. Research across healthcare, labor, immigration, and reentry systems consistently documents these patterns of institutional harm.

Extensive research shows that through racialized healthcare, inaccessible workplaces, immigration courts, or discriminatory housing policies, the systems meant to support healing often deepen harm. Recovery is not only about managing symptoms or triggers; it is also about confronting the structures that reproduce injury and deciding what is required for safety to be more than an individual accomplishment. Every survivor's folder, literal or metaphorical, contains layers of systemic harm: denied claims, unanswered appeals, notices written in inaccessible language, and policies that assume a level of stability many survivors do not have. Trauma recovery is not simply clinical; it is political. Survivors are not only asking for grounding techniques or validation. They are asking for help navigating institutions that wound them, for someone to bear witness to the politics of their healing, and for interventions that shift the conditions of survival rather than asking them to adapt to injustice.

Operationalizing trauma-informed care through a social justice lens is therefore essential. Advocacy, policy, and activism are not adjuncts to recovery; they are ethical imperatives. As Bowen and Murshid (2016) argue, trauma-informed practice must include systemic advocacy to address the structural conditions that produce and perpetuate trauma. Without this engagement, practitioners risk reinforcing the very inequities that harm survivors, offering care that soothes in the moment while leaving the systems that continue to injure intact. A clinician who supports a survivor in coping with panic symptoms but remains silent about the housing policy that keeps them in a dangerous environment may inadvertently communicate that the problem lies within the survivor's reactions rather than the conditions they endure.

Intersectionality provides the critical lens for understanding how overlapping systems of oppression, racism, sexism, ableism, transphobia, xenophobia, and classism compound trauma and complicate recovery. A Black trans woman navigating homelessness or a disabled immigrant worker facing exploitation encounters forms of harm that cannot be reduced to a single axis of identity. Matthews et al. (2022) emphasize that trauma-informed care must be explicitly intersectional and culturally responsive, grounding clinical practice in an awareness of how structural inequities shape both risk and healing. Intersectionality is not an abstract concept in this context; it is a practical tool for understanding why some survivors face repeated exposure to violence, surveillance, or neglect even after engaging in services. Crenshaw's foundational work (1989) reminds us that identities do not exist in isolation, and that legal and institutional systems are often designed around single-axis categories that erase people whose lives intersect. Contemporary applications in trauma care underscore the need for culturally responsive, justice-oriented approaches that recognize how policies, policing practices, labor conditions, and immigration regimes distribute vulnerability unevenly. Bryant-Davis and Ocampo (2005) note that recovery from psychosocial trauma occurs within a cultural context of inequity and dehumanization, particularly for those at the margins whose experiences of racism and structural violence are too often pathologized rather than contextualized.

Scholars of trauma-informed care argue that operationalizing the model through a social justice lens means asking different questions. Instead of only "What happened to you?" practitioners must also ask, "What systems failed you?" "Who benefited from those failures?", and "How can we intervene collectively?" These questions reorient responsibility away from individual coping and toward shared accountability for the conditions that made the trauma possible and its aftermath so enduring. In this way, advocacy becomes more than support; it becomes solidarity. It is the practice of standing with survivors against the institutions that harm them, recognizing that healing requires both intrapsychic work and systemic change. To claim a trauma-informed stance without engaging these political dimensions is to offer care that soothes symptoms while leaving the machinery of harm untouched. A social justice lens insists that trauma-informed care must be both clinically skillful and structurally aware, committed not only to helping survivors endure unjust conditions but to transforming them.

ADVOCACY IN PRACTICE

Trauma-informed care literature consistently identifies advocacy as the bridge between survival and stability. It operates across multiple levels, direct and indirect, clinical and community, individual and institutional, and is always about helping survivors navigate systems that can feel opaque, hostile, or overwhelming. Advocacy is not an optional enhancement to trauma work; it is a core expression of trauma-informed principles, translating values like safety, empowerment, and collaboration into concrete action.

Consider the range of possibilities:

- A clinician writes a letter to a landlord invoking housing protections, preventing eviction for a survivor of domestic violence.
- A social worker accompanies a disabled employee to human resources meetings, ensuring Americans with Disabilities Act accommodations are honored.
- An advocate helps an immigrant family prepare documentation for asylum hearings, translating bureaucratic language into accessible steps.
- A community organizer connects formerly incarcerated residents to housing coalitions, challenging discriminatory rental practices.

Work across advocacy and social support consistently illustrates that what may look like small acts often carry far-reaching impact; micro-level support can reshape a survivor's sense of agency and strengthen the resilience of the communities around them. Advocacy is not only about resolving immediate crises; it is about dismantling barriers and amplifying voices that institutions too often silence. A single letter or clarified right can interrupt cycles of harm that have persisted for years, offering survivors a sense of possibility that extends beyond the moment of crisis.

For practitioners, advocacy often begins with small, concrete actions that help survivors navigate systems affecting their safety and stability. Studies of trauma-informed practice show that this may involve identifying which institutions are shaping a survivor's options, clarifying which rights or protections may apply, and collaborating with the survivor to determine what support feels both empowering and safe. Simple steps such as drafting a verification letter, making a warm referral, or helping a survivor prepare documentation can significantly reduce barriers without overstepping professional boundaries. These everyday acts translate trauma-informed principles into tangible support and communicate a powerful message: the survivor does not have to face dehumanizing systems alone.

Advocacy must be collaborative, consent-based, and paced with care for a survivor's readiness. Knight (2015) emphasizes that trauma-informed practice requires practitioners to navigate these decisions with attention to role boundaries, power dynamics, and the potential for inadvertently replicating coercive systems. For survivors with intersecting marginalized identities, this often means navigating systems never designed with their safety or dignity in mind. Advocacy, therefore, must be grounded in humility and guided by the survivor's own assessment of risk, capacity, and desire for engagement. This aligns with broader research emphasizing that trauma-informed practice requires attention to power, role clarity, and the risk of replicating coercive dynamics.

Empowering survivors to influence systems safely requires balance. As Knight (2015) cautions, practitioners must remain attuned to power dynamics and avoid replicating coercive structures. DePrince et al. (2016) argue that advocacy and social support are crucial buffers against the adverse effects of trauma. DePrince et al. (2016) note that victim advocates play a key role in connecting survivors with necessary resources and social support networks, often serving as the connective tissue between fragmented systems.

Advocacy also looks different across practice contexts. Clinicians in healthcare or mental health settings may focus on documentation, safety planning, or navigating insurance barriers, while social workers and case managers often engage directly with housing systems, public benefits, or legal protections. Community organizers and peer specialists may work at the level of collective action, resource mobilization, or community education. Educators and campus-based practitioners may advocate through policy interpretation, accommodation processes, or institutional accountability. Each role carries distinct opportunities and constraints shaped by licensure requirements, organizational culture, and the populations served.

Regardless of setting, however, the ability to engage in advocacy is shaped by the institutional contexts practitioners must navigate. Research on organizational trauma-informed care shows that these contexts include the policies, expectations, and role boundaries that define the environment in which practitioners operate. Documentation requirements, mandated reporting laws, billing structures, supervisory hierarchies, and agency protocols all influence what kinds of support are formally sanctioned. These conditions are not neutral; they reflect organizational cultures and regulatory histories that determine how much flexibility, creativity, or risk-taking a practitioner can safely engage in.

Within these institutional contexts, practitioners also encounter barriers: distinct but related constraints that limit their ability to act, even when they recognize a survivor's need. Barriers may include liability concerns, restrictive documentation rules, unclear role expectations, punitive supervision, or fear of institutional retaliation. These barriers often arise from the very structures in which practitioners work, creating tension between ethical commitments to survivors and practical realities of agency life. They can make even straightforward acts of advocacy feel fraught, especially for practitioners who hold marginalized identities or work in under-resourced settings.

These constraints do not negate the importance of advocacy; rather, they highlight the need for trauma-informed organizations that support ethical action, clarify role expectations, and create pathways for practitioners to engage in systemic work without risking professional repercussions. When organizations acknowledge both the contexts and the barriers practitioners face, they make it possible for advocacy to be sustainable rather than heroic and integrated rather than improvised.

Scholars of trauma-informed evaluation note that traditional clinical outcome measures often fail to capture the effects of reduced bureaucratic stress, increased safety, or improved access to resources. More meaningful indicators include whether a survivor gains clarity about their rights, experiences fewer system-related crises, or reports feeling more empowered and less alone when navigating institutions. Organizational outcomes such as improved coordination with community partners, reduced service barriers, or increased use of trauma-informed policies also signal effective advocacy. These forms of evaluation shift the focus from symptom reduction to systemic change, aligning measurement with the realities of trauma-informed, justice-oriented practice.

When practiced through a social justice lens, advocacy becomes more than support; it becomes solidarity. It is a collective commitment to justice, grounded in the recognition that trauma recovery requires not only individual healing but also the transformation of the systems that shape survivors' lives.

POLICY AS A DRIVER OF RECOVERY

Analyses of trauma and social policy show that while policy is commonly viewed as a bureaucratic backdrop, it in fact plays a central role in determining the conditions of survivors' daily lives. Policy determines who has access to safety, stability, and care; who is believed; who is surveilled; and who is repeatedly exposed to harm. It influences everything from housing eligibility to healthcare access, employment protections, immigration pathways, and the availability of community resources. For many survivors, policy is not abstract but provides the architecture of their survival. Understanding trauma recovery through a social justice lens requires recognizing policy as a living system that can either reinforce cycles of harm or create conditions in which healing becomes possible.

Studies of social policy show that policies operate at multiple levels: federal, state, local, and organizational. At each level, they shape the environments in which survivors attempt to rebuild their lives. Housing policies determine whether a survivor can leave an unsafe home without risking homelessness. Healthcare policies dictate whether trauma treatment is accessible or financially prohibitive. Employment policies influence whether a survivor can take time off for court hearings, medical appointments, or recovery without risking job loss. Immigration policies determine whether a survivor can seek protection without fear of detention or deportation. Even organizational policies such as documentation requirements, confidentiality rules, or eligibility criteria can either support or undermine a survivor's sense of safety and agency.

Bowen and Murshid (2016) argue that trauma-informed care must include systemic advocacy to address the structural conditions that produce and perpetuate trauma. Bowen and Murshid (2016) note that policies that appear neutral on paper often have disparate impacts on marginalized communities, reinforcing inequities that shape both exposure to trauma and access to recovery. For example, policies governing public benefits may require documentation that survivors do not have, impose work requirements that are unrealistic during a crisis, or create waiting periods that leave families without support during critical moments. These policy structures can retraumatize survivors by forcing them to repeatedly justify their needs, recount their trauma, or navigate systems designed without their realities in mind.

Intersectionality research demonstrates that policies distribute vulnerability. Crenshaw's (1989) work shows that laws and institutional systems often fail to account for the lived experiences of people whose identities intersect across race, gender, class, disability, and immigration status. Matthews et al. (2022) extend this insight to trauma-informed practice, emphasizing that culturally responsive, justice-oriented care must account for how policies disproportionately harm survivors at the margins. A policy that appears equitable in design may still produce inequitable outcomes when applied to communities facing structural racism, xenophobia, transphobia, or economic precarity. Trauma recovery cannot be disentangled from these policy landscapes.

Research on trauma-informed organizations shows that policies also shape the conditions under which practitioners operate. Organizational policies determine what clinicians can document, how they can communicate with external systems, and what forms of advocacy are formally sanctioned. These policies influence whether practitioners feel supported in challenging harmful systems or constrained by liability concerns and administrative expectations. Hopper et al. (2010) highlights the importance of trauma-informed organizational policies in homelessness services, noting that system-level change is necessary to prevent cycles of harm and support long-term stability. When organizations adopt trauma-informed policies such as flexible documentation practices, collaborative decision-making structures, or survivor-centered confidentiality protocols, they create environments where advocacy is not only possible but expected.

Policy engagement can take many forms. At the micro level, practitioners may help survivors understand their rights, complete applications, or navigate appeals processes. At the mezzo level, they may collaborate with community partners to address systemic gaps or advocate for organizational policy changes. At the macro level, practitioners may participate in coalitions, provide testimony, or contribute to policy development informed by lived experience. Each level of engagement reflects a commitment to addressing the structural determinants of trauma and expanding pathways to safety and healing.

Scholars of trauma-informed evaluation note that evaluating the impact of policy on trauma recovery requires attention to both individual and systemic outcomes. Traditional clinical measures may not capture the significance of a survivor securing stable housing, gaining access to healthcare, or receiving workplace accommodations. More meaningful indicators include reductions in bureaucratic stress, increased access to resources, improved coordination across systems, and greater alignment between policy and the lived realities of survivors. These forms of evaluation shift the focus from individual symptom reduction to structural change, aligning with the broader goals of trauma-informed, justice-oriented practice.

When viewed through a social justice lens, policy becomes more than a set of rules; it becomes a site of intervention. Trauma-informed practitioners recognize that healing requires not only individual support but also the transformation of the policies that shape survivors' lives. Engaging with policy is therefore an ethical imperative, grounded in the understanding that recovery is not solely a personal journey but a collective responsibility.

ACTIVISM AS COLLECTIVE HEALING

Across work on collective trauma and social movements, it becomes clear that while activism is frequently cast as political action, it also serves as a powerful site of collective healing for many survivors and communities. When trauma is rooted in systemic violence, racism, misogyny, xenophobia, homophobia, transphobia, ableism, and economic exploitation, individual recovery cannot be separated from the conditions that produced the harm. Activism becomes a way to transform personal pain into collective power, shifting the focus from "What happened to me?" to "What is happening to us, and how do we change it?" Through this lens, activism is not an optional extension of trauma-informed care; it is a pathway through which communities reclaim agency, dignity, and possibility.

Studies of collective healing show that activism creates spaces where survivors can see their experiences reflected, validated, and contextualized within broader patterns of injustice. Movements such as Black Lives Matter, #MeToo, disability justice organizing, immigrant rights coalitions, and Indigenous land and sovereignty movements demonstrate how collective action can interrupt the isolation that trauma often produces. These movements offer survivors a sense of belonging and solidarity, reminding them that their experiences are not the result of individual failure but responses to structural harm. In this way, activism becomes a counternarrative to the shame and self-blame that trauma can generate.

Research on social movements describes collective efficacy as the shared belief that change is possible. This belief is itself healing. When survivors participate in movements that challenge oppressive systems, they experience themselves not only as recipients of harm but as agents of transformation. This shift in identity can be deeply reparative, particularly for those whose trauma involved powerlessness, silencing, or erasure. Activism offers opportunities to reclaim voice, assert boundaries, and participate in shaping the conditions of one's community.

Community resilience shows that activism also functions as a form of community care. Mutual aid networks, grassroots organizing, and community-led safety initiatives often emerge in response to institutional failures. These efforts provide material support like food, housing assistance, transportation, childcare as well as emotional and relational support. They demonstrate that healing is not solely an individual endeavor but a collective responsibility. For communities disproportionately affected by trauma, activism becomes a means of building infrastructures of care that institutions have neglected or denied.

Activism is not limited to public protest or large-scale mobilization. It includes quieter forms of resistance: storytelling, art, cultural preservation, community education, and the creation of alternative spaces where marginalized identities are affirmed. These practices challenge dominant narratives and expand the possibilities for healing. They also honor the cultural and historical knowledge that communities carry, which has often been dismissed or pathologized within traditional systems of care.

Within trauma-informed organizing, one principle is constant: activism must be shaped by sustainability, consent, and an honest reckoning with the emotional labor of confronting systemic harm. Movements can reproduce the same inequities they seek to dismantle if they do not attend to power dynamics, accessibility, and the well-being of participants. Trauma-informed principles of safety, trustworthiness, collaboration, empowerment, and cultural humility offer a framework for building movements that are not only effective but also healing. When activism is grounded in these principles, it becomes a space where survivors can engage at their own pace, contribute in meaningful ways, and step back when needed without shame.

Historical analyses of social movements show that activism also plays a critical role in shaping policy and institutional change. Survivor-led movements have historically driven major shifts in public awareness, legal protections, and social norms. From domestic violence and sexual assault reforms to disability rights legislation and immigration protections, activism has been a catalyst for structural transformation. These changes, in turn, create conditions that support individual and collective recovery. In this way, activism and policy are intertwined: activism identifies the harm, articulates the need, and mobilizes the will for change; policy codifies that change into lasting structures.

When viewed through a social justice lens, activism becomes a form of collective healing that extends beyond individual recovery. It is a practice of imagining and building a world in which safety, dignity, and justice are not exceptional outcomes but shared realities. For survivors and communities impacted by trauma, activism offers not only a means of resistance but a pathway to reclaiming wholeness together.

INTEGRATING THE THREE LENSES

Scholarship on trauma-informed systems shows that advocacy, policy, and activism are often discussed as separate domains, but in trauma-informed, justice-oriented practice, they are deeply interconnected. Each lens illuminates a different dimension of how trauma is produced, sustained, and healed. When integrated, they offer a comprehensive framework for understanding recovery not only as an individual process but as a collective and structural one. This integration is essential for practitioners who aim to support survivors in ways that honor both their lived experiences and the systemic forces shaping their lives.

Advocacy addresses the immediate, concrete barriers survivors face as they navigate systems that can retraumatize or exclude them. It focuses on the micro and mezzo levels, helping individuals access resources, assert their rights, and move through institutional landscapes that are often hostile or confusing. Policy scholarship demonstrates that policy shapes the structural conditions that determine whether those resources and protections exist in the first place. It operates at the macro level, influencing the distribution of safety, stability, and opportunity across communities. Activism bridges these levels by mobilizing collective power to challenge harmful systems, shift public narratives, and demand policy changes rooted in lived experience. Together, these lenses create a feedback loop: advocacy reveals systemic gaps, activism mobilizes to address them, and policy codifies the changes needed to prevent future harm.

Scholars of trauma-informed care argue that integrating these lenses requires practitioners to adopt a broader understanding of their role. Trauma-informed care is not limited to symptom reduction or individual coping strategies; it involves recognizing how structural inequities shape exposure to trauma and access to recovery. Bowen and Murshid (2016) contend that trauma-informed practice must include systemic engagement to address the social determinants of health. Without this engagement, practitioners risk offering care that soothes in the moment while leaving intact the conditions that perpetuate harm. Similarly, Matthews et al. (2022) emphasize that culturally responsive, intersectional approaches are essential for understanding how overlapping systems of oppression, racism, sexism, ableism, and xenophobia compound trauma and complicate recovery. Integrating advocacy, policy, and activism ensures that trauma-informed care remains grounded in this intersectional reality.

A clinician may support a survivor in managing panic symptoms, but if the survivor remains in unsafe housing due to discriminatory policies, their recovery will be limited. A case manager may help a survivor access public benefits, but if those benefits are governed by punitive eligibility criteria, the survivor may remain trapped in cycles of instability. Activism and policy engagement expand the scope of what practitioners can influence, allowing them to address the root causes of harm rather than only its symptoms. This does not mean that every practitioner must become a policy expert or organizer; rather, it means recognizing that trauma recovery is shaped by systems and that practitioners have a role, however small, in shaping those systems in return.

Work on coordinated, trauma-informed systems underscores that integrating the three lenses strengthens collaboration across sectors. Trauma-informed care cannot be siloed within mental health or social services; it requires partnerships with legal advocates, housing organizations, healthcare providers, educators, community organizers, and policymakers. These collaborations create pathways for survivors to access comprehensive support and for practitioners to share knowledge about systemic barriers and opportunities for change. Hopper et al. (2010) highlight the importance of system-level alignment in homelessness services, demonstrating that meaningful change requires coordination across agencies and sectors. When practitioners work together across these boundaries, they create a more cohesive and responsive network of care.

Scholars of trauma-informed systems note that integrating advocacy, policy, and activism reframes trauma recovery as a collective responsibility. It challenges the notion that survivors must adapt to unjust conditions and instead asks what systems must change to support healing. This shift aligns with the core principles of trauma-informed care safety, trustworthiness, collaboration, empowerment, and cultural humility by recognizing that these principles cannot be fully realized within systems that perpetuate harm. Integrating the three lenses ensures that trauma-informed care is not only compassionate but also transformative, committed not only to helping survivors endure unjust conditions but to reshaping those conditions in pursuit of justice.

SUSTAINING THE WORK

Sustaining trauma-informed, justice-oriented practice requires more than individual commitment; it requires structures, relationships, and communities that make the work possible over time. Practitioners who engage in advocacy, policy, and activism often do so while navigating their own histories, identities, and vulnerabilities. They carry the emotional weight of witnessing systemic harm, supporting survivors through institutional failures, and confronting inequities that cannot be resolved through clinical skill alone. Without intentional practices of sustainability, the work can become overwhelming, leading to burnout, moral distress, or disengagement. Sustaining the work is therefore both an ethical responsibility and a collective endeavor.

Sustainability begins with recognizing that no single practitioner can hold the full burden of systemic change. Trauma-informed, justice-oriented care must be shared across teams, organizations, and communities. This includes building collaborative relationships, distributing responsibilities, and creating spaces where practitioners can reflect, debrief, and receive support. Organizational cultures play a critical role in this process. Policies that prioritize manageable caseloads, reflective supervision, interdisciplinary collaboration, and staff well-being are not luxuries; they are prerequisites for ethical practice. When organizations fail to support practitioners, the burden shifts onto individuals in ways that are neither sustainable nor just.

Sustaining the work also requires attending to the emotional and relational dimensions of advocacy, policy engagement, and activism. Practitioners must navigate the tension between hope and frustration, progress and setback, and possibility and limitation. This emotional labor is often invisible, yet it shapes the capacity to remain engaged. Practices such as reflective consultation, peer support, community care, and intentional rest help practitioners maintain connection to their values and to one another. These practices are not signs of weakness or retreat; they are strategies for resilience that honor the complexity of the work.

At the same time, sustainability demands humility and clear boundaries. Practitioners must recognize the limits of their roles and resist the pressure to compensate for systemic failures through personal overextension. Trauma-informed care is not about heroic individual effort; it is about collective responsibility and structural change. As Burstow (2003) argues, trauma work must account for the social and political conditions that produce harm, rather than locating trauma solely within the individual. When practitioners overidentify with the work or attempt to take on responsibilities beyond the scope of their role, they risk replicating the very dynamics of overwork, scarcity, and self-sacrifice that oppressive systems rely on. Sustainable practice requires pacing, discernment, and a commitment to working within one's scope while contributing to broader efforts for change. Sustaining the work also involves cultivating a long view of justice. Advocacy, policy change, and activism unfold over years, sometimes decades. Progress is often nonlinear and marked by setbacks, resistance, and slow-moving institutional shifts. Practitioners who remain grounded in community, connected to purpose, and supported by collective structures are better able to sustain engagement over time. This long view honors the reality that trauma recovery, whether individual or collective, is not a quick process but a sustained commitment to creating conditions in which healing is possible.

Ultimately, sustaining the work requires recognizing that trauma-informed, justice-oriented practice is not only about what practitioners do but about the systems they help shape. It is about building organizations that embody trauma-informed principles, policies that promote equity and safety, and movements that center the voices and leadership of survivors. When advocacy, policy, and activism are integrated and supported, they create pathways for both practitioners and survivors to move toward healing, dignity, and justice.

Sustaining the work is not the end of the story; it is the ongoing commitment that makes the story possible. It is the recognition that healing is a collective endeavor, and that justice is not a destination but a practice that requires courage, collaboration, and care over time.

A CALL TO STEWARDSHIP

The stories traced throughout this chapter, from the mother navigating racialized healthcare, to the disabled worker denied accommodations, to the immigrant family facing deportation, to the formerly incarcerated man struggling for housing, remind us that trauma recovery is inseparable from systemic engagement. Advocacy, policy, and activism are not adjuncts to care; they are ethical imperatives. We must also acknowledge that these stories are aspirational rather than representative. For every survivor who finds safety and a voice, countless others remain unheard, with their letters unanswered, their protections unenforced, and their trauma met with bureaucracy instead of care.

This chapter does not offer a blueprint but a possibility a glimpse of what could be if care were resourced, if policy were just, if activism were sustained. Our task is not to replicate outcomes but to multiply conditions and pose questions. What made recovery possible in these stories? Who showed up? What protections were implemented? What movements reached survivors? How can we make those answers more common?

Operationalizing trauma-informed care through a social justice lens means recognizing that every practitioner, educator, organizer, policymaker, and community member holds a sphere of influence. Within that sphere, we can challenge inequities, amplify survivor voices, and co-create conditions for healing. Stewardship does not require doing everything. It requires doing something that shifts the balance toward justice, dignity, and repair.

Start where you are. Learn the policies that shape your practice. Build relationships with advocates and organizers. Reflect on your own boundaries, biases, and capacities. And above all, remember that trauma-informed care is not only about what we do but also about what we are willing to change. Recovery is neither linear nor solitary. It is braided through relationships, institutions, and movements. Stewardship means tending to those braids, ensuring they hold, and weaving new strands where gaps remain.

The call is not to perfection but to presence. Not to heroism but to solidarity. Not to resilience alone but to justice. In answering this call, we move from containment to transformation and from intervention to liberation. We become stewards of healing not only for individuals but for the systems that shape their lives.

REFERENCES

Bowen, E. A., & Murshid, N. S. (2016). Trauma-informed social policy: A conceptual framework for policy analysis and advocacy. *American Journal of Public Health, 106*(2), 223–229. DOI: 10.2105/AJPH.2015.302970 PMID: 26691122

Bryant-Davis, T., & Ocampo, C. (2005). The trauma of racism: Implications for counseling, research, and education. *The Counseling Psychologist, 33*(4), 574–578. DOI: 10.1177/0011000005276581

Burstow, B. (2003). Toward a radical understanding of trauma and trauma work. *Violence Against Women, 9*(11), 1293–1317. DOI: 10.1177/1077801203255555

Crenshaw, K. (1989). Demarginalizing the intersection of race and sex: A Black feminist critique of antidiscrimination doctrine, feminist theory and antiracist politics. *University of Chicago Legal Forum, 1989*(1), 139–167. https://chicagounbound.uchicago.edu/uclf/vol1989/iss1/8

DePrince, A. P., Combs, M. D., & Shanahan, M. E. (2016). Victim advocacy, social support, and trauma recovery: Practice, research, and policy. *Journal of Interpersonal Violence, 31*(1), 110–118.

Hopper, E. K., Bassuk, E. L., & Olivet, J. (2010). Shelter from the storm: Trauma-informed care in homelessness services. *The Open Health Services and Policy Journal, 3*, 80–100. htttps://DOI: 10.2174/1874924001003020080

Knight, C. (2015). Trauma-informed social work practice: Practice considerations and challenges. *Clinical Social Work Journal, 43*(1), 25–37. DOI: 10.1007/s10615-014-0481-6

Matthews, C., Leary, K., & Ricks, E. (2022). Intersectionality and trauma-informed care: A framework for culturally responsive practice. *Journal of Counseling Psychology, 69*(3), 215–229. DOI: 10.1080/10926771.2019.1572403

Chapter 10
Building Trauma-Informed Systems:
Implementation and Evaluation

Samantha Swift
http://orcid.org/0009-0009-7690-3752
National Louis University, USA

ABSTRACT

This chapter explores the critical transition from individual trauma-informed clinical practice to the development of trauma-informed systems. While trauma-informed care is widely endorsed, the author argues that meaningful change requires institutional accountability and structural transformation across counseling, healthcare, and human service sectors. The chapter examines the organizational readiness and cultural foundations necessary to support trauma-informed values, emphasizing leadership commitment, workforce sustainability, and the mitigation of secondary traumatic stress. An intersectional lens examines how systems can actively prevent retraumatization for marginalized populations, particularly women and gender-diverse individuals. By distinguishing between program, organization, and system-level implementation, this chapter provides a practical roadmap for embedding safety and equity into policy. The author proposes specific evaluation strategies to move institutions beyond symbolic language toward measurable, sustainable, and transformative standards of care.

INTRODUCTION

The preceding chapters underscored how trauma is frequently embedded in systems of privilege and power. While trauma is traditionally viewed through the

DOI: 10.4018/979-8-3373-8597-6.ch010

lens of individual loss or displacement, it is frequently intensified by structural forces such as prejudice, detention, and institutional exclusion that reinforce vulnerability across intersecting identities (Middleton et al., 2019; Substance Abuse and Mental Health Services Administration [SAMHSA], 2014).

For marginalized communities, particularly women, Transgender and Gender Non-conforming (TGNC) individuals, and those navigating intersecting inequities of race, disability, and socioeconomic status, trauma is further compounded by a legacy of institutional betrayal and cultural invalidation. In these contexts, the systems intended to provide care can become sites of retraumatization (Peeren et al., 2025). As a result, trauma-informed care cannot remain confined to individual clinical skills. It must extend to systemic accountability and organizational transformation. As trauma-informed approaches continue to gain momentum across counseling and human service settings, an essential question emerges: how can institutions move beyond trauma-informed language to create trauma-informed systems that actively resist retraumatization, confront inequity, and sustain environments of safety, dignity, and empowerment?

THE IMPLEMENTATION GAP: RHETORIC VS. REALITY

A persistent challenge in current scholarship is the symbolic implementation of Trauma-Informed Care (TIC), in which organizations adopt trauma-informed language without operationalizing it at the structural level (Bargeman et al., 2022). This lack of conceptual clarity often leads to fragmented implementation and a failure to differentiate between individual program shifts and broader system-wide transformation (Avery et al., 2021). Such systemic failure often manifests as medical gaslighting, an ethical threat to patient autonomy where institutional norms invalidate the lived experience of service users (Bokek-Cohen & Gabay, 2025). In healthcare and child welfare, retraumatization frequently occurs not through malice, but through institutional norms that prioritize procedural efficiency over relational safety (Huo et al., 2023). Whether through coercive medical practices or the systemic disbelief of gender-based violence survivors, these dynamics highlight that trauma-informed change must move beyond staff training to address the institutional legacies that perpetuate harm (O'Dwyer et al., 2019).

ROADMAP FOR TRANSFORMATION

Sustainable transformation requires a shift from awareness to actionable infrastructure. While brief training may improve provider knowledge and comfort, meaningful outcomes depend on leadership engagement, financial investment, and intentional policy revision (Bills et al., 2023; Powers et al., 2024). Evaluation remains a missing link; without systematic measurement tools that look beyond staff satisfaction, TIC initiatives remain performative rather than transformative (Bargeman et al., 2022).

This chapter provides a practical and ethically grounded roadmap for building trauma-informed systems. By integrating systemic support, ethical accountability, and intersectional awareness, it explores how organizations can:

- Cultivate institutional readiness and transition from individual intent to consistent organizational enactment.
- Address power imbalances through community collaboration and service-user autonomy.
- Establish evaluation frameworks that measure safety and engagement for historically underserved populations.

Operationalizing these systems requires a shift from individual clinical competence to institutional accountability. This is not simply a philosophical shift; it is a structural mandate that ensures equity for both service users and the workforce.

Across the literature and applied examples presented in this chapter, three priorities emerge as central to trauma-informed systems transformation: (1) alignment between policy and practice, ensuring that organizational procedures consistently reflect trauma-informed values; (2) workforce sustainability as a structural condition of care, recognizing that staff well-being is essential to maintaining relational safety; and (3) evaluation frameworks that center service-user experience, particularly for those most impacted by systemic inequities. These priorities provide a guiding structure for translating trauma-informed principles into sustainable systems-level change.

FROM CLINICAL SENSITIVITY TO SYSTEMIC ACCOUNTABILITY

While clinical sensitivity is an essential entry point for trauma-informed care, it cannot serve as the endpoint. Lasting transformation requires a movement toward institutional accountability. Trauma-informed care (TIC) is fundamentally defined by a commitment to safety, trustworthiness, and cultural responsiveness (SAMHSA, 2014). However, as TIC transitions from a clinical trend to an institutional obligation, a critical disconnect has emerged. While individual providers are increasingly trained in the "Four Rs" (realizing, recognizing, responding, and resisting retraumatization), these efforts are often confined to interpersonal skills. While clinical sensitivity and relational attunement are foundational, they remain fragile if the broader organizational environment is rigid, under-resourced, or inequitable (Bargeman et al., 2022; Purtle, 2020).

THE INTEGRATION MANDATE: VERTICAL AND HORIZONTAL ALIGNMENT

Sustainable systemic change requires more than trauma-informed language. It demands structural alignment across three levels: program (clinical practices), organization (infrastructure and policy), and system (cross-sector networks) (Bargeman et al., 2022). To prevent institutional retraumatization, these levels must be synchronized through two forms of alignment:

- **Vertical Integration:** This ensures consistency across the organizational hierarchy. A system fails vertically when clinicians are trained in trauma-responsiveness, but intake protocols remain shaming, or administrative policies prioritize productivity over relational safety.
- **Horizontal Integration:** This addresses the fragmentation of care across intersecting sectors, such as healthcare, child welfare, and legal systems. For a survivor of intimate partner violence, a lack of horizontal integration results in a "retraumatization loop," where conflicting agency requirements and repeated disclosures act as barriers to safe access (Cronholm & Dichter, 2018).

The necessity of horizontal alignment is most visible when examining the trajectory of service users navigating multiple bureaucracies. For example, a woman experiencing intimate partner violence (IPV) may seek counseling for anxiety and trauma symptoms while simultaneously interacting with primary healthcare, law enforcement, housing services, family court, and community advocacy organizations. If these systems operate independently, she is often forced into a "retraumatization loop," where she must repeatedly disclose traumatic experiences, navigate conflicting agency recommendations, and encounter institutional responses that feel dismissive or coercive (Cronholm & Dichter, 2018; Bargeman et al., 2022). In contrast, horizontal integration involves coordinated referral pathways and shared trauma-informed protocols that allow services to respond in ways that promote safety and continuity of care. Without this structural mandate, individuals experience inconsistent standards of care, increasing the likelihood of institutional betrayal.

The Cost of Symbolic Implementation

When organizations adopt TIC language without building the necessary infrastructure, the ethical burden of care falls on individual providers. This performative adoption leads to a crisis of sustainability marked by vicarious trauma and burnout. Ultimately, TIC must move from a personal clinical responsibility to a systems-level accountability process.

The following table highlights the critical priorities for transitioning from traditional, compliance-based models to empowerment-based systems.

Table 1. Realignment from compliance to accountability

Feature	Traditional/Compliance System	Trauma-Informed/Accountable System
Primary Goal	Clinical stability; rule adherence	Safety, trust, and autonomy (SAMHSA, 2014)
Power Dynamics	Hierarchical; provider-led	Collaborative; service-user sovereignty (Elliott et al., 2005)
"No-Show" Policy	Punitive; discharge or fees	Analytical; inquiry into systemic barriers (Stanton et al., 2025)
Evaluation	Volume-focused (Output metrics)	Experience-focused (Safety outcomes) (Goldstein et al., 2024)

OPERATIONALIZING CHANGE: FROM INDIVIDUAL CARE TO SYSTEMIC ACCOUNTABILITY

A trauma-informed system is defined by the consistent enactment of values—safety, transparency, collaboration, and empowerment—across every organizational layer. This shift moves beyond procedural adjustments toward a fundamental cultural realignment (Bargeman et al., 2022; SAMHSA, 2014). To achieve this, institutions must examine how existing institutional practices, such as policies that restrict autonomy or environments that compromise privacy, unintentionally replicate dynamics of powerlessness and control.

Meaningful transformation requires an organization-wide commitment that extends to every staff role. Because the first point of contact for a service user is often a receptionist, security officer, or billing representative, these early interactions dictate whether an individual experiences safety or institutional betrayal (Bills et al., 2023). Without structural support for workforce resilience, including reflective supervision and manageable workloads, these initiatives remain fragile and prone to surface-level implementation rather than lasting change (Elisseou et al., 2024; Purtle, 2020).

INTERSECTIONAL CONSIDERATIONS AND INSTITUTIONAL TRUST

Trauma-informed systems must be grounded in equity, recognizing that trauma is intensified by racism, sexism, and social marginalization. These forces do not merely exist alongside trauma; they shape both the exposure to harm and the subsequent access to supportive services. To move beyond a universalized model, systems must incorporate justice-oriented practices that address how power imbalances manifest during help-seeking.

For example, consider the trajectory of a Black woman seeking care after intimate partner violence (IPV) in a hospital emergency department. If staff focus narrowly on physical injuries while failing to provide relational safety, the system risks misinterpreting her guardedness or mistrust as "noncompliance" or "aggression." This lack of intersectional awareness can lead to shorter interactions, less information offered, or security involvement, effectively transforming a site of care into a site of surveillance and judgment (Cronholm & Dichter, 2018; Peeren et al., 2025). For women and transgender/gender non-conforming (TGNC) individuals and those navigating the compounding inequities of racism, disability, and socioeconomic marginalization, a trauma-informed system must actively resist these institutional legacies by:

- **Prioritizing Relational Safety:** Ensuring staff are trained in cultural humility to recognize how historical bias shapes current behavior.
- **Safeguarding Autonomy:** Revising invasive procedures and documentation practices to prioritize consent and choice over procedural efficiency (Peeren et al., 2025).
- **Centering Service-User Sovereignty:** Incorporating feedback from those most impacted by systemic harm to ensure safety definitions are grounded in lived reality rather than dominant cultural assumptions (Clements et al., 2020; Elliott et al., 2005).

SUSTAINING THE STRUCTURAL MANDATE

Ultimately, the transition from trauma-informed *care* to trauma-informed *systems* reflects a shift from individual to institutional responsibility. Success in this realignment is not measured by the presence of a "trauma-informed" mission statement, but by the policies, leadership practices, and accountability mechanisms that determine whether safety and empowerment are consistently enacted across all professional roles.

ENGINEERING CHANGE: THE ARCHITECTURE OF INSTITUTIONAL READINESS

Organizational readiness is the bridge between adopting trauma-informed language and sustaining systemic change. It is not a static status, but a dynamic measure of an institution's infrastructure and its cultural capacity to absorb transformation (Robey et al., 2021; Yatchmenoff et al., 2017). To move beyond surface-level policies, organizations must evaluate readiness across three primary domains: Cultural Foundations, Structural Integrity, and Macro-Level Resource Alignment.

1. Cultural Foundations and Leadership Commitment

Readiness begins with a shift in the organizational culture. This requires leadership to move beyond mission statements and embed trauma-informed values into the actual mechanics of supervision and communication.

- **Active Alignment:** Leadership commitment is demonstrated when executive decisions prioritize relational safety over rigid compliance. This includes revising intake protocols to ensure privacy and dignity and ensuring that communication norms across all staff reflect a shared language of respect and transparency (Bills et al., 2023; Purtle, 2020).
- **Reflective Accountability:** A ready system fosters an environment where power dynamics are regularly evaluated through reflective supervision. This ensures that the organization remains responsive to the needs of both service users and the workforce, laying a foundation for systemic safety to take root (Robey et al., 2021).

2. Structural and Financial Integrity

Readiness at this level is defined by the tangible realignment of resources to support systemic integrity. Because systemic failure is often a function of macro-level constraints rather than a lack of institutional will (Purtle, 2020), organizations must transition from figurative support to material investment.

- **Workforce Infrastructure:** This involves formalizing protected training time and integrating trauma-informed metrics into standard performance reviews. Sustainable systems move beyond one-time workshops to ongoing, multi-role training that is structurally supported by manageable caseload expectations (Bills et al., 2023; Robey et al., 2021).
- **Environmental Safety:** Readiness includes the physical and fiscal capacity to modify service environments. This ensures that privacy, accessibility, and relational safety are embedded into the organization's capital and operational budgets (Bargeman et al., 2022).
- **Supervisory Support:** A structurally ready system invests in reflective supervision models that address vicarious trauma as a collective organizational responsibility rather than an individual provider's self-care task (Elisseou et al., 2024).

3. A Synthesis of Readiness: The Implementation Framework

To synthesize these requirements for practitioners, organizational readiness can be evaluated through the following hierarchy of needs:

- **Level 1: Foundational Readiness (Culture):** Leadership buy-in, psychological safety for staff, and a shift from punitive to restorative policy.
- **Level 2: Structural Readiness (Capacity):** Financial investment in training, adequate staffing levels, and physical environments that promote safety.
- **Level 3: Strategic Readiness (Accountability):** Ongoing performance evaluation and feedback loops that incorporate service-user voices (Bargeman et al., 2022; SAMHSA, 2014).

THE HUMAN INFRASTRUCTURE: SUSTAINING WORKFORCE AND CULTURE

For a trauma-informed system to move beyond a procedural adjustment, staff well-being must be a structural necessity. When organizations fail to address the systemic roots of secondary traumatic stress, a dangerous mirroring occurs: the institution expects clinicians to provide relational safety while forcing them to operate in a state of chronic overwhelm and zero control (Elisseou et al., 2024; Robey et al., 2021). Consider a therapist in a high-volume clinic who must transition immediately from a session involving severe violence to a new appointment due to rigid productivity quotas. When forced to shut down emotionally as a survival mechanism, the clinician inadvertently creates a lack of safety for the next client. In this scenario, the organizational policy has authored the retraumatizing environment (Elisseou et al., 2024). True sustainability requires a transition from individual "self-care" to collective organizational responsibility. This involves:

- **Structural Buffers:** Implementing buffer time between high-acuity sessions and maintaining manageable caseloads.
- **Reflective Supervision:** Normalizing emotional processing and psychological safety within internal workplace relationships (Bills et al., 2023).
- **Unified Frontline Engagement:** Ensuring that relational safety is enacted at every touchpoint, preventing the breakdown of trauma-informed principles at the system's most vulnerable points of entry (SAMHSA, 2014).

MEASURING SUCCESS: FROM RHETORIC TO ACCOUNTABILITY

To ensure trauma-informed implementation moves beyond surface-level language and behaviors, organizations must utilize structured assessment processes that bridge the gap between rhetoric and reality (Kim et al., 2021). Emerging research on trauma-informed care training initiatives in healthcare settings suggests that while training improves provider knowledge and attitudes, sustained change depends on ongoing structural support and evaluation (Choi et al., 2024). Success in a trauma-informed system is evidenced when evaluation metrics shift from traditional, volume-based outputs (e.g., number of clients served) to relational outcomes, such as:

- **Service-User Safety Ratings:** Explicitly measuring whether clients felt a sense of choice, dignity, and psychological safety during high-vulnerability points, such as intake or crisis intervention.
- **Policy-Practice Alignment:** Utilizing organizational self-assessment tools to identify and revise punitive behavioral policies or surveillance-based routines that contradict trauma-informed values (Yatchmenoff et al., 2017).
- **Long-term Stability:** Monitoring the retention of master's-level clinicians and the continuity of care as primary indicators of a healthy, sustainable organizational climate.

STRATEGIC ALIGNMENT: POLICY, EQUITY, AND CROSS-SECTOR DESIGN

If institutional readiness is the foundation, then strategic alignment is the construction of the trauma-informed system. This requires moving beyond general principles toward a justice-oriented design that addresses the specific barriers faced by marginalized communities (Peeren et al., 2025; SAMHSA, 2014).

1. Policy Review and Procedural Justice

Meaningful transformation often occurs through routine procedures. Implementation is strongest when organizations move to establish a shared operational definition of care and clarify measurable goals (Berring et al., 2024). This requires a systematic audit of high-vulnerability points:

- **Intake and Documentation:** Organizations must evaluate whether intake requirements, such as requiring disclosure of trauma in public waiting rooms, unintentionally replicate surveillance dynamics. Transitioning to choice-based disclosure and transparent confidentiality protocols is a primary step in resisting institutional gaslighting (Bokek-Cohen & Gabay, 2025).
- **Compliance vs. Inquiry:** Rather than labeling clients who miss appointments as "noncompliant," trauma-informed systems adopt an analytical inquiry into systemic barriers, such as housing instability or transportation barriers (Stanton et al., 2025).
- **Relational Safety in Healthcare:** As noted in healthcare settings, technical competence is insufficient without relational safety. For survivors of sexual violence, this means revising medical protocols (e.g., pelvic exams) to prioritize explicit consent-checking and trauma-responsive communication (Peeren et al., 2025).

2. Cross-Sector Integration and Community Sovereignty

Trauma-affected individuals frequently move between disconnected bureaucracies, healthcare, legal, and social services. Fragmented care leads to repeated disclosure and inconsistent safety standards (Bargeman et al., 2022).

- **The Continuity Mandate:** For survivors of intimate partner violence, implementation success depends on coordinated referral pathways that prevent the "retraumatization loop" previously discussed (Cronholm & Dichter, 2018).

- **Service-User Sovereignty:** Equity-centered design requires the meaningful inclusion of those most impacted by systemic harm. Trauma-informed systems are strengthened only when service-user perspectives shift from feedback to active roles in program planning and evaluation (Clements et al., 2020; Elliott et al., 2005).

3. Long-Term Sustainability and Policy Environments

Finally, the transition to a trauma-informed system must be durable. Sustainability research emphasizes that large-scale change requires coordinated planning that outlasts the initial rollout (Sebton et al., 2025). This includes:

- **Onboarding and Professional Development:** Embedding TIC into the DNA of the organization through onboarding and continuing education, rather than one-time workshops (Powers et al., 2024).
- **Policy-Level Support:** Recognizing that organizational efforts are often limited by broader funding and policy environments. Trauma-informed systems must advocate for macro-level shifts in reimbursement and staffing structures to prevent the ethical burden from falling solely on individual providers (Purtle, 2020).

THE MACRO-LEVEL LANDSCAPE: POLICY AND REGULATORY DRIVERS

While individual organizations may commit to trauma-informed transformation, they do not operate in a vacuum. Systemic change is often throttled by macro-level policy environments that prioritize risk mitigation and cost-containment over relational safety.

- **The Policy-Practice Friction:** Reimbursement structures in community mental health frequently use "Fee-for-Service" models that pay only for direct, face-to-face clinical time. This fiscal policy creates an active barrier to the human infrastructure; it leaves no billable room for reflective supervision or buffer time. To resolve this, trauma-informed systems must advocate for value-based care models that incentivize long-term wellness and workforce stability over high-volume throughput (Purtle, 2020).
- **Regulatory Surveillance vs. Trauma-Informed Values:** In sectors like child welfare, state-level oversight often defaults to a surveillance framework. When policy dictates that safety is measured by the absence of incidents rath-

er than the presence of empowerment, institutions are structurally incentivized to maintain an infrastructure of control. Moving beyond this requires shifting policy to a systems-level accountability framework where funding is tied to safety outcomes and staff retention (Bills et al., 2023)

THE ACCOUNTABILITY FRAMEWORK: MECHANISMS OF SYSTEMIC EVALUATION

To move from awareness to action, organizations must implement a multi-layered evaluation strategy that audits system reliability (Berring et al., 2024; Purtle, 2020). Specific mechanisms required to measure organizational transformation are as follows:

1. The Infrastructure Audit

This evaluates whether the system's routines align with trauma-informed values. It requires a formal review of the previously discussed organizational structure.

- **Procedural Scrub:** A systematic review of intake and discharge bylaws. This involves identifying and removing punitive defaults, such as automatic discharge for missed appointments, and replacing them with mandatory analytical inquiry into systemic barriers, such as housing or transportation (Stanton et al., 2025).
- **The Resource Allocation Check:** A quantitative audit of staff schedules and budgets. A ready system must demonstrate protected time for reflective supervision and post-crisis debriefing. If these minutes are not formally accounted for in the operational budget, the system is structurally failing despite its mission statement (Huo et al., 2023).

2. Relational Safety Assessments

Meaningful evaluation must prioritize the voices of those historically harmed by institutional systems (Clements et al., 2020). This audit moves from "satisfaction" to relational safety metrics.

- **Autonomy Verification:** Implementation of setting-specific indicators that measure service-user choice. For survivors of sexual violence, success is measured by direct data on whether they felt they were explicitly asked for consent for any procedure or exam, could pause or decline a medical exam or procedure, or refuse a specific documentation question without consequence (Peeren et al., 2025).

- **Engagement Tracking:** Shifting metrics from "compliance" (program completion) to relational engagement. If a specific department shows high disengagement after crisis-level interventions, that protocol is flagged for an immediate trauma-informed redesign (Goldstein et al., 2024).

Case Illustration: Intersectional Safety in Women's Healthcare

Consider the experience of "Elena," a transgender woman of color and survivor of sexual violence, entering a large urban health center. In a compliance and productivity-based model, Elena's safety is compromised before she ever sees a provider. The system's intake protocol, a productivity-first triage model, requires her to disclose her trauma and gender history on a standardized form in a high-traffic waiting room. When she enters the exam room, the provider, pressured by rigid volume-based quotas, defaults to a clinical compliance mode. The pelvic exam is conducted with minimal communication, and the provider misinterprets Elena's physical guardedness as difficult behavior. Because the system prioritizes procedural efficiency over relational safety, Elena experiences medical gaslighting and disengages from care, feeling processed rather than seen (Peeren et al., 2025; Bokek-Cohen & Gabay, 2025).

To resolve this, the center transitions to an accountable system using justice-oriented design. They move Elena's trauma-history disclosure to a choice-based model, where initial screenings are conducted privately and at the patient's pace. Most significantly, the clinic formalizes a pause protocol. Before any invasive procedure, the providers are trained to establish a non-verbal stop signal to build safety and trust. This allows Elena autonomy and control over her own care. By shifting the power dynamic and giving her absolute sovereignty over the pace of the exam, the clinic honors her intersectional identity as a survivor who requires bodily autonomy. This case demonstrates that safety is not an abstract feeling, but a procedural outcome of giving the patient actual control (Goldstein et al., 2024).

3. The Mirroring Metric (Workforce Sustainability)

Because a system cannot ensure client safety if it fails to offer the same to its staff, workforce health is a primary indicator of system health (Stanton et al., 2025).

- **Turnover and Stability:** Treating high turnover in master's-level clinicians as a systemic failure of the human infrastructure rather than an HR issue.

- **Climate Feedback Loops:** Using regular, anonymous psychological safety surveys to determine if staff feel empowered to report institutional errors without fear of retaliation, a key indicator of a restorative vs. a punitive culture (Elisseou et al., 2024).

CASE ILLUSTRATION: NAVIGATING STRUCTURAL PATERNALISM IN RURAL CARE

Amara, a first-generation West African immigrant living in an isolated rural county, is navigating both significant language barriers and severe socioeconomic instability. Amara seeks support at a local community health center for symptoms of complex trauma. Under a system of structural paternalism, Amara's care is dictated by rigid institutional requirements that ignore her lived reality. The center's attendance policy, one based on compliance, mandates that two missed appointments result in an automatic administrative closure of her file. This policy fails to account for Amara's reliance on a fragmented rural bus system, or for her low-SES status, which means she cannot afford the no-show fees the clinic uses to recoup costs.

In this environment, Amara's clinician is also overburdened by an inequitable system. Carrying an unrealistically large caseload and lacking any buffer time for cultural consultation, the clinician misinterprets Amara's missed appointments as a lack of motivation or resistance to treatment. Because the system is designed for surveillance and rule-following rather than relational safety, Amara is discharged from the program during a period of high vulnerability, reinforcing her mistrust of Western institutional systems (Stanton et al., 2025).

To transform this, the center's leadership implements a sustainability framework. They move away from structural paternalism by eliminating the two-strike discharge rule and replacing it with a mandatory analytical inquiry. Now, when Amara misses an appointment, the system's default is not a penalty, but a collaborative outreach. The clinic also reallocates a portion of its administrative budget to fund a part-time community health liaison who understands Amara's cultural context and transportation barriers.

By treating workforce health as a mirroring metric, the clinic also reduces clinician caseloads, enabling paid, reflective supervision. This structural shift provides Amara's clinician the psychological bandwidth necessary to move beyond a compliance-only mindset toward a practice of cultural humility. In this space, the clinician is no longer simply performing a technical assessment; they are engaging in a continuous process of self-critique and power-redressing, acknowledging how their own institutional position may unintentionally mirror the systemic barriers Amara faces as an immigrant.

Rather than aiming for a static cultural competence, which often risks stereotyping intersectional identities, the clinician utilizes this protected time to listen for the specific survival needs Amara expresses. For Amara, this transition means she is no longer being managed by a bureaucracy but is supported by an infrastructure that treats her cultural context and safety as primary clinical outcomes rather than administrative hurdles (Bills et al., 2023; Elisseou et al., 2024).

SUSTAINING THE SHIFT: FROM IMPLEMENTATION TO INSTITUTIONAL PERMANENCE

Many TIC initiatives fail because they rely on the extraordinary effort of a few dedicated staff members who lack the systemic authority to sustain the work. When these individuals leave, the initiative often suffers a decay effect. To move beyond this, sustainability requires a policy anchor. This includes the legal and contractual mechanisms that ensure trauma-informed values survive leadership turnover and budget cycles. TIC principles must be written into the organization's bylaws, personnel manuals, and union contracts. When trauma-responsiveness is a contractual expectation rather than a philosophy, it becomes immune to budget cuts

The Three Bolts of the Policy Anchor

1. The Governance Bolt (Bylaws & Charters)

Institutional permanence begins by writing TIC principles into the organization's primary governing documents and bylaws. This ensures that relational safety is a foundational mandate that the Board of Directors must uphold, making the initiative immune to shifting administrative priorities. This bolt is reinforced by data-feedback loops, such as permanent service-user councils (e.g., involving individuals like Elena and Amara), ensuring safety definitions remain grounded in lived reality rather than administrative assumptions (Yatchmenoff et al., 2017; Sebton et al., 2025).

2. The Workforce Bolt (HR & Successor Strategy)

TIC must shift from a philosophy to a contractual expectation. This involves integrating trauma-informed competencies into job descriptions, personnel manuals, and union contracts. Furthermore, a successor strategy ensures that new leadership is vetted specifically for their ability to maintain the human infrastructure, preventing the initiative from fading when key advocates depart (Elisseou et al., 2024).

3. The Fiscal Bolt (Resource Allocation)

Sustainability is a financial decision. A policy anchor requires that reflective supervision and buffer time are not disposable and are embedded into the core operating budget. By transitioning to value-based oversight, the system rewards long-term engagement and safety outcomes rather than just volume-based outputs (Purtle, 2020).

NAVIGATING SYSTEMIC TENSIONS: BARRIERS TO SUSTAINED TRANSFORMATION

While the principles of trauma-informed care (TIC) are rarely disputed, the implementation gap persists due to three primary systemic tensions. Navigating these requires addressing the structural misalignment between institutional mandates and trauma-responsive values (Huo et al., 2023; Robey et al., 2021).

1. The Productivity vs. Presence Paradox

A significant barrier to implementation is treating TIC as an add-on task rather than an integrated operational model. When clinicians are mandated to provide empowering care while simultaneously meeting rigid, volume-based productivity quotas, the result is chronic workforce strain and secondary traumatic stress (Eliseou et al., 2024). This often manifests as a barrier where staff may bypass trauma assessments because they lack the structural buffer time to ethically manage a disclosure (Huo et al., 2023).

2. Structural Depletion and Rural Disparity

In rural and safety-net systems, chronic underfunding creates a depletion effect, in which implementation fades once initial training funds are exhausted (Purtle, 2020). Without a dedicated financial infrastructure for ongoing supervision and staff coverage, trauma-informed initiatives remain fragile and susceptible to implementation fatigue (Bills et al., 2023).

3. Institutional Legacy and the Infrastructure of Control

In sectors such as child welfare, justice, and restricted psychiatric settings, a fundamental tension exists between the institutional mandate of surveillance and the trauma-informed value of autonomy (Middleton et al., 2019). In these environments, the system's perceived need for control often overrides the survivor's requirement for relational safety, leading to a cultural resistance that cannot be solved by training alone (O'Dwyer et al., 2019).

CONCLUSION

The transition from trauma-informed *care* to trauma-informed *systems* represents an ethical shift from clinical sensitivity to institutional accountability. As this chapter has argued, moving past surface-level implementation requires a practical investment in the human infrastructure, reflective supervision, manageable workloads, and the formal embedding of TIC into the organization's DNA through onboarding and performance metrics (SAMHSA, 2014; Purtle, 2020).

Ultimately, a trauma-informed system is defined by its equitable enactment. It requires a proactive commitment to addressing power imbalances for those whose trauma is compounded by institutional mistrust, specifically women, transgender and gender-nonconforming (TGNC) individuals, and those navigating intersecting identities (Peeren et al., 2025).

True transformation is not found in a mission statement, but in the moments of service delivery: the intake call, the discharge decision, the billing interaction, and the supervisory response to a crisis. When organizations move beyond rhetoric and anchor their work in measurable accountability and justice-oriented design, trauma-informed care ceases to be a specialized initiative. It becomes the woven-in, expected, and sustainable standard of care for all (Bargeman et al., 2022; Yatchmenoff et al., 2017). Ultimately, trauma-informed systems are defined not by intention, but by consistent enactment. Safety, autonomy, and dignity must be experienced across every level of service delivery.

REFERENCES

Avery, J. C., Morris, H., Galvin, E., Misso, M., Savaglio, M., & Skouteris, H. (2021). Systematic review of school-wide trauma-informed approaches. *Journal of Child & Adolescent Trauma*, *14*(3), 381–397. DOI: 10.1007/s40653-020-00321-1 PMID: 34471456

Bargeman, M., Abelson, J., Mulvale, G., Niec, A., Theuer, A., & Moll, S. (2022). Understanding the conceptualization and operationalization of trauma-informed care within and across systems: A critical interpretive synthesis. *The Milbank Quarterly*, *100*(3), 785–853. DOI: 10.1111/1468-0009.12579 PMID: 36161340

Berring, L. L., Holm, T., Hansen, J. P., Delcomyn, C. L., Søndergaard, R., & Hvidhjelm, J. (2024). Implementing trauma-informed care—Settings, definitions, interventions, measures, and implementation across settings: A scoping review. *Health Care*, *12*(9), 908. Advance online publication. DOI: 10.3390/healthcare12090908 PMID: 38727465

Bills, L. J., Hutchison, S. L., Snider, M. D. H., Skrzypek, B. E., Minnich, C. L., Korney, J. M., Taylor, R. M., & Herschell, A. D. (2023). Implementing a trauma-informed system of care: An analysis of learning collaborative outcomes. *Journal of Traumatic Stress*, *36*(2), 433–443. DOI: 10.1002/jts.22931 PMID: 36995179

Bokek-Cohen, Y., & Gabay, G. (2025). Medical gaslighting as a threat to beneficence and patient autonomy: A qualitative study. *BMC Medical Ethics*, *27*(1), 5. Advance online publication. DOI: 10.1186/s12910-025-01324-z PMID: 41272715

Choi, J., Gabay, E. K., Rachel, A., Brown, A., Cruz, R., Yan, Q., & Cuccaro, P. M. (2024). Evaluation of a trauma-informed care (TIC) training program across community health centers in Texas: A qualitative study. *BMC Health Services Research*, *24*(1), 1360. Advance online publication. DOI: 10.1186/s12913-024-11813-3 PMID: 39511566

Clements, A. D., Haas, B., Cyphers, N. A., Hoots, V., & Barnet, J. (2020). Creating a communitywide system of trauma-informed care. *Progress in Community Health Partnerships*, *14*(4), 499–507. DOI: 10.1353/cpr.2020.0055 PMID: 33416770

Cronholm, P. F., & Dichter, M. E. (2018). The need for systems of care and a trauma-informed approach to intimate partner violence. *American Family Physician*, *97*(11). https://www.aafp.org/pubs/afp/issues/2018/0601/p717.html PMID: 30215942

Elisseou, S., Shamaskin-Garroway, A., Kopstick, A. J., Potter, J., Weil, A., Gundacker, C., & Moreland-Capuia, A. (2024). Leading organizations from burnout to trauma-informed resilience: A vital paradigm shift. *The Permanente Journal*, *28*(1), 198–205. DOI: 10.7812/TPP/23.110 PMID: 38332699

Elliott, D. E., Bjelajac, P., Fallot, R. D., Markoff, L. S., & Reed, B. G. (2005). Trauma-informed or trauma-denied: Principles and implementation of trauma-informed services for women. *Journal of Community Psychology*, *33*(4), 461–477. DOI: 10.1002/jcop.20063

Goldstein, E., Chokshi, B., Melendez-Torres, G., Rios, A., Jelley, M., & Lewis-O'Connor, A. (2024). Effectiveness of trauma-informed care implementation in health care settings: Systematic review of reviews and realist synthesis. *The Permanente Journal*, *28*(1), 135–150. DOI: 10.7812/TPP/23.127 PMID: 38444328

Huo, Y., Couzner, L., Windsor, T., Laver, K., Dissanayaka, N. N., & Cations, M. (2023). Barriers and enablers for the implementation of trauma-informed care in healthcare settings: A systematic review. *Implementation Science Communications*, *4*(1), 49. Advance online publication. DOI: 10.1186/s43058-023-00428-0 PMID: 37147695

Kim, J., Aggarwal, A., Maloney, S., & Tibbits, M. (2021). Organizational assessment to implement trauma-informed care for first responders, child welfare providers, and healthcare professionals. *Professional Psychology, Research and Practice*, *52*(6), 569–578. DOI: 10.1037/pro0000408

Middleton, J. S., Bloom, S. L., Strolin-Goltzman, J., & Caringi, J. (2019). Trauma-informed care and the public child welfare system: The challenges of shifting paradigms. *Journal of Public Child Welfare*, *13*(3), 235–244. DOI: 10.1080/15548732.2019.1603602

O'Dwyer, C., Tarzia, L., Fernbacher, S., & Hegarty, K. (2019). Health professionals' experiences of providing care for women survivors of sexual violence in psychiatric inpatient units. *BMC Health Services Research*, *19*(1), 839. Advance online publication. DOI: 10.1186/s12913-019-4683-z PMID: 31727056

Peeren, S., Montgomery, E., Sweeney, A., Spaducci, G., Kaul, A., Smeeth, D., & Oram, S. (2025). Trauma-informed healthcare from the perspectives of women who have experienced sexual violence in adulthood: A systematic review and meta-ethnography. *BMC Health Services Research*, *26*(1), 13. Advance online publication. DOI: 10.1186/s12913-025-13584-x PMID: 41310653

Powers, A., Langhinrichsen-Rohling, R. A., Sonu, S. C., Haynes, T., & Lathan, E. C. (2024). Brief trauma-informed care training to enhance health care providers' knowledge, comfort, and implementation of trauma-informed care in primary care clinics: A pilot effectiveness study. *Psychological Services*, *21*(4), 792–796. DOI: 10.1037/ser0000823 PMID: 37956055

Purtle, J. (2020). Systematic review of evaluations of trauma-informed organizational interventions that include staff trainings. *Trauma, Violence & Abuse*, *21*(4), 725–740. DOI: 10.1177/1524838018791304 PMID: 30079827

Robey, N., Margolies, S., Sutherland, L., Rupp, C., Black, C., Hill, T., & Baker, C. N. (2021). Understanding staff- and system-level contextual factors relevant to trauma-informed care implementation. *Psychological Trauma: Theory, Research, Practice, and Policy*, *13*(2), 249–257. DOI: 10.1037/tra0000948 PMID: 32915041

Sebton, S. A., Bridger, C. M., Arias, P. A., Okeibunor, C. K., Spencer, S. R., Willis, R. E., Taylor, S. E., & Alsip, B. J. (2025). Comprehensive trauma-informed organizational change at an academic medical center in South Texas. *BMC Health Services Research*, *25*(1), 1433. Advance online publication. DOI: 10.1186/s12913-025-13381-6 PMID: 41185002

Stanton, M. C., Ali, S., McCormick, K. A., Stanley, M., Traylor, M., Johnson, V., & Scruggs, L. (2025). Implementation outcomes of trauma-informed organizational change among HIV service organizations in the Southern United States. *SSM. Mental Health*, *8*, 100500. Advance online publication. DOI: 10.1016/j.ssmmh.2025.100500

Substance Abuse and Mental Health Services Administration. (2014). *SAMHSA's concept of trauma and guidance for a trauma-informed approach* (HHS Publication No. SMA 14-4884). https://ncsacw.acf.hhs.gov/userfiles/files/SAMHSA_Trauma.pdf

Yatchmenoff, D. K., Sundborg, S. A., & Davis, M. A. (2017). Implementing trauma-informed care: Recommendations on the process. *Advances in Social Work*, *18*(1), 167–185. DOI: 10.18060/21311

Chapter 11
Boundaries, Representation, and Advocacy in Ethical Practice

Maritza Azucena Salazar Cha
http://orcid.org/0000-0002-1079-9982
Claremont Graduate University, USA

Yuridia Carrete
La Sierra University, USA

ABSTRACT

This chapter reframes professional ethics through an intersectional, trauma-informed lens, emphasizing that "neutral" approaches often overlook how trauma, oppression, and structural inequities shape client experiences and ethical decision-making. The chapter invites readers to map power across interpersonal, organizational, policy, and historical levels, inviting practitioners to engage in reflexivity through positionality tools and to navigate common tensions. The chapter offers practical guidance on confidentiality, safety-forward documentation, technology security, culturally responsive collaboration, and disability justice.

DOI: 10.4018/979-8-3373-8597-6.ch011

INTRODUCTION

When "Neutral" Ethics Cause Harm

María is a bilingual Latina mother seeking counseling support after experiencing workplace harassment. During intake, she hesitates before answering questions about her immigration history, family composition, and prior interactions with authorities. The clinician, trained to value transparency and neutrality, presses for "complete disclosure," reassuring María that these questions are standard and ethically required. When María becomes guarded, the clinician documents her as "resistant" and "avoidant."

What is missing from this interaction is not ethics—it is context. María's hesitation is not a lack of insight or cooperation; it is a survival strategy shaped by historical surveillance, institutional betrayal, and real fears of family separation (Freyd, 2013; Menjívar & Abrego, 2012). An ethical framework that treats all clients as if they enter systems on equal footing fails to recognize how power, trauma, and identity shape what safety actually means.

The **American Counseling Association (ACA) Code of Ethics (2014)** emphasizes client autonomy, beneficence, and nonmaleficence; however, when applied without cultural and systemic awareness, these principles may unintentionally produce harm. For example, Standard A.2.a (Informed Consent) assumes that clients can freely disclose information without fear of consequences—an assumption that may not hold true for undocumented or mixed-status families.

For Latina/x women, ethics are never neutral. They are experienced through gendered racism, cultural expectations of compliance, and the constant negotiation between self-protection and being perceived as "appropriate," "grateful," or "non-threatening" (Crenshaw, 1989; Delgado & Stefancic, 2017).

WHY ETHICS MUST BE INTERSECTIONAL

Traditional ethical frameworks often assume a universal subject: autonomous, resourced, fluent in institutional norms, and safe to self-disclose. This assumption collapses under an intersectional lens. Intersectionality highlights how overlapping systems of oppression shape lived experience and access to power (Crenshaw, 1989).

For Latina/x women, ethical interactions are filtered through:

- Racialization and gendered stereotypes (e.g., emotionality, passivity, hyper-sexualization) (Hurtado, 1996)
- Immigration-related fears (personal or familial) (Menjívar & Abrego, 2012)

- Language-based power differentials (Flores, 2020)
- Cultural expectations around respect, silence, and deference (familismo, respeto) (Castillo et al., 2010)
- Historical and contemporary mistrust of institutions (Freyd, 2013)

An ethics model that ignores these realities risks replicating harm under the guise of professionalism. What is considered "ethical" for a dominant-group client may be coercive, unsafe, or retraumatizing for a Latina/x woman navigating layered vulnerabilities.

Intersectional ethics demand recognition that trauma does not exist in isolation—it is compounded by oppression, surveillance, and repeated experiences of being disbelieved or disciplined for self-advocacy (Crenshaw, 1989; Substance Abuse and Mental Health Services Administration, 2014).

Trauma-Informed Principles as Ethical Commitments

Trauma-informed care is often discussed as a clinical enhancement. In this chapter, it is reframed as an **ethical obligation**, particularly when working with marginalized communities (Substance Abuse and Mental Health Services Administration, 2014).

The core trauma-informed principles can be translated into the following ethical commitments:

- **Safety** → Actively assessing emotional, cultural, and institutional safety, not assuming it exists
- **Trustworthiness & Transparency** → Explaining why information is requested and how it will be used
- **Choice** → Respecting selective disclosure as an ethical right, not a clinical barrier
- **Collaboration** → Sharing power in decision-making rather than enforcing compliance
- **Empowerment** → Valuing survival strategies rather than pathologizing them
- **Cultural Humility** → Ongoing self-reflection and acknowledgment of systemic power (Hook et al., 2013)

These commitments align with ethical standards such as **ACA A.4.a (Avoiding Harm)** and **A.2.c (Developmental and Cultural Sensitivity)**, but extend them by requiring practitioners to actively interrogate how systems shape client safety.

For Latina/x women, these commitments are not abstract ideals. They are the difference between ethical care and institutional harm.

LATINA/X WOMANHOOD AND ETHICAL COMPLEXITY

Ethical dilemmas for Latina/x women are rarely "standard." They are shaped by intersecting pressures, including:

- **Respectability politics:** Pressure to conform to dominant norms to be perceived as credible (Higginbotham, 1993)
- **Familismo and collectivism:** Ethical decisions prioritize family safety over individual disclosure (Castillo et al., 2010)
- **Gendered power dynamics:** Assertiveness may be misread as hostility (Hurtado, 1996)
- **Language and accent bias:** Fluency is often conflated with intelligence or credibility (Flores, 2020)

As a result, Latina/x women are often forced to choose between ethical self-protection and institutional approval. Trauma-informed intersectional ethics recognize this bind and refuse to penalize clients or professionals for navigating it.

Ethics, when stripped of context, become tools of control rather than care. An intersectional, trauma-informed ethical framework insists that *how* we practice matters as much as *what* we follow. For Latina/x women, ethical practice must account for history, power, and survival—not as exceptions, but as the standard.

MAPPING POWER: PRACTITIONERS, INSTITUTIONS, AND SYSTEMS

Scenario: When Credibility Is Racialized

Early in my career as a high school counselor, I encountered an ethical rupture that clarified how power operates across identity, hierarchy, and institutional culture. A male administrator accused me of improperly placing a student in coursework that was allegedly not aligned with graduation requirements. The concern itself was not unethical; accountability and student advocacy are essential parts of educational practice. What made the situation ethically fraught was *how* the concern was handled.

Rather than approaching me directly, reviewing the student record, or following established due process, the administrator relied solely on statements made by two white colleagues. Their accounts were accepted at face value. Mine was not. I was neither consulted nor given the opportunity to explain my clinical reasoning, documentation, or prior administrative oversight before assumptions were made about my competence.

When the matter was formally reviewed, my case notes told a different story. The student had been appropriately placed. Multiple documented conversations with the student and family supported the decision, and a previous administrative review had already occurred. The evidence was clear. The harm, however, had already been done.

At the time, I was young, new to the counseling team, and the only Mexican counselor on a predominantly white staff in a predominantly white school. My professional judgment was questioned not because of a lack of documentation or ethical lapse, but because credibility itself was unevenly distributed. This was not simply a misunderstanding between colleagues; it was an example of how power, race, gender, and institutional hierarchy intersect to create ethical vulnerability.

This experience illuminated how ethical tensions rarely exist only at the interpersonal level. They are embedded within organizational cultures that privilege some voices over others, within policies that are unevenly enforced, and within historical patterns that frame women of color as needing oversight rather than being trusted as experts. What appeared on the surface as a concern about student placement was, in practice, a lesson in gatekeeping, surveillance, and the racialized politics of professional legitimacy.

How This Scenario Maps Power

This vignette illustrates how ethical tensions operate across multiple, overlapping levels of power:

- Interpersonal power: Credibility was shaped by race, gender, age, and tenure rather than evidence. Trust was extended selectively.
- Organizational power: Due process was bypassed. Informal channels and alliances carried more weight than documentation and policy.
- Policy and legal power: Counseling records—intended to protect students and practitioners—became tools that *had* to be mobilized defensively to prove legitimacy.
- Historical and colonial power: Longstanding narratives about authority, expertise, and professionalism positioned a young Mexican woman counselor as a suspect within a white-dominant institutional culture.

This experience reflects how ethical decision-making is embedded within systems of power, not just individual actions (Foucault, 1980). The ACA Code of Ethics (2014) emphasizes fairness and equity; however, without structural awareness, ethical processes such as consultation, documentation, and supervision may reproduce inequities.

Ethical Tensions Exposed

This scenario reflects several recurring ethical dilemmas in trauma-informed and intersectional practice:

- Gatekeeping of professional credibility and resources
- The misuse of documentation as surveillance rather than protection (Foucault, 1977)
- Power imbalances that constrain practitioner voice
- Disproportionate emotional labor placed on marginalized practitioners (Padilla, 1994)

REFLEXIVITY IN PRACTICE: MAPPING POWER BEYOND INTENT

Ethical practice requires more than good intentions; it requires structured ethical decision-making.

One applicable model is the Forester-Miller & Davis (1996) ethical decision-making model, which includes:

1. Identify the problem
2. Apply the ACA Code of Ethics
3. Determine the nature of the dilemma
4. Generate potential courses of action
5. Consider consequences
6. Choose and evaluate action

When applied through an intersectional lens, this model must include an additional step:

EXPLICIT ANALYSIS OF POWER, IDENTITY, AND SYSTEMIC INEQUITIES INFLUENCING THE SITUATION

Reflexivity Exercise: Identity Wheel and Power Ledger

Step 1: Identity Wheel (Individual and Institutional)

Practitioners and supervisors are invited to map both their *personal* and *professional* identities, including but not limited to:

- Race and ethnicity
- Gender and gender expression
- Age and career stage
- Role and positional authority
- Institutional longevity

Professional credentials and perceived expertise

Participants then reflect on the following prompts:

- Which of my identities are most likely to be read as "credible" or "authoritative" in this setting?
- Which identities may require additional labor to establish trust or legitimacy?
- How does my role amplify or constrain my voice in ethical decision-making?

Step 2: Power and Privilege Ledger (Case-Based)

Using the vignette as a case example, institutions can implement a power ledger that tracks:

- Who raised the concern?
- Whose account was accepted without verification?
- Who was excluded from the initial decision-making process?
- What formal processes were bypassed or upheld?
- Who bore the emotional, professional, or reputational risk?

This exercise shifts ethics from abstract principle to lived reality, revealing how power circulates through everyday decisions.

FROM INCIDENT TO INSIGHT: ETHICAL COMMITMENTS FOR SUPERVISORS AND ADMINISTRATORS

This scenario highlights ethical responsibilities that extend beyond individual counselors to leadership practice. Ethical supervision must be proactive, not merely corrective.

Ethical Commitments

Supervisors and administrators committed to trauma-informed, intersectional ethics must ask themselves:

- Due Process as an Ethical Obligation:
  - Are concerns addressed through transparent, consistent procedures regardless of the practitioner's identity?
  - Are informal reports treated as hypotheses rather than conclusions?
- Credibility Is Not Neutral
  - How do race, gender, age, and tenure influence whose judgment is trusted?
  - What safeguards exist to prevent credibility from being racialized or gendered?
- Documentation as Protection, Not Surveillance
  - Are case notes used to support ethical practice—or to retroactively justify suspicion?
  - Who is most often required to "prove" their competence through documentation?
- Supervision as Accountability, Not Policing
  - Does supervision create psychological safety for dialogue and clarification?
  - Or does it function as a mechanism of control that disproportionately impacts marginalized staff?

These commitments require institutions to examine not only *what* decisions are made, but *how* and *by whom.*

Additionally, these commitments align with:

- ACA F.1.a (Client Welfare in Supervision)
- ACA F.2.b (Multicultural Competence in Supervision)

Yet, trauma-informed supervision extends beyond compliance toward psychological safety and equity (Substance Abuse and Mental Health Services Administration, 2014).

Aligning the Scenario With Trauma-Informed Principles at the Systems Level

Trauma-informed care is frequently framed as an interpersonal skill set. This scenario demonstrates why such a narrow framing is insufficient. Trauma-informed principles must be embedded in institutional behavior.

Safety

Psychological safety applies not only to students but to practitioners. When counselors fear being undermined without consultation, ethical decision-making becomes constrained. Systems that bypass due process erode safety and invite defensive practice.

Systemic question: Do staff feel safe raising questions, clarifying decisions, or disagreeing with authority without fear of retaliation?

Trustworthiness

Trustworthiness requires consistency, fairness, and transparency. Selectively believing some professionals over others fractures trust and reinforces inequity.

Systemic question: Are concerns handled consistently across staff, or does trust shift based on identity and status?

Transparency

Ethical transparency demands that concerns be communicated directly, with clear processes and opportunities for response.

Systemic question: Are decisions made through open dialogue, or behind closed doors that exclude those most affected?

Accountability

True accountability is institutional, not individual scapegoating. In this case, the eventual confirmation of ethical practice did not negate the initial harm caused by procedural failures.

Systemic question: When harm results from biased processes, how does the institution repair trust and prevent recurrence?

Trauma-informed care must move beyond interpersonal interactions and into organizational ethics (Bloom, 2013).

Systems that fail to ensure due process, transparency, and equity risk perpetuating institutional betrayal, even when individual practitioners act ethically (Freyd, 2013).

REFRAMING ETHICS AS STRUCTURAL PRACTICE

This vignette demonstrates that ethical tensions are rarely about isolated mistakes. They emerge at the intersection of interpersonal bias, organizational culture, and historical inequity.

Mapping power is therefore not optional in ethical work; it is foundational, because power is most tangibly enacted through the boundaries institutions and practitioners create, communicate, and enforce. A trauma-informed, intersectional ethic requires recognizing that boundaries are not merely interpersonal tools but structured expressions of authority that can either reinforce hierarchy or cultivate safety. Counseling scholarship has increasingly challenged universalized ethical frameworks by centering intersectionality and systemic power in ethical decision-making, demonstrating that "neutral" approaches often obscure the lived realities of marginalized communities (Shin et al., 2017). These perspectives are further supported by relational approaches to boundary-setting, which argue that boundaries are culturally situated and can function as sites of solidarity and repair rather than rigid professional distance. This aligns with the American Counseling Association's ACA Code of Ethics, which explicitly requires counselors to avoid harm (A.4.a), practice with cultural and developmental sensitivity (A.2.c), and intentionally manage boundaries in ways that protect client dignity and well-being (A.6).

When institutions fail to interrogate how boundaries are constructed and enacted, they risk reproducing the very conditions of unpredictability, exclusion, and powerlessness that underlie trauma. In contrast, ethical boundary-setting becomes a site of repair when it is transparent, collaborative, and responsive to context, particularly for individuals navigating layered forms of marginalization. For those who have experienced chronic, systemic, or relational trauma, boundaries are not neutral; unclear expectations, sudden rule changes, or inconsistently enforced limits can replicate earlier experiences of betrayal. Trauma-aligned boundaries, therefore, prioritize clarity, predictability, and collaborative limit-setting, ensuring that boundaries function not as mechanisms of control, but as relational frameworks that promote trust, accountability, and dignity.

BOUNDARIES THAT HEAL (NOT HARM)

People attend counseling and are often encouraged to create boundaries to protect their well-being; however, without explicit guidance, this recommendation can remain abstract and difficult to implement in practice. The American Psychological Association's APA Ethics Code emphasizes the ethical responsibility to avoid harm and provide competent, developmentally and culturally appropriate services

(Principles A; Standards 2.01, 3.04), underscoring that boundary-setting must be actively taught rather than assumed. Unfortunately, some counselors do not provide clients with explicit tools for establishing healthy boundaries. As a developing clinical skill, counselors must therefore be intentional and explicit in defining what healthy boundaries look like in practice. When thoughtfully constructed, boundaries can be relational, transparent, and reparative rather than distant or punitive. They create safety not through separation, but through clarity, predictability, and mutual respect (Zur, 2007).

For individuals who have experienced trauma, particularly chronic, systemic, or relational trauma, boundaries are not neutral. Trauma theory highlights that inconsistent or ambiguous limits can mirror earlier experiences of instability, powerlessness, or betrayal (van der Kolk, 2014). Unclear expectations, sudden rule changes, or inconsistently enforced limits can replicate earlier experiences of powerlessness or betrayal. Trauma-aligned boundaries prioritize clarity, predictability, and collaborative limit-setting, aligning with ethical mandates to minimize harm and promote client welfare (American Psychological Association (APA) Ethics Code, Standard 3.04).

Clarity involves explicitly naming roles, expectations, and limits in language that is accessible and culturally responsive. Ethical standards require practitioners to ensure informed understanding and adapt communication to clients' contexts and identities (APA Ethics Code, Standard 3.10). Rather than assuming students or clients understand institutional norms, trauma-aligned practitioners explain *why* boundaries exist and *how* they function. For example, stating, "I don't communicate about crises over social media because I want to make sure you get support right away," frames the boundary as a safety measure rather than a rejection.

Predictability means that boundaries are applied consistently over time and across situations. Consistency is central to ethical practice because it reinforces fairness, trust, and professional integrity (APA Ethics Code, Principle B). Predictability builds trust, especially for individuals whose prior experiences with adults or systems were marked by arbitrariness or punishment. When exceptions are necessary, practitioners name them explicitly and explain the rationale, reducing the risk that flexibility is misinterpreted as favoritism or unpredictability.

Collaboration shifts boundary-setting from a unilateral act of authority to a shared process. When appropriate, practitioners can invite dialogue about what feels safe and supportive while still holding ethical and professional limits. Phrases such as "Here's what I'm able to do, and here's what I'm not, let's talk about what support would feel most helpful within those limits," reinforce agency without abandoning responsibility.

Trauma-aligned boundaries are about *transparent containment*: clients and students know what to expect, what is possible, and where support continues beyond the practitioner.

DUAL RELATIONSHIPS AND SMALL-COMMUNITY REALITIES

Ethical codes often caution against dual or multiple relationships, yet these guidelines may be unrealistic in some communities. The American Psychological Association's (APA) Ethics Code (Standard 3.05) and the American Counseling Association's ACA Code of Ethics (A.5.c) both caution against dual relationships when there is a risk of harm or impaired objectivity; however, they also acknowledge that not all multiple relationships are inherently unethical if they are managed with careful attention to client welfare. For example, in rural communities, college campuses, immigrant communities, and lesbian, gay, bisexual, transgender, queer/questioning, intersex, asexual, and other sexual and gender-diverse identities (LGBTQIA+) spaces, overlapping roles are often unavoidable (Schank & Skovholt, 2006). The question is not whether dual relationships exist, but how practitioners navigate them ethically and intentionally.

In small or close-knit communities, a counselor may also be a neighbor, faith community member, or family friend. On campuses, practitioners may encounter students at cultural events, protests, or shared community spaces. For immigrant and LGBTQIA+ communities, shared identity can be a source of trust and access—but also heightened vulnerability if boundaries are unclear.

Mitigating harm in these contexts requires proactive strategies rather than denial. These include:

- **Early acknowledgment** of potential overlap (e.g., "Because this is a small community, we may see each other outside of this space. Let's talk about how you'd like me to handle that.") consistent with informed consent practices (APA Ethics Code, Standard 3.10; ACA Code of Ethics, A.2.a).
- **Informed consent**, revisited over time, rather than a one-time disclosure.
- **Documentation and consultation** when navigating complex boundary decisions (ACA Code of Ethics, I.2.c; APA Ethics Code, Standard 4.01).
- **Avoidance of secrecy**, which can increase power imbalances and risk.

Shared identity does not eliminate the need for boundaries; in many cases, it heightens it. Practitioners must continually assess whether a dual role benefits the client or primarily meets the practitioner's needs. When the latter is true, ethical realignment is required.

DIGITAL BOUNDARIES

Digital communication has expanded access to care while simultaneously complicating professional boundaries. Texting, direct messages, telehealth platforms, and social media increasingly blur distinctions between personal and professional space. The American Psychological Association's (APA) Ethics Code (Standards 3.04, 4.01, 6.02) and the American Counseling Association's (ACA) Code of Ethics (H.2.a, H.4.b) emphasize the ethical obligation to protect client welfare, confidentiality, and professional boundaries in technology-assisted services. Trauma-aligned digital boundaries therefore center safety, informed consent, and data protection as core components of ethical care (Barnett, 2011; Reamer, 2015).

Practitioners should clearly communicate which digital platforms are used, for what purposes, and within what time frames. Ethical guidelines stress the importance of informed consent in digital contexts, including risks, benefits, and limits of electronic communication (APA Ethics Code, Standard 3.10; ACA Code of Ethics, H.2.a). For example, texting may be appropriate for scheduling but not for crisis support. Social media boundaries should be explicit, including policies around following, friending, or responding to messages as these interactions can create unintended dual relationships or confidentiality risks (Kolmes, 2012).

Telehealth introduces additional considerations related to privacy, encryption, and environmental safety. Ethical standards require psychologists and counselors to take reasonable precautions to protect confidential information transmitted through digital means (APA Ethics Code, Standard 4.01; ACA Code of Ethics, H.2.d). Practitioners should use secure, HIPAA-compliant platforms and educate clients about safeguarding their own digital privacy, particularly when working with individuals impacted by intimate partner violence, stalking, or technology-facilitated abuse (Freed et al., 2017). Safety planning in digital contexts may include:

- Discussing the risk of stalkerware or shared device access
- Identifying safe devices or locations for telehealth sessions
- Establishing code words or backup plans if a session becomes unsafe

Digital boundaries are not merely professional preferences; they are part of the ethical duty of care. Failure to attend to digital safety can expose clients to real-world harm.

VICARIOUS TRAUMA AND ETHICAL SELF-CARE

Boundaries also protect practitioners. Chronic exposure to trauma narratives, systemic injustice, and high-stakes decision-making can lead to vicarious trauma, burnout, or impairment. The American Psychological Association's (APA) Ethics Code (Standard 2.06) and the American Counseling Association's (ACA) Code of Ethics (C.2.g) explicitly require practitioners to monitor their own physical, mental, and emotional well-being and to refrain from providing services when impaired. Ethical practice requires ongoing self-monitoring and a willingness to seek support.

Counselor impairment becomes an ethical concern when it interferes with clinical judgment, emotional presence, or professional responsibilities. Research on vicarious trauma and compassion fatigue identifies warning signs such as emotional numbing, irritability, boundary drift, over-identification with clients, and avoidance behaviors (Bride, 2007; Figley, 2002). These indicators not only affect practitioner well-being but can also compromise client care, underscoring the ethical obligation to engage in preventative and responsive self-care (APA Ethics Code, Standard 3.04; ACA Code of Ethics, A.4.a). Ethical self-care is not ancillary to practice; it is integral to maintaining competence and safeguarding clients.

Supervision and peer consultation are essential boundary-sustaining practices. Ethical standards emphasize the importance of consultation and supervision as mechanisms for ensuring competent and ethical care (APA Ethics Code, Standard 2.05; ACA Code of Ethics, C.2.e). These spaces allow practitioners to process the emotional impact of their work, examine decision-making, and receive accountability and support. In such contexts, peer consultation groups or community-based supervision models may be especially vital.

Practitioners must also recognize when stepping back is ethically necessary—whether through reducing caseloads, making referrals, or taking temporary leave. Ethical codes mandate appropriate steps when personal problems or impairment may interfere with professional duties, including limiting, suspending, or terminating services when needed (APA Ethics Code, Standard 2.06; ACA Code of Ethics, C.2.g). Modeling healthy boundaries around capacity not only protects clients but also communicates a critical message about sustainability, professionalism, and inherent worth. In this way, practitioner self-regulation becomes both an ethical obligation and a relational intervention that reinforces the importance of limits, care, and accountability.

REPRESENTATION ETHICS: STORIES, IMAGES, AND DATA

Narrative sovereignty

Narrative sovereignty refers to the right of individuals and communities to control how their stories are told, by whom, and for what purpose. Historically marginalized communities, particularly Black, Indigenous, and People of Color (BIPOC), immigrant, undocumented, LGBTQIA+, and low-income communities, have often been positioned as subjects of stories rather than authors of them. These stories are frequently extracted for institutional gain, whether through research publications, grant reports, marketing materials, or professional advancement.

Avoiding extractive storytelling begins with interrogating intent. Practitioners and researchers must ask: *Who benefits from this story being told? Who bears the risk?* Ethical storytelling centers community-defined goals rather than institutional convenience. This may mean declining to share a compelling narrative if it cannot be done safely or with genuine consent.

Practices that support narrative sovereignty include:

- Inviting individuals to tell their own stories in their own words, when and if they choose
- Offering editorial control or the right to review how stories are used
- Being transparent about where, how long, and in what formats stories will appear
- Accepting a "no" without pressure or penalty

Importantly, not every story needs to be told publicly to be valued. Silence can also be a form of agency.

ANONYMITY VS. RECOGNIZABILITY

Traditional ethical guidance often frames anonymity as a sufficient safeguard. In small or close-knit communities, rural districts, campuses, immigrant neighborhoods, or LGBTQIA+ spaces, anonymity may be rarely absolute. Even when names are changed, details such as role, age, migration pathway, or family structure can make individuals recognizable.

Ethical representation, therefore, requires assessing *recognizability*, not just anonymity. Composite vignettes, which intentionally blend details from multiple individuals, can reduce risk while still conveying essential themes. When using direct quotes, practitioners should obtain explicit consent that addresses potential recognizability and downstream risks.

Social media introduces additional complexity. A quote or image shared online can be screenshot, reshared, or taken out of context indefinitely. Ethical consent must include discussion of these realities, including the inability to fully retract content once it is public.

Key practices include:

- Explaining the limits of anonymity clearly and honestly
- Using composite or fictionalized examples when risk is high
- Obtaining specific consent for quotes, images, and social media use (not blanket consent)
- Revisiting consent over time, especially for long-term projects

AVOIDING TOKENISM AND TRAUMA-PORN

Tokenism occurs when individuals or communities are included symbolically rather than substantively, often to signal diversity without redistributing power. Trauma-porn refers to the overexposure of pain, suffering, or crisis in ways that strip individuals of complexity and agency, often to evoke sympathy or justify intervention.

Ethical representation resists both by adopting strength-based framing that acknowledges harm without centering identity solely on trauma. This does not mean ignoring need or inequity; rather, it means holding an *asset-plus-need* lens. Communities are not only sites of deficit—they are sources of resilience, knowledge, resistance, and care.

Practitioners can ask:

- Does this representation reduce someone to their worst experience?
- Are we showing people as passive recipients of help or active agents in their lives?
- Would this portrayal feel respectful if it were about my own community?

When stories of trauma are shared, they should be contextualized within systems and structures, not individualized as personal failure.

PHOTOGRAPHY AND MEDIA

Images can humanize, but they can also place people in danger. Photography and media use require careful consideration of safety, culture, and consent, particularly in an era of facial recognition, geotagging, and digital permanence.

Protective strategies may include face blurring, voice masking, silhouette photography, or using images of hands, spaces, or symbolic objects rather than identifiable faces. Practitioners should also be aware of geotagging and metadata embedded in photos, which can reveal locations even when names are withheld.

Cultural considerations are equally critical. In some communities, being photographed may carry spiritual, political, or familial implications. Consent processes should be culturally responsive and, when appropriate, involve family or community consultation rather than assuming individual consent is sufficient.

Ethical media practices include:

- Explaining exactly where and how images will be used
- Avoiding images that reinforce stereotypes or voyeurism
- Respecting cultural norms related to visibility, modesty, and representation
- Prioritizing safety over aesthetics or marketing appeal

RESEARCH AND EVALUATION

Ethical representation extends to how data are collected, analyzed, and shared. Community-led and community-engaged research models challenge extractive traditions by positioning communities as partners rather than subjects.

Key principles include:

- Community-defined questions: Research agendas should emerge from community priorities, not solely institutional interests.
- Fair compensation: Lived experience is expertise and should be compensated accordingly.
- Data ownership and access: Communities should have a say in who owns the data, how it is stored, and how it is used in the future.
- Review and accountability: In addition to formal IRB processes, community review boards or advisory groups can provide culturally grounded ethical oversight.

Evaluation findings should be shared back with communities in accessible formats, not only academic journals or funder reports. Transparency and reciprocity are essential to ethical data practice.

WORKING ACROSS CULTURES, LANGUAGES, AND MODALITIES

Interpreters and Cultural Brokers

Language access is a legal requirement in many settings, but ethical practice demands more than literal translation. Interpreters and cultural brokers play a critical role in meaning-making, trust-building, and safety, particularly for immigrant, refugee, Deaf/Hard of Hearing, and linguistically marginalized communities.

Qualified interpreters should have formal training in interpretation ethics, trauma-informed practice, and confidentiality. Whenever possible, practitioners should avoid using children, family members, or untrained staff as interpreters, as this can distort information, compromise consent, and exacerbate power imbalances. Cultural brokers who may provide context beyond language require even clearer role definition to prevent boundary confusion.

Key ethical practices include:

- **Clear role clarification**: Distinguishing interpretation from advocacy, counseling, or decision-making
- **Confidentiality agreements**: Explicit, documented, and explained to all parties
- **Pre- and post-session briefings**: Aligning on terminology, goals, and emotional impact
- **Attention to power dynamics**: Recognizing that interpreters may hold social, immigration, or community power over clients

Practitioners must also be attentive to how institutional authority interacts with language. Speaking "through" an interpreter does not absolve counselors of responsibility for tone, pacing, or relational presence. Direct eye contact, respectful pauses, and inclusive body language communicate dignity across languages.

DISABILITY JUSTICE IN PRACTICE

Disability justice frameworks challenge practitioners to move beyond accommodation toward access, autonomy, and collective care. Ethical practice recognizes disability not as an individual deficit, but as a product of environments, systems, and norms that exclude.

Accessible practice includes providing materials in multiple formats (plain language, large print, captions, screen-reader compatible documents) and proactively asking about access needs rather than waiting for disclosure. Sensory considerations such as lighting, noise, seating, and virtual platform features are essential, particularly for neurodivergent individuals and trauma survivors.

Supported decision-making is a core ethical principle within disability justice. Rather than defaulting to substitute decision-making, practitioners should explore how individuals can make their own choices with appropriate support. This may include visual aids, additional time, trusted support persons, or alternative communication methods.

Ethical questions to consider include:

- Are we prioritizing efficiency over accessibility?
- Do our policies assume a narrow definition of competence or participation?
- Are disabled individuals involved in designing the services meant to support them?

Disability justice reminds practitioners that access is not an add-on—it is foundational to ethical care.

SPIRITUAL/FAITH CONTEXTS

For many individuals and communities, spirituality and faith are central sources of meaning, resilience, and healing. Ethical practice requires respecting these dimensions without imposing beliefs or allowing spiritual frameworks to override client autonomy.

Practitioners should create space for clients to name spiritual or religious identities if they choose, while remaining clear that participation is voluntary and client-led. Respect does not require agreement, nor does collaboration require endorsement of all practices.

Navigating collaborations between clergy and clinicians can be particularly complex. Clear boundaries, role clarification, and informed consent are essential. Ethical collaboration involves:

- Ensuring clients understand the distinct roles and confidentiality limits of clergy versus clinicians
- Avoiding coercion, particularly when services are embedded in faith-based institutions
- Addressing conflicts when spiritual guidance contradicts clinical recommendations or client safety

Practitioners must be especially vigilant in contexts where faith has been used to justify harm, exclusion, or conversion practices.

COMMUNITY CARE NETWORKS

Community care networks, including mutual aid groups and peer support models, have long filled gaps left by formal systems, particularly for marginalized communities. These networks often operate outside traditional professional frameworks, offering relational, culturally grounded support.

Ethical engagement with community care requires honoring their strengths while acknowledging limitations. Practitioners should avoid professionalizing or co-opting mutual aid in ways that undermine its autonomy. At the same time, clear ethical guardrails are necessary when harm risk is present.

Considerations include:

- **Scope and role clarity**: Distinguishing peer support from clinical intervention
- **Risk awareness**: Knowing when referral or escalation is necessary
- **Consent and transparency**: Ensuring participants understand what support is—and is not—being offered
- **Reciprocity and respect**: Valuing community knowledge without extraction

When practitioners partner with community networks, the goal should be complementarity, not control.

COMMON PITFALLS AND HOW TO AVOID THEM

Even the most well-intentioned counselors can cause harm when ethical commitments are treated as checklists rather than living practices. In trauma-informed, culturally responsive, and justice-oriented work, harm often occurs not through overt misconduct, but through subtle patterns that go unexamined. The goal is not perfection. It is accountability, reflection, and a willingness to change course when practice drifts away from values.

Performative Inclusion Without Power-Sharing

One of the most pervasive pitfalls is performative inclusion: the appearance of diversity, equity, or community engagement without any meaningful redistribution of power. This can look like advisory boards with no decision-making authority, tokenized representation on panels, or the use of community voices to validate predetermined agendas.

Performative inclusion often benefits institutions more than communities. It signals progress while leaving underlying hierarchies intact. For individuals from marginalized communities, this dynamic can feel extractive and disillusioning, particularly when their labor, stories, or identities are visible, but their influence is not.

How to avoid it:

- Move beyond consultation toward shared decision-making.
- Compensate community members for their time, expertise, and emotional labor.
- Be transparent about which decisions are negotiable and which are constrained by policy or funding.
- Build feedback mechanisms that can lead to real change, not just acknowledgment.

Inclusion without power-sharing is not neutral; it reinforces the very inequities it claims to address.

Over-Documentation That Endangers Clients

Documentation is often framed as a protective practice for clinicians, schools, and institutions. Yet over-documentation, particularly when it includes unnecessary detail about trauma, immigration status, legal vulnerability, or family dynamics, can place clients and students at risk.

Records can be subpoenaed, accessed by multiple systems, or misinterpreted outside of their original context. For undocumented individuals, survivors of violence, or those navigating child welfare or criminal legal systems, documentation can become a site of surveillance rather than support.

How to avoid it:

- Document purposefully, recording what is necessary for continuity of care and ethical accountability—not curiosity or liability anxiety.
- Avoid speculative language, moral judgments, or excessive trauma detail.
- Understand who can access records and under what circumstances.
- Discuss documentation limits and risks as part of informed consent.

Ethical documentation balances professional responsibility with harm reduction.

"Cultural Competence" Claims Without Accountability

The language of "cultural competence" is widespread, yet often unexamined. Claiming competence can falsely suggest mastery over cultures that are dynamic, diverse, and internally complex. Worse, it can be used to shield practitioners from feedback or accountability.

Without structures for reflection and correction, cultural competence becomes a static label rather than an ethical practice. Communities experience this as dismissal: "I've had the training" replaces listening, and intent is prioritized over impact.

How to avoid it:

- Shift from competence to cultural humility, emphasizing ongoing learning and self-interrogation.
- Build accountability systems, such as supervision, peer consultation, and community feedback.
- Treat harm disclosures as data, not defensiveness triggers.
- Recognize that shared identity does not eliminate the need for accountability.

Ethical practice is demonstrated through responsiveness, not self-ascribed expertise.

Boundary Collapses Framed as "Community Care"

Community care is often invoked to justify boundary crossings that would otherwise raise ethical concerns of excessive self-disclosure, dual relationships without safeguards, or practitioners meeting needs outside their role or capacity. While mutual aid and relational support are vital, boundary collapse can place both practitioners and community members at risk.

When boundaries dissolve, power dynamics do not disappear. Instead, they become less visible and harder to navigate. Clients may feel pressure to accept care that blurs roles, or practitioners may unconsciously seek validation, belonging, or purpose through overextension.

How to avoid it:

- Distinguish clearly between community care and professional responsibility.
- Name roles, limits, and expectations explicitly—even in informal or identity-based spaces.
- Use supervision and consultation to examine urges to "do more" that may signal burnout or over-identification.
- Remember that saying no can be an act of care.

Ethical community care is sustainable, reciprocal, and bounded.

One-Time Consent for Ongoing Storytelling

Consent is often treated as a single event rather than an evolving process. This is especially risky in storytelling, research, media, and advocacy work, where narratives may be reused, reshared, or reframed over time.

Individuals may consent under conditions of urgency, trust, or perceived obligation, without fully anticipating future consequences. Over time, their circumstances, safety, or comfort with visibility may change while their story continues to circulate.

How to avoid it:

- Treat consent as ongoing and revisitable, not permanent.
- Re-check consent when stories are reused, adapted, or shared in new contexts.
- Provide clear pathways for withdrawing consent without penalty.
- Avoid tying access to services or support to willingness to share personal narratives.

Ethical storytelling respects people's right to change their minds.

CONCLUSION

For practitioners working within systems, ethics cannot be reduced to individual behavior or compliance with codes alone. Ethical practice must also involve recognizing how institutions themselves produce harm and how practitioners with less institutional power are often the first to absorb its impact.

REFERENCES

American Counseling Association. (2014). *ACA code of ethics*. Author. https://www.counseling.org/resources/aca-code-of-ethics.pdf

American Psychological Association. (2017). *Ethical principles of psychologists and code of conduct*. https://www.apa.org/ethics/code

American School Counselor Association. (2022). *ASCA ethical standards for school counselors*. Author. https://www.schoolcounselor.org/Standards-Positions/Ethical-Standards

Barnett, J. E. (2011). Utilizing technology to provide clinical supervision: Opportunities and challenges. *The Clinical Supervisor, 30*(1), 59–77.

Bloom, S. L. (2013). *Creating sanctuary: Toward the evolution of sane societies* (2nd ed.). Routledge.

Bride, B. E. (2007). Prevalence of secondary traumatic stress among social workers. *Social Work, 52*(1), 63–70. DOI: 10.1093/sw/52.1.63 PMID: 17388084

Castillo, L. G., Perez, F. V., Castillo, R., & Ghosheh, M. R. (2010). Construction and initial validation of the Marianismo Beliefs Scale. *Counselling Psychology Quarterly, 23*(2), 163–175. DOI: 10.1080/09515071003776036

Crenshaw, K. (1989). Demarginalizing the intersection of race and sex: A Black feminist critique of antidiscrimination doctrine, feminist theory, and antiracist politics. *University of Chicago Legal Forum, 1989*(1), 139–167.

Delgado, R., & Stefancic, J. (2017). *Critical race theory: An introduction* (3rd ed.). NYU Press.

Figley, C. R. (2002). Compassion fatigue: Psychotherapists' chronic lack of self-care. *Journal of Clinical Psychology, 58*(11), 1433–1441. DOI: 10.1002/jclp.10090 PMID: 12412153

Flores, N. (2020). From academic language to language architecture: Challenging raciolinguistic ideologies in research and practice. *Theory into Practice, 59*(1), 22–31. DOI: 10.1080/00405841.2019.1665411

Forester-Miller, H., & Davis, T. (1996). *A practitioner's guide to ethical decision making*. American Counseling Association.

Foucault, M. (1977). *Discipline and punish: The birth of the prison*. Pantheon.

Foucault, M. (1980). *Power/knowledge: Selected interviews and other writings.* Pantheon.

Freed, D., Palmer, J., Minchala, D., Levy, K., Ristenpart, T., & Dell, N. (2017). "A stalker's paradise": How intimate partner abusers exploit technology. *Proceedings of the ACM on Human-Computer Interaction, 1*(CSCW), 1–27.

Freyd, J. J. (2013). Preventing betrayal. *Journal of Trauma & Dissociation, 14*(2), 119–124. PMID: 24060032

Higginbotham, E. B. (1993). *Righteous discontent: The women's movement in the Black Baptist church, 1880–1920*. Harvard University Press.

Hook, J. N., Davis, D. E., Owen, J., Worthington, E. L., & Utsey, S. O. (2013). Cultural humility: Measuring openness to culturally diverse clients. *Journal of Counseling Psychology, 60*(3), 353–366. DOI: 10.1037/a0032595 PMID: 23647387

Hurtado, A. (1996). *The color of privilege: Three blasphemies on race and feminism.* University of Michigan Press. DOI: 10.3998/mpub.9839

Kolmes, K. (2012). Social media in the future of professional psychology. *Professional Psychology, Research and Practice, 43*(6), 606–612. DOI: 10.1037/a0028678

Menjívar, C., & Abrego, L. J. (2012). Legal violence: Immigration law and the lives of Central American immigrants. *American Journal of Sociology, 117*(5), 1380–1421. DOI: 10.1086/663575

Padilla, A. M. (1994). Ethnic minority scholars: Research, and mentoring. *Educational Researcher, 23*(4), 24–27.

Reamer, F. G. (2015). Clinical social work in a digital environment: Ethical and risk-management challenges. *Clinical Social Work Journal, 43*(2), 120–132. DOI: 10.1007/s10615-014-0495-0

Schank, J. A., & Skovholt, T. M. (2006). Multiple relationships and boundary challenges for therapists in rural practice. *Journal of Clinical Psychology, 62*(4), 505–512.

Shin, R. Q., Smith, L. C., Welch, J. C., & Ezeofor, I. (2017). Is Allison more likely than Lakisha to receive a callback from counseling professionals? A racism audit study. *Journal of Counseling Psychology, 64*(1), 41–52. DOI: 10.1037/cou0000179 PMID: 28068130

Substance Abuse and Mental Health Services Administration. (2014). *SAMHSA's concept of trauma and guidance for a trauma-informed approach* (HHS Publication No. SMA 14-4884). https://ncsacw.samhsa.gov/userfiles/files/SAMHSA_Trauma.pdf

van der Kolk, B. A. (2014). *The body keeps the score: Brain, mind, and body in the healing of trauma*. Viking.

Zur, O. (2007). *Boundaries in psychotherapy: Ethical and clinical explorations*. American Psychological Association. DOI: 10.1037/11563-000

KEY TERMS AND DEFINITIONS

Ableism in Care: Practices that privilege neurotypical, physically able, or emotionally "regulated" presentations often pathologize trauma responses or disabilities.

Deportation Fear: Chronic anxiety related to immigration enforcement that affects disclosure, help-seeking behavior, and trust in institutions, even for individuals who are citizens or legal residents.

Gaslighting: A form of psychological manipulation in which a person's lived experience is dismissed or reframed to cause self-doubt, often occurring in institutional or professional contexts.

Institutional Betrayal: Harm that occurs when institutions fail to protect, respond appropriately to, or actively harm those who depend on them for safety or care.

Respectability Pressures: Implicit or explicit expectations that marginalized individuals must conform to dominant norms of behavior to be deemed credible, deserving, or ethical.

Chapter 12
Future Directions in Trauma, Feminism, and Intersectionality

Yolanda Loften Sims
http://orcid.org/0009-0009-6402-9666
National Louis University, USA

ABSTRACT

Culturally responsive contemplative practices offer transformative pathways of healing for women navigating trauma within contexts of systemic oppression. Grounded in intersectionality and trauma-informed care, these approaches extend beyond symptom reduction to restore dignity, cultural identity, and collective agency. This chapter examines how contemplative practices, when rooted in cultural reclamation and relational accountability, disrupt reductionist wellness models and resist epistemic hierarchies. While emerging neuroscience suggests meaningful shifts in attention and regulation, healing must also be understood through lived experience, community knowledge, and justice-centered sustainability. Ultimately, culturally responsive contemplative practice is advanced not merely as a clinical intervention but as an epistemological shift that reorients counseling, education, and research toward equity, relational care, and collective flourishing.

INTRODUCTION

Mindfulness, meditation, and yoga are increasingly offered as tools in counseling and related helping professions. However, when faced with the realities of systemic oppression and deep-seated historical trauma, they are never simply neutral (Hargons, 2022; Polinska, 2018). To overlook a person's cultural world or the power structures

DOI: 10.4018/979-8-3373-8597-6.ch012

that shape their lived experience is not simply an oversight; it risks deepening those wounds rather than fostering meaningful healing.

From a counseling perspective, healing is not solely an internal process; it is relational, embodied, and culturally situated, grounded in connection, belonging, and mutual strength (Crenshaw, 1991; Herman, 1992). Rather than an isolated journey, it unfolds through relationships, cultural identity, and lived experience. Culturally responsive contemplative practices extend beyond stress reduction, functioning as pathways that restore dignity, cultivate agency, and foster meaningful connection (Harrell & Malebranche, 2025; Watson-Singleton et al., 2019). Within this space, contemplative practice becomes both a clinical and ethical endeavor in which healing is inseparable from justice.

Justice-oriented contemplative practice requires more than cultural awareness; it demands a critical interrogation of how knowledge is constructed, validated, and disseminated within counseling and psychology. Intersectionality, as articulated by Crenshaw (1991), is not merely an analytic tool but a challenge to single-axis thinking that flattens lived experience. When contemplative practices are applied without this lens, they risk replicating the very systemic hierarchies they seek to alleviate. Thus, culturally responsive contemplative work must confront not only trauma but also the epistemic structures that determine whose trauma is legible, whose healing is measurable, and whose wisdom is recognized.

This chapter advances an integrated, justice-oriented framework that brings together intersectionality, feminist praxis, Sankofa-informed healing, and intersectional neuroscience. Within this framework, healing is conceptualized as relational, culturally grounded, and structurally informed, in which contemplative practice serves as both an intervention and an ethical engagement (Collins, 2019; Harrell & Malebranche, 2025). By centering culturally meaningful contemplative traditions, engaging neuroscientific insight with critical awareness, and emphasizing community-driven approaches to healing, this chapter offers a justice-oriented direction for counseling practice, education, and research (Bhambhani & Gallo, 2021; Weng et al., 2020). In doing so, it calls the profession toward forms of care that are ethically grounded, culturally responsive, and accountable to the lived experiences of those it seeks to serve.

In counseling spaces, this may involve counselors intentionally integrating culturally grounded rituals, narrative reflection, or communal practices that align with participants' lived experiences rather than relying solely on standardized contemplative techniques.

The Evidence Base: Scope, Strengths, and Limitations

Morales and Burnett-Zeigler (2024) highlight that our understanding of culturally responsive contemplative practices is drawn from diverse methodologies, disciplines, and sources of knowledge, yet remains incomplete. Community narratives, collaborative scholarship, programmatic work, and neuroscience collectively suggest that these practices are most effective and ethical when cultural respect is foundational rather than peripheral. At the same time, persistent barriers and tensions reveal deeper inequities in how knowledge is produced and disseminated. Access to research findings remains uneven, and neuroscientific studies frequently rely on White participant samples, reflecting broader disparities in research funding, representation, and legitimacy. These patterns shift the focus from simply asking what works to examining how power shapes what is recognized as evidence and whose knowledge is legitimized.

Beyond issues of representation, the evidence base reveals deeper epistemological tensions. Much of contemplative research privileges randomized controlled trials and symptom reduction as primary indicators of legitimacy. While these approaches offer valuable insight, they can inadvertently marginalize relational, communal, and spiritually grounded dimensions of healing that do not lend themselves easily to standardized measurement (Kwah & Fellner, 2020). For women navigating layered trauma shaped by race, gender, spirituality, and class, healing is rarely reducible to a numerical decrease in distress. Instead, it is often experienced as restored dignity, renewed belonging, and reclaimed cultural meaning, outcomes that resist narrow operationalization and call for broader interpretive frameworks. In applied settings, this may translate into shifting evaluation away from symptom checklists toward narrative, relational, or community-defined indicators of change.

Morales and Burnett-Zeigler's (2024) scoping review further highlights that many culturally adapted mindfulness interventions remain surface-level modifications rather than structural transformations. Adjustments to language or imagery may enhance engagement, yet without confronting systemic inequities or integrating culturally grounded epistemologies, such adaptations risk becoming cosmetic. In this way, the evidence base reflects both promise and limitation: promise in the demonstrated benefits of contemplative practices across diverse communities, and limitation in the continued dominance of Western frameworks that define what counts as evidence and how healing is measured.

These patterns call for a more contextual and justice-oriented understanding of evidence. Effectiveness cannot be disentangled from power. Certain questions must be asked: Whose stress is framed as pathological? Whose coping strategies are labeled maladaptive? Whose spiritual traditions are recognized only when translated into Western clinical language? These inquiries move the field beyond effectiveness toward ethical accountability, positioning evidence not as neutral, but as shaped by cultural, historical, and structural forces.

A justice-centered evidence model must expand rather than replace existing paradigms. It positions community-defined outcomes as central rather than supplemental and recognizes mixed-method and participatory approaches as rigorous forms of inquiry capable of capturing relational and cultural dimensions of healing (Kwah & Fellner, 2020; La Scala et al., 2023). Within this extended framework, the question shifts from whether culturally responsive contemplative practices work in isolation to how they transform relational systems, restore cultural continuity, and restructure psychological safety within communities.

Emerging trends within the field reflect this broader shift. There is a movement away from individual symptom reduction toward collective and relational models of healing that prioritize belonging and cultural affirmation (Bhambhani & Gallo, 2021; Collins, 2019). Research is increasingly grounded in participatory and community-based approaches that center lived experience as a valid and necessary form of evidence (Kwah & Fellner, 2020; La Scala et al., 2023). At the same time, contemplative practices are being reframed as justice-oriented interventions that explicitly engage power, oppression, and systemic inequities rather than remaining culturally neutral (Hargons, 2022; Morales & Burnett-Zeigler, 2024). Together, these developments signal a broader reorientation of the field, one that moves toward ethical accountability, cultural grounding, and relationally informed care.

ADAPTING EASTERN CONTEMPLATIVE PRACTICES WITH CULTURAL INTEGRITY

Scholars consistently note that when Western contexts adopt contemplative practices, they often strip them of their cultural and spiritual richness, particularly within mindfulness traditions shaped by dominant White, middle-class norms (Polinska, 2018). When race-related stress, spiritual meaning, and systemic oppression are overlooked, these practices can feel imposed, irrelevant, or even harmful for marginalized communities, undermining their capacity to support meaningful healing (Morales & Burnett-Zeigler, 2024). In this way, what is often presented as universally beneficial can, in practice, reproduce disconnection when cultural context is not centered.

Ethical adaptation requires more than surface-level modification. It demands a fundamental shift in how contemplative practices are understood and implemented. While adjustments to language or imagery may enhance accessibility, deeper adaptations are necessary to meaningfully engage ancestral knowledge, collective memory, spiritual identity, and lived experiences of oppression (Watson-Singleton et al., 2019; Harrell & Malebranche, 2025). For women navigating intersecting identities, trauma is not isolated but cumulative and socially embedded. Separating symptoms from this broader context risks obscuring lived realities and sustaining the inequities these practices seek to address (Herman, 1992).

Polinska (2018) cautions that when mindfulness is detached from its philosophical and ethical roots, it can become complicit in what she terms "white ignorance," a condition in which structural harm remains unnamed while individuals are encouraged to regulate themselves within unjust systems. This invites further examination of how contemplative practices are adapted in relation to power. The question is not simply whether these practices are accessible, but whether they are being used to help individuals endure inequity or to cultivate critical consciousness and collective agency.

Within this context, cultural integrity becomes a central ethical commitment. Contemplative traditions cannot be ethically engaged when they are extracted from their lineages and repackaged as culturally neutral commodities. Tsomo (2024) reminds us that Buddhist identity is both racialized and historically situated, highlighting the importance of honoring diasporic histories, spiritual frameworks, and community contexts. Acknowledging these foundations does not preclude adaptation. Instead, it ensures that adaptation occurs in dialogue rather than erasure.

Expanding beyond Western frameworks also invites engagement with Indigenous and Afro-diasporic contemplative traditions that center relational, communal, and spiritually grounded approaches to healing (Hargons, 2022). These traditions challenge individualistic and decontextualized models of mindfulness by emphasizing connection, cultural continuity, and collective care as essential components of well-being.

For women navigating intersecting forms of marginalization, contemplative spaces must explicitly validate race-related stress, gendered violence, and spiritual plurality. Watson-Singleton et al. (2019) demonstrate that culturally responsive adaptations for African American communities include facilitator congruence, collective dialogue, and the explicit naming of racism as a stressor. These are not peripheral enhancements. They are central ethical commitments. Without them, contemplative practice risks reinforcing isolation rather than alleviating it.

This invites a reorientation of contemplative practice. At its core, this shift moves beyond adaptation as technique and toward adaptation as ethical engagement. This takes shape through co-creating contemplative exercises with participants, incorporating culturally familiar forms such as storytelling, music, or movement rather than imposing silence-based meditation as a universal starting point.

When grounded in cultural integrity, relational awareness, and a critical understanding of power, contemplative practices can more closely align with their intended purpose. They do not simply regulate distress. They support healing that is culturally meaningful, relationally grounded, and aligned with justice.

Sankofa and Reclaiming Cultural Joy as Healing Praxis

Harrell and Malebranche (2025) describe Sankofa as a framework rooted in African philosophy, emphasizing return, retrieval, and revitalization. Sankofa is more than a concept; it is a way of understanding healing that centers cultural reclamation, collective memory, and liberation. It invites movement beyond surface-level adaptation toward deeper reconnection with cultural knowledge, relational grounding, and ways of knowing disrupted over time.

Within this framework, trauma is not understood solely as psychological injury. Instead, it is experienced as a disruption of cultural continuity. Healing, then, becomes a process of returning, remembering, and restoring connection to ancestral knowledge, communal memory, and embodied practices that affirm identity and belonging (Harrell & Malebranche, 2025). Rather than positioning contemplative practice as an inward retreat, Sankofa invites presence as an act of collective remembrance. Presence becomes reclamation.

Sankofa-informed contemplative work is not prescribed; rather, it is co-created and grounded in culturally meaningful ways of being. Soulfulness, for example, cultivates inner dignity and resilience through connection to communal histories and spiritual traditions (Chatters et al., 2008; Draper-Clarke & Green, 2024). Ancestral storytelling and oral traditions, including call-and-response, create space for collective wisdom to be shared and sustained (Covington-Ward & Jouili, 2021). Movement and dance, rooted in Afro-centric traditions, offer pathways for emotional expression, spiritual renewal, and relational connection, while strengthening cultural identity (Chatters et al., 2008). Communal rituals and ceremonies further deepen this work by fostering a sense of belonging, shared meaning, and collective presence.

Water-based contemplative practices add another dimension by honoring water as sacred, as a source of purification, renewal, and life across many African spiritual traditions (Kgatle & Qiki, 2023). Rituals of cleansing and renewal, whether through intentional use of water or engagement with natural bodies such as rivers and oceans, support grounding, release, and reconnection (Wepener & Müller, 2012; Mboweni & Crom, 2016). These practices reflect a broader understanding of healing that is not separate from nature but is deeply interconnected with it.

What becomes clear within Sankofa is that contemplative practice is not limited to silence or stillness. Movement, sound, storytelling, and ritual are all contemplative when they cultivate attunement, relational presence, and embodied awareness. This expands dominant Western constructions of contemplation and affirms that healing can take many forms, especially when grounded in culture and community.

Sankofa reframes healing from colonial trauma and cultural disconnection as a relational and decolonial process. Regulation and presence are not the end goal. They are pathways toward agency, connection, and collective dignity (Hargons, 2022). When held alongside feminist praxis, Sankofa also disrupts narratives of individual resilience that are disconnected from history. Survival is not isolated. It is collective, inherited, and shaped through community.

Seen through this lens, joy is not positioned as superficial or disconnected from struggle. It emerges as something more enduring and expansive. Cultural joy, when shared and ritualized, becomes a form of resistance. It restores dignity in ways that symptom-focused interventions alone cannot achieve.

In this space, the question becomes how these practices are thoughtfully brought into clinical work in ways that remain aligned with cultural meaning and lived experience.

Table 1. Practices of care: Culturally rooted pathways of contemplative healing

Community Context	Contemplative Practice	Cultural adaptation focus	Mode of community engagement
Racially minoritized communities	Mindfulness-based practices	Cultural reclamation and spiritual lineage	Collaborative autoethnography
African american women	Mindfulness (Buddhist traditions)	Spiritual congruence and cultural values	Focus groups and interviews
Racially diverse communities	MBSR / MBCT	Trauma-informed and culturally responsive design	Ongoing community feedback
Marginalized populations	Mindfulness and compassion practices	Person-centered and inclusive adaptations	Community-based participatory research
Women of color (students)	Buddhist meditation and visual arts	Creative resistance and cultural meaning	Participatory learning spaces

Note. Table created by the author illustrating culturally responsive contemplative adaptations that honor cultural integrity and spiritual lineage (Collins, 2019; Hargons, 2022; Tsomo, 2024).

Clinical Application of Culturally Rooted Practices

As illustrated in Table 1, culturally responsive contemplative practices vary across community contexts, yet share a common emphasis on relational engagement, cultural reclamation, and community collaboration. For example, mindfulness-based practices within racially minoritized communities are most effective when paired with participatory approaches such as collaborative autoethnography or community-based dialogue, reinforcing that practice must emerge from context rather than be universally applied.

Building on this foundation, translating culturally rooted contemplative practices into clinical and community-based settings requires more than technical adaptation; it calls for intentional alignment with cultural meaning, relational context, and lived experience (Hargons, 2022; Watson-Singleton et al., 2019). Rather than introducing contemplative practices as pre-structured interventions, counselors are invited to co-construct these practices alongside participants, allowing culture, story, and embodiment to guide how healing unfolds (Harrell & Malebranche, 2025).

For example, when working with African American women navigating race-related stress and cumulative trauma, a counselor may begin with narrative-centered grounding rather than silence-based meditation. Sessions may open with reflective prompts that invite participants to name sources of strength, ancestral resilience, or moments of cultural pride. These narratives can then be integrated with breath-based practices that incorporate rhythm, music, or movement, allowing regulation to emerge through culturally familiar forms rather than imposed stillness (Watson-Singleton et al., 2019; Hargons, 2022).

In group contexts, contemplative practice can be facilitated through communal processes such as call-and-response dialogue, shared reflection circles, or embodied practices like gentle movement or expressive arts. These approaches support co-regulation and collective meaning-making, shifting the focus from individual symptom management to relational healing (Bhambhani & Gallo, 2021; Collins, 2019). Participants are not positioned as recipients of care, but as contributors to a shared healing space where cultural knowledge and lived experience are central (La Scala et al., 2023).

CULTURAL RESPONSIVENESS IN PRACTICE

For contemplative practices to be effective for African American women and other marginalized communities, they must align with lived experience, cultural values, and relational context (Morales & Burnett-Zeigler, 2024).

Effective culturally responsive practices, as stated by Watson-Singleton et al. (2019), involve facilitators who share cultural backgrounds, promote empowerment, storytelling, and use familiar language. Addressing faith conflicts is essential, highlighting that ethical practice demands spiritual and cultural alignment. This is necessary for women navigating trauma across multiple identities, given trauma's link to social structures determining whose suffering is acknowledged (Crenshaw, 1991). For marginalized women, healing encompasses their bodies, relationships, and social development, not just an internal shift (Collins, 2019).

Within this context, cultural responsiveness in practice is not simply about representation; it is about meaning. Participants must feel that their lived realities are not minimized or pathologized within contemplative space. This includes explicitly naming race-related stress, validating spiritual plurality, and allowing practices to be shaped by community feedback rather than imposed through standardized manuals (Watson-Singleton et al., 2019).

Facilitator identity and positionality also play a critical role. When facilitators acknowledge their own social locations and power dynamics, contemplative spaces become more transparent and trustworthy. Silence around difference can inadvertently reinforce exclusion. In contrast, reflexive dialogue fosters relational safety. Hence, cultural responsiveness extends beyond technique into relational ethics.

To grasp how contemplative practice offers both healing and resistance, we must move beyond general trauma models. Focusing on women's embodied experiences, relationships, and structural challenges is key. Healing through an intersectional lens becomes a collective process grounded in culture, community, and justice. Contemplative practice then develops as a spiral of recognition, reconnection, and shared dignity, transcending mere recovery (Hargons, 2022).

This spiral metaphor underscores that cultural responsiveness is ongoing rather than achieved. Programs must remain adaptable, continually engage community input, and adjust to evolving social conditions. Cultural congruence is not static; it requires constant dialogue, humility, and accountability.

Illustrative Case Example

This becomes visible through lived and relational engagement. Consider a community-based group intervention designed for women of color navigating chronic stress, relational trauma, and experiences of marginalization. The group begins not with silence, but with connection. The facilitator opens with culturally familiar music and a reflective prompt such as, "What has helped you carry yourself through difficult moments?"

Participants share brief narratives rooted in personal and cultural resilience. These narratives are not treated as separate from the reflective work, but rather as its foundation. Breathwork is then introduced in a way that aligns with rhythm and voice, allowing regulation to emerge through familiarity rather than imposition.

As the group develops, sessions incorporate embodied practices such as movement, storytelling, and creative expression. Participants are invited to co-create the space, offering input on what feels grounding, meaningful, and supportive. Emotional expressions such as grief, anger, and resistance are not redirected, but honored as valid responses to lived experience.

Over time, participants describe shifts not only in stress but in connection. Healing is expressed through language such as "I feel seen," "I feel more like myself," and "I'm not carrying this alone." Through this process, contemplative practice becomes a space for reclaiming identity, restoring a sense of belonging, and cultivating collective dignity.

Avoid Appropriation through Community Partnership

Adapting contemplative practices bereft of genuine community partnership can be unethical, risking cultural appropriation and silencing local wisdom (Hargons, 2022; Polinska, 2018). True collaboration is needed to preserve dignity and cultural integrity. The Intersectional Neuroscience model shows ethical alliance by partnering with diverse communities at every research step, from design to revision (Weng et al., 2020). This joint approach turns research into a mutual, empowering process, validating community knowledge and promoting justice (Hargons, 2022; Weng et al., 2020).

Appropriation often occurs subtly, when traditions are abstracted from their historical and spiritual contexts, stripped of lineage, and repackaged for commercial or institutional use. Polinska (2018) warns that such decontextualization can reproduce white ignorance by rendering practices culturally neutral while ignoring the communities from which they emerged. Ethical adaptation, therefore, requires crediting origins, engaging lineage holders when possible, and resisting commodification.

Community partnership must extend beyond advisory roles. It requires shared decision-making power, transparent communication, and equitable resource distribution. When communities are positioned merely as participants rather than collaborators, research risks extractive dynamics. In contrast, participatory models redistribute authority and foster mutual investment (La Scala et al., 2023).

In counseling contexts, this translates into co-created programming, community-led facilitation, and mechanisms for ongoing feedback. Ethical contemplative practice honors that cultural knowledge is not supplementary to clinical expertise; it is central to it.

Women's Trauma as Contextual, Layered, and Relational

It is important to recognize that while trauma-informed care has become widely accepted across mental health, education, and healthcare, many prevailing approaches regularly do not thoroughly capture how women's trauma is profoundly formed by overlapping systems of oppression and societal injustice (Crenshaw, 1991; Herman,

1992; Collins, 2019). For women, trauma is not a singular, separate event that can be neatly resolved or simply left in the past.

Feminist and intersectional scholars remind us that to understand women's trauma, we must situate it within power, social context, and lived history, rather than attempting to separate it from these shaping forces (Collins, 2019). Intersectionality clarifies that trauma is experienced differently as multiple aspects of identity intersect within a lived context, including race, culture, gender, and spiritual beliefs (Crenshaw, 1991). These intersections themselves affect how trauma shows up in their bodies, how they express distress, and how they seek help. If trauma-informed care doesn't consider these unique combinations, it risks treating all women's experiences as if they're the same. This oversight can obscure what women genuinely need and might even unintentionally cause more pain, especially for women of color and those facing multiple challenges (Hargons, 2022).

Herman (1992) reminds us that prolonged and repeated trauma often restructures relational expectations, bodily safety, and self-concept. For many women, particularly those situated at multiple marginalized intersections, trauma is cumulative, relational, and historically patterned. It is not simply a cognitive memory; it is embodied. It is transmitted through families, shaped by institutions, and reinforced by ongoing inequities. An intersectional lens reveals that trauma does not occur in isolation from racism, sexism, economic precarity, or spiritual invalidation. Rather, these forces interact, intensify, and compound vulnerability over time.

Collins (2019) extends this analysis by framing intersectionality as critical social theory, emphasizing that systems of domination are interlocking rather than additive. Thus, trauma experienced by women of color cannot be understood by stacking categories of oppression. It must be understood through structural arrangements that simultaneously shape vulnerability, resilience, and access to care. This theoretical grounding moves trauma-informed care beyond compassion into structural critique.

This deeper, intersectional understanding reveals why healing is never a simple, straight line towards being fixed. As illustrated in Figure 1, healing is more like a continuous journey of returning to oneself and evolving, nurtured by care that deeply understands culture, is informed by trauma, and is built on collective strength. As Herman (1992) reminds us, a woman's trauma often builds up over time and through relationships, permeating through families, communities, and generations, deeply affected by ongoing unfairness and constantly being dismissed, rather than just being about a few isolated events.

Within this cyclical model, regulation is not an endpoint but a doorway. Stabilization creates space for narrative reconstruction, relational repair, and cultural reconnection. Healing unfolds through iterative movements, recognition, reclamation, and reimagining, rather than a linear progression from pathology to health.

This spiral framework aligns with feminist understandings of growth as nonlinear, relational, and historically informed.

Culturally responsive contemplative practices offer a powerful way to engage with life's complexities, connecting body, mind, and relationships so healing can unfold through presence (Harrell & Malebranche, 2025). When thoughtfully adapted, these practices become safe havens that honor women's various experiences without reducing or dismissing them. This supports reconnection with the body and acknowledges cultural connections to emotion, spirituality, and healing, thereby combating feelings of disconnection (Watson-Singleton et al., 2019).

Grounded in cultural understanding and genuine community partnership, contemplative practices transform emotions such as grief, anger, and even resistance into meaningful responses to lived realities rather than simple symptoms to be corrected (Hargons, 2022). This approach to contemplative practice truly champions personal healing, collective dignity, and justice-driven transformation, much like the continuous spiral depicted in Figure 1 (Harrell & Malebranche, 2025; Watson-Singleton et al., 2019).

Notably, this reframing resists the medicalization of emotional expression. Grief may represent mourning for ancestral loss. Anger may signal the violation of dignity. Resistance may embody ethical refusal. When contemplative practice validates these emotions within a cultural context, it shifts from pacification to empowerment. Healing does not mean erasing intensity; it means integrating it with agency and community-centered belonging.

Contemplative Practice as a Feminist Praxis

From a feminist perspective, contemplative practice is much more than just self-regulation; it is a deeply relational and ethical act, recognizing that a woman's healing often blossoms using shared understanding, collective support, and mutual care rather than in isolation (Collins, 2019). Feminist praxis insists that personal transformation and social transformation are inseparable. Within this orientation, contemplative practice becomes political, not because it is partisan, but because it refuses neutrality in the face of injustice. When women gather to breathe, reflect, move, or ritualize together, they are not merely calming their nervous systems; they are reclaiming space in environments that often marginalize their voices. Presence becomes both restoration and resistance. Clinically, this may be reflected in group-based practices that prioritize shared reflection, voice, and collective meaning-making over individual inward focus alone.

We must remember that practices like meditation or profound reflection are not always safe for everyone, especially for those who have experienced significant trauma, as stillness can sometimes trigger painful memories instead of calm

(Treleaven, 2018). This is why trauma-informed contemplative approaches wisely emphasize individual choice, gentle pacing, cultural appropriateness, and strong, supportive connections rather than rigid techniques, empowering women to discover what genuinely feels grounding, meaningful, and caring in their unique healing journeys. Treleaven's (2018) trauma-sensitive framework emphasizes that choice is foundational. For survivors of interpersonal or systemic violence, enforced silence or prolonged inward focus may replicate dynamics of powerlessness. Feminist contemplative praxis, therefore, centers consent, relational attunement, and adaptive flexibility. It privileges safety not as avoidance, but as collaborative co-creation.

Contemplative healing unfolds as an ongoing cycle of returning and becoming, where personal restoration and collective dignity remain interwoven. Regulation serves as a vital foundation for reclaiming agency, rebuilding connections, and strengthening cultural continuity (Harrell & Malebranche, 2025). It is within this praxis that embodiment is reclaimed as sacred rather than surveyed. Women whose bodies have been politicized, commodified, or regulated through oppressive systems are invited to experience their bodies as sources of wisdom rather than sites of deficit. Feminist contemplative work actively challenges dominant narratives that separate cognition from embodiment and self-care from collective care.

Figure 1. Healing unfolds through presence, culture, and collective care

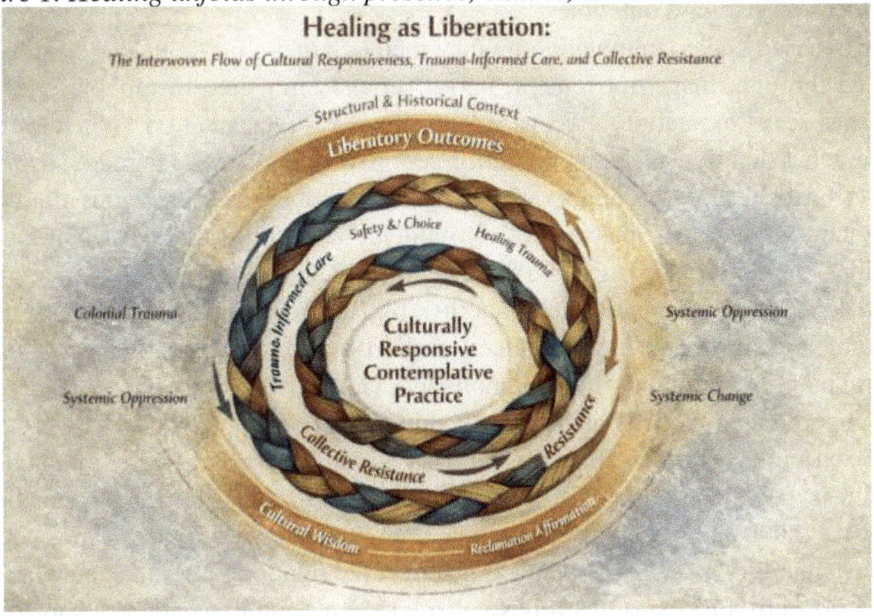

Note. Conceptual figure created by the author illustrating culturally responsive contemplative practice as a cyclical, relational process integrating personal healing and collective resistance (Crenshaw, 1991; Harrell & Malebranche, 2025).

Gaps in Assessment, Neuroscience, and Sustainability

Even with the growing research on culturally responsive contemplative practices, important gaps remain that prevent this work from truly helping people heal in ways that foster fairness and justice. These gaps frequently reflect bigger issues in how we create and evaluate knowledge in counseling and psychology. For example, many assessment tools tend to focus solely on reducing individual symptoms, often missing the key roles that relationships, culture, and community play in healing (Morales & Burnett-Zeigler, 2024).

Standardized instruments often prioritize anxiety reduction, depressive symptom decline, or physiological regulation as primary endpoints. While meaningful, these indicators do not fully capture communal belonging, restored cultural identity, or strengthened collective agency. Healing for marginalized women may manifest as increased boundary-setting, renewed spiritual connection, or participation in community ritual, outcomes that challenge narrow psychometric frameworks.

Kwah and Fellner (2020) highlight that it is important to use approaches that actively involve people and combine different ways of understanding things. This means truly attending to their stories, respecting their reflections, and valuing what well-being means to their own communities. Without these kinds of approaches, a woman's own understanding of what healing looks like can be overlooked by systems that focus on standard outcomes.

Arts-based and contemplative inquiry methods invite participants to represent healing through image, movement, narrative, and embodied metaphor. Such approaches resist extraction and instead privilege co-interpretation. When women define what dignity, safety, or liberation feel like in their own language, research shifts from evaluation to collaboration. These methodological extensions align with community-based participatory research models that intentionally redistribute power and focus on lived experience (La Scala et al., 2023).

Making these practices last is another big, interconnected challenge. Often, contemplative programs are introduced as short-term fixes rather than becoming a natural part of community life (Bhambhani & Gallo, 2021). When local leaders do not support these practices, shared ownership, and cultural inclusion, that beautiful, unbroken journey of healing (like the spiral in Figure 1) can get cut short. Sustainability is not just about maintaining programs; it is about honoring an ethical responsibility to ensure that healing remains accessible, community-centered, and lasting.

Sustainability must be reframed as an ethical obligation rather than an administrative concern. Programs that rely solely on external funding cycles or short-term grant initiatives risk reinforcing instability. When initiatives that integrate contemplative practice into existing cultural, spiritual, or educational institutions are fostered, continuity is strengthened. Shared leadership, facilitator training within communities, and adaptable program structures increase long-term practicability (Bhambhani & Gallo, 2021).

In practice, evaluation can be expanded through culturally responsive and participatory methods such as reflective journaling, narrative interviews, arts-based expressions, and community-defined indicators of well-being. These approaches allow participants to articulate shifts in dignity, belonging, and agency in their own language, offering a more holistic and contextually grounded understanding of healing beyond standardized measures.

For example, outcomes such as dignity and belonging may be operationalized through participant-defined indicators, including increased boundary-setting, willingness to engage in community dialogue, expressions of cultural pride, or shifts in relational language such as "I feel seen" or "I feel connected." These indicators, while not always captured through standardized instruments, offer meaningful insight into relational and culturally grounded healing.

Beyond how healing is understood and evaluated, sustainability intersects with epistemic justice. When marginalized communities are positioned merely as recipients rather than co-creators, programs often dissolve once external experts depart. Ethical sustainability requires capacity building, leadership cultivation, and collective ownership. Healing must remain accessible, connected, and enduring, rather than dependent on temporary institutional attention.

NEUROSCIENCE, TRAUMA, AND CONTEMPLATIVE HEALING

Expanding this perspective, neuroscience offers insight into how contemplative practices may enhance attention and self-awareness, with various studies suggesting improved brain integration. However, these outcomes call for careful interpretation, as diverse individual insights and healing outcomes often transcend standardized neuroscientific measures (Katyal et al., 2023). Existing research frequently relies on small, homogeneous samples, limiting our understanding of diverse healing processes (Morales & Burnett-Zeigler, 2024). Over-privileging neuroscience as the sole metric of progress risks disrupting the holistic healing journey by overlooking crucial relational, cultural, and contextual meanings (Hargons, 2022). For communities facing chronic stress and inequity, neuroscience alone cannot fully define or dictate how healing unfolds.

The growing field of contemplative neuroscience has produced compelling findings regarding attentional networks, emotional regulation, and neural plasticity (Weng et al., 2020). However, when neuroscientific evidence is positioned as the ultimate arbiter of legitimacy, it can inadvertently reproduce epistemic hierarchies. Communities whose healing traditions predate neuroimaging technologies do not require neural validation to establish credibility. The risk lies not in neuroscience itself, but in its elevation above cultural knowledge systems.

Weng et al. (2020) suggest that a fairer, trauma-informed, contemplative neuroscience develops when research embraces healing's spiral nature rather than fixed outcomes. Individualized, participatory methods recognize that attentional patterns during practice vary and are shaped by culture, trauma, and lived experiences. These differences are not flaws, but natural aspects of adaptation. When neuroscience supports healing rather than controlling it, it can engage with cultural wisdom, allowing scientific insight to prosper alongside equity, relational care, and justice (Collins, 2019; Weng et al., 2020).

An intersectional neuroscience framework requires methodological humility. Recruitment strategies must intentionally include racially diverse participants. Interpretation must avoid pathologizing divergence from normative baselines. Language must reflect person-centered respect rather than reductionist categorization. When grounded in ethical practice, neuroscience can offer insight into contemplative experience while honoring, rather than replacing participants' lived expertise.

Moving forward, contemplative neuroscience must adopt methodological transparency regarding sampling, interpretation, and cultural framing. Researchers should explicitly report demographic limitations and avoid universalizing findings derived from homogeneous samples (Weng et al., 2020). Furthermore, integrating qualitative participant narratives alongside neuroimaging data would contextualize neural findings within lived experience. Neural change without relational meaning risks abstraction; relational meaning without structural awareness risks romanticization. Ethical integration requires holding both simultaneously. When neuroscience is situated within community partnerships rather than positioned above them, it can contribute insights without eclipsing cultural knowledge systems.

The Intersectional Neuroscience Framework in Practice

The Intersectional Neuroscience framework guides us toward more responsible research by directly challenging biases in traditional neuroscience (Weng et al., 2020). It champions including diverse, often overlooked groups in studies, moving past the narrow focus of past research (Weng et al., 2020). This approach meaningfully involves community members from start to finish, using methods like community-based participatory research to ensure equal power between researchers and the communities they serve (La Scala et al., 2023). This commitment ensures that research remains culturally relevant, even in the interpretation of neuroimaging data. It calls for person-centered language that honors how individuals understand and define themselves (Weng et al., 2020).

This framework encourages researchers to interrogate baseline assumptions about normal neural functioning. Neural variability shaped by chronic stress or culturally specific attention patterns should not automatically be framed as a deficit. Intersectional neuroscience emphasizes contextual interpretation, recognizing that neural adaptation reflects lived environments. More importantly, this framework promotes interdisciplinary integration. This includes cultivating collaboration between neuroscientists, community scholars, clinicians, and cultural leaders that fosters richer interpretation and guards against reductionism. These partnerships not only broaden methodological rigor but also mandate ethical accountability.

HEALING AS COLLECTIVE AND RELATIONAL

For communities navigating systemic oppression, healing extends beyond individual symptom reduction and emerges through shared regulation, cultural affirmation, and collective meaning-making (Collins, 2019). These approaches not only lessen distress but also augment cultural identity, foster belonging, and boost collective efficacy (Bhambhani & Gallo, 2021). Safety in these spaces demands cultural affirmation and conscious attention to power, countering the exclusion commonly felt in mainstream settings by overtly addressing oppression and honoring full identities (Hargons, 2022). This ensures that healing unfolds through connection, sustaining the vital spiral of returning and becoming. Within counseling practice, this may involve structuring interventions around group dialogue, co-regulation, and culturally affirming spaces that emphasize shared experience rather than isolated coping.

Collective healing disrupts the privatization of suffering. Rather than positioning trauma as an individual burden, it acknowledges that harm often arises from shared structural conditions. Community-based contemplative spaces create opportunities for co-regulation, mutual witnessing, and communal affirmation. These relational processes strengthen resilience not as solitary endurance but as shared capacity.

Bhambhani and Gallo (2021) demonstrate that group-based mindfulness programs adapted for racially marginalized communities enhance social cohesion while reducing stress. Participants report increased trust, relational warmth, and collective efficacy. These outcomes illustrate that healing within the community can simultaneously address emotional and social dimensions of well-being.

Collective healing also reframes belonging as therapeutic. For women, whose identities have been marginalized within dominant institutions, contemplative spaces that affirm culture, spirituality, and lived experience restore relational safety. Belonging becomes both an outcome and a mechanism of healing.

Resistance as Therapeutic Intervention

In culturally responsive contemplative practice, resistance is not peripheral; it is integral to healing (Hargons, 2022). Sankofa-oriented approaches link regulation with cultural reclamation and collective dignity, seeing resistance and reimagining as essential healing movements (Harrell & Malebranche, 2025). Community-engaged mindfulness fosters critical consciousness of systemic racism rather than passive coping. Arts-based contemplative methods show how healing and resistance can unfold together through creative expression, allowing self-care and political refusal. These practices affirm that grief, anger, and hope can coexist, sustaining healing as a justice-oriented process rather than a return to neutrality.

Hargons (2022) argues that contemplative practice divorced from material realities risks becoming a mechanism of accommodation rather than transformation. When women are encouraged to regulate without simultaneously questioning injustice, coping replaces critical engagement. Notably, contemplative spaces that validate anger at racism or grief over gendered violence transform emotional expression into political awareness. Regulation becomes a resource for sustained advocacy rather than withdrawal.

Creative resistance, as illustrated through arts-based contemplative modalities (Kwah & Fellner, 2020), allows embodied expression to carry sociopolitical meaning. Movement, poetry, painting, and rituals become agents for reclaiming narrative authority. Within these spaces, participants are not pathologized for intensity; they are affirmed for moral clarity. Healing, then, is not about returning to a prior state of normalcy but about cultivating the capacity to endure, imagine, and organize within unjust conditions.

This reframing aligns with Collins' (2019) assertion that intersectionality requires linking personal experience with structural exploration. Contemplative practice that integrates resistance affirms that emotional well-being and social justice are not competing aims. Rather, psychological regulation can sustain long-term engagement in liberation efforts. Hope, within this model, is disciplined and communal; it is not naïve optimism, but joint commitment.

BARRIERS AND PATHWAYS FORWARD

For culturally responsive contemplative practices to genuinely thrive, they require a foundation that values both intersectionality and trauma, and that clearly accounts for how power systems influence access, engagement, and sustained viability. Intersectionality, as articulated by Crenshaw (2018), urges us to move past mere demographic inclusion, designing instead with the intention to recognize how race, gender, sexuality, disability, class, and spirituality intricately intertwine to form lived experience. In contemplative practice, this means acknowledging that identities are not separate pieces yet are deeply interwoven. This highlights that healing unfolds uniquely based on one's social location and lived experience.

Crenshaw's (1991) framework cautions against single-axis interventions that isolate one dimension of identity while neglecting others. Programs designed solely around gender without attending to race, or solely around race without attending to sexuality or disability, risk reproducing exclusion within marginalized groups. Pathways forward require intersectional implementation, not simply intersectional rhetoric.

The Intersectional Neuroscience framework illustrates how to put these principles into action. Weng et al. (2020) show this ethical research model actively tackles biases in traditional neuroscience. It does so through inclusive recruitment, person-centered language, and individualized analysis, often utilizing community-based participatory research to equalize power dynamics (Weng et al., 2020), thereby moving beyond single-axis approaches that isolate identity dimensions. This framework respects the full complexity of people's lives and trauma-informed values, viewing diverse responses as natural adaptations, not pathology.

However, barriers remain rooted. Historical mistrust of medical and psychological institutions, shaped by exploitation and neglect, inhibits engagement. Religious incongruence may arise when contemplative practices are perceived as incompatible with faith traditions. Economic constraints limit access to sustained programming. Institutional practices often shape which voices are heard, frequently favoring researchers affiliated with well-resourced universities (Morales & Burnett-Zeigler, 2024). These structural barriers cannot be resolved through individual adaptation alone; they require systemic accountability.

Implementing trauma-informed contemplative practices entails thoughtfully considering pacing, choice, predictability, embodiment, and contextual awareness, especially for racially and economically marginalized communities. Programs developed with these communities emphasize versatile scheduling, extended durations, and modular skill-building to truly accommodate chronic stressors, caregiving, and systemic limitations (Bhambhani & Gallo, 2021). Crucially, trauma-informed care within these communities must openly acknowledge colonial, racialized, and intergenerational trauma, focusing on cultural reclamation and shared meaning rather than just symptom reduction, recognizing many responses as natural coping mechanisms rather than flaws (Harrell & Malebranche, 2025). However, major obstacles persist, including cultural mismatches, historical mistrust, religious incongruence, and reduced access. Institutional inequities in research funding and academic publishing further restrict which practices are recognized and whose knowledge is valued, deepening disparities in what's considered legitimate evidence (Morales & Burnett-Zeigler, 2024).

Pathways forward include embedding contemplative education into counselor training programs, integrating cultural humility coursework, and developing co-created assessment tools with communities. Ethical implementation also demands transparent dialogue about power, funding, and representation. The future of this work depends not solely on clinical refinement but on structural transformation within the profession (Watson-Singleton et al., 2019).

When programs weave contemplative practice into existing spiritual traditions, honor local stories, and empower participants as co-creators, they develop a stronger sense of continuity and shared ownership of the healing journey (Bhambhani & Gallo, 2021). This illustrates a spiral logic in which trauma-informed, intersectional implementation is an ongoing, relational process that requires reflection, accountability, and responsiveness to what healing means to the community. These pragmatic aspects make clear that advancing culturally responsive contemplative practice is not simply a technical responsibility but a profound ethical and professional commitment that directs how we engage with healing, equity, and justice in our work.

SIGNIFICANCE FOR COUNSELING, EDUCATION, AND RESEARCH

For counselors and educators, culturally responsive contemplative practice demands humility, self-reflection, and a firm commitment to justice. Practitioners must critically examine their positionality, resist appropriation, and nurture authentic community partnerships. Training programs must prepare catalysts for race-related stress, spiritual diversity, and collective healing.

Counselor education programs must move beyond elective diversity modules and embed intersectional contemplative frameworks across the curriculum. This includes training in trauma-sensitive facilitation, race-related stress responsiveness, and ethical adaptation of contemplative traditions (Treleaven, 2018; Polinska, 2018; Watson-Singleton et al., 2019). Supervision models should incorporate reflective dialogue around cultural identity, power dynamics, and embodied countertransference.

For researchers, urgent priorities include culturally grounded assessments, inclusive neuroscience, and evaluations reflecting community-defined outcomes. Healing must be measured by dignity, belonging, and collective empowerment, not just symptom reduction. This practice implores the field to accept its ethical responsibility, recognizing that implementing healing is inseparable from upholding justice, dignity, and collective care (Collins, 2019).

Future research must expand participatory designs, longitudinal sustainability studies, and mixed-method approaches that integrate narrative, embodied, and quantitative data. Researchers must interrogate whose knowledge is cited, whose language is privileged, and whose methodologies are validated. Publication practices must widen to include community scholarship and collaborative authorship. Without such shifts, the field risks perpetuating epistemic exclusion while claiming inclusivity.

Framework for Implementation in Practice

To translate these ideas into action, the following framework outlines key considerations for implementation in practice:

1. *Cultural Grounding Through Identity and Context Exploration:* Implementation begins with intentional exploration of participants' cultural identities, spiritual beliefs, relational contexts, and lived experiences. Counselors invite individuals to define what healing, safety, and connection mean within their own cultural frameworks. This process centers on participant voice and ensures that contemplative practices align with identity, history, and community rather than with assumed universality.
2. *Relational Entry Through Dialogue and Co-Construction:* Rather than introducing contemplative practices as predetermined techniques, counselors begin with relational engagement. Dialogue serves as the entry point, allowing participants to express preferences, hesitations, and cultural considerations. Practices are then co-constructed, fostering trust and ensuring that the process emerges from a relationship rather than rigid protocol.
3. *Adaptation of Practices Using Culturally Meaningful Forms:* Contemplative practices are adapted to reflect cultural expression, including storytelling, music, movement, spiritual rituals, or communal practices. Stillness is not assumed to be the primary pathway to regulation. Instead, practices are shaped to align with participants' ways of knowing and being, allowing healing to unfold through culturally resonant forms.
4. *Integration of Community and Collective Healing Processes:* Healing is intentionally expanded beyond the individual to include relational and collective dimensions. Group-based engagement, shared reflection, and community involvement are integrated to support co-regulation and mutual witnessing. Participants are positioned as contributors to the healing space, reinforcing that healing is both individual and collective.
5. *Ongoing Reflexive Evaluation and Community Feedback:* Implementation remains dynamic through continuous reflection and feedback. Counselors engage in reflexivity, examining how their positionality and facilitation impact

the process. Participants are invited to share what feels meaningful and what needs to shift. This ongoing dialogue ensures that practices remain responsive, culturally aligned, and ethically grounded over time.

CONCLUSION

Across this chapter, a unifying insight emerges: contemplative practice is not simply an intervention, but a reorientation of how healing is understood. Rather than positioning healing as an individual, internal process, this framework situates it within relational, cultural, and structural contexts that shape lived experience. Intersectionality reveals trauma as layered and structurally embedded; feminist praxis situates healing within relational accountability and challenges neutrality in the face of injustice; Sankofa centers cultural memory and reclamation as integral to restoration; and intersectional neuroscience calls into question dominant definitions of evidence while inviting more inclusive and contextually grounded interpretations of healing. Together, these perspectives converge to form a coherent, justice-oriented framework in which contemplative practice functions not as a tool for adaptation to inequity, but as an ethical engagement that restores dignity, cultivates agency, and sustains collective care. This chapter contributes to the field by offering an integrated, justice-oriented framework that moves beyond surface-level cultural adaptation toward co-constructed, relationally grounded contemplative practices rooted in intersectionality, feminist praxis, and community engagement.

Furthermore, integrating contemplative neuroscience into this framework requires a careful balance. Neuroscientific insight offers valuable contributions to understanding attention, emotion regulation, and neural plasticity (Weng et al., 2020). Yet these contributions must remain accountable to lived experience and community knowledge. When evidence hierarchies privilege laboratory validation over embodied wisdom, epistemic inequities persist. A justice-centered contemplative science must therefore hold relational meaning and empirical inquiry in dynamic dialogue rather than competition.

Sustainability further clarifies that healing cannot be episodic. Programs rooted in community partnership, facilitator congruence, and cultural resonance endure beyond funding cycles and institutional trends (Bhambhani & Gallo, 2021). Such sustainability is not simply logistical; it is ethical. It signals a commitment to collective dignity and long-term relational repair. Intersectionality reframes trauma as interlocking rather than isolated; feminist praxis situates healing within relational accountability; Sankofa grounds contemplative work in cultural reclamation; and intersectional neuroscience challenges epistemic hierarchies. Together, these strands converge into a coherent framework in which regulation supports agency, presence restores dignity, and community sustains transformation.

To move forward, the profession must embrace contemplative practice as both intervention and ideology. Healing cannot be abstracted from power, nor can resilience be abstracted from context. Intersectionality calls the field to confront the systems that produce trauma, not simply soothing their consequences. Progress, therefore, requires evolving beyond symptom-focused solutions that inadvertently perpetuate systemic injustices. Counselors, educators, researchers, and policymakers are called to deeper ethical accountability, honoring cultural wisdom alongside empirical research, valuing community-defined meanings of healing, and designing contemplative spaces that boldly confront oppression while cultivating collective power (Hargons, 2022; Morales & Burnett-Zeigler, 2024).

To engage in contemplative practice without acknowledging culture, power, and history risks perpetuating the very inequities such practices seek to resolve. True healing is sustained through ethical presence, relational responsibility, and authentic community partnership. In this vision, contemplative practice becomes both remembrance and reimagining. It remembers ancestral wisdom, communal resilience, and embodied knowledge. It reimagines counseling not as isolated symptom management but as relational liberation work. When trauma-informed care, intersectional analysis, and culturally rooted contemplative practice converge, healing unfolds not only within individuals but within communities. This convergence marks the future direction of trauma, feminism, and intersectionality, an integrated commitment to dignity, accountability, and collective flourishing.

REFERENCES

Bhambhani, Y., & Gallo, L. (2021). Developing and adapting a mindfulness-based group intervention for racially and economically marginalized patients in the Bronx. *Cognitive and Behavioral Practice, 28*(2), 265–277. DOI: 10.1016/j.cbpra.2021.04.010

Chatters, L. M., Taylor, R. J., Bullard, K. M., & Jackson, J. S. (2008). Spirituality and subjective religiosity among African Americans, Caribbean Blacks, and Non-Hispanic Whites. *Journal for the Scientific Study of Religion, 47*(4), 725–737. DOI: 10.1111/j.1468-5906.2008.00437.x PMID: 21052481

Collins, P. H. (2019). *Intersectionality as Critical Social Theory*. Duke University Press.

Covington-Ward, Y., & Jouili, J. S. (2021). *Embodying Black Religions in Africa and Its Diasporas*. Duke University Press.

Crenshaw, K. W. (1991). Mapping the Margins: Intersectionality, Identity Politics, and Violence Against Women of Color. *Stanford Law Review, 43*(6), 1241–1299. DOI: 10.2307/1229039

Draper-Clarke, L., & Green, C. (2024). Cultivating well-being, community cohesion, and a sense of purpose through African contemplative practices. *Creative Arts in Education and Therapy, 10*(2), 235–252. DOI: 10.15212/CAET/2024/10/19

Hargons, C. N. (2022). Mindfulness and matter. In Purser, R. E., Forbes, D., & Burke, A. (Eds.), *Beyond white mindfulness: Critical perspectives on race, power, and meditation* (pp. 133–150). North Atlantic Books. DOI: 10.4324/9781003090922-8

Harrell, S. P., & Malebranche, D. A. (2025). Reclamation and emancipation in mindfulness and nature-based contemplative practice: A Sankofa-oriented collaborative autoethnography. *The American Journal of Orthopsychiatry, 95*(1), 1–15. DOI: 10.1037/ort0000860 PMID: 41166194

Herman, J. (1992). Complex PTSD: A Syndrome in survivors of prolonged and repeated trauma. *Journal of Traumatic Stress, 5*(3), 377–391. DOI: 10.1002/jts.2490050305

Katyal, S., Lumma, A. L., Goldin, P., & Roy, S. K. (2023). Editorial: The varieties of contemplative experiences and practices. *Frontiers in Psychology, 14*, 1156937. Advance online publication. DOI: 10.3389/fpsyg.2023.1232999 PMID: 37408976

Kgatle, M. S., & Qiki, V. (2023). The commercialisation of anointed water in two ministries: An African theological perspective. *In die Skriflig*, *57*(1), a2937. DOI: 10.4102/ids.v57i1.2937

Kwah, H., & Fellner, G. L. (2020). Contemplative, visual arts–based research methods for self-care and transformation. *Qualitative Research in Psychology*, *17*(4), 533–550. DOI: 10.1163/9789004446885_009

La Scala, S., Mullins, J. L., Firat, R. B., & Michalska, K. J. (2023). Equity, diversity, and inclusion in developmental neuroscience: Practical lessons from community-based participatory research. *Frontiers in Integrative Neuroscience*, *16*, 1007249. Advance online publication. DOI: 10.3389/fnint.2022.1007249 PMID: 37007188

Mboweni, T. J., & De Crom, E. P. (2016). A narrative interpretation of the cultural impressions on water of the communities along the Vaal River, Parys, Free State. *The Journal for Transdisciplinary Research in Southern Africa*, *12*(1), a345. DOI: 10.4102/td.v12i1.345

Morales, A., & Burnett-Zeigler, I. E. (2024). A scoping review of culturally adapted mindfulness-based interventions for communities of color. *Journal of Integrative and Complementary Medicine*, *30*(3), 214–226. DOI: 10.1089/jicm.2023.0457 PMID: 39093941

Polinska, W. (2018). Mindfulness meditation as a remedy to "white ignorance" and its consequences. *Journal of Applied Philosophy*, *35*(4), 683–697. DOI: 10.1111/japp.12308

Treleaven, D. A. (2018). *Trauma-sensitive mindfulness: Practices for safe and transformative healing*. WW Norton & Company.

Tsomo, K. L. (2024). Being Black and Buddhist. *Religious Studies Review*, *50*(1), 12–15. DOI: 10.1111/rsr.17079

Watson-Singleton, N. N., Black, A. R., & Spivey, B. N. (2019). Recommendations for a culturally-responsive mindfulness-based intervention for African Americans. *Complementary Therapies in Clinical Practice*, *34*, 132–138. DOI: 10.1016/j.ctcp.2018.11.013 PMID: 30712717

Weng, H. Y., Ikeda, M. P., Lewis-Peacock, J. A., Chao, M., Fullwiley, D., Goldman, V., Skinner, S., Duncan, L. G., Gazzaley, A., & Hecht, F. M. (2020). Toward a compassionate intersectional neuroscience: Increasing diversity and equity in contemplative neuroscience. *Frontiers in Psychology*, *11*, 573594. Advance online publication. DOI: 10.3389/fpsyg.2020.573134

Wepener, C., & Müller, B. (2012). Water rituals as a source of (Christian) life in an African Independent Church: To be healed and (re)connected. *Studia Liturgica, 42*(1–2), 255–269. DOI: 10.1177/0039320712042001-216

Compilation of References

Abuhassan, Q., Al-Assi, G., Rekha, M. M., Chanania, K., Bavanilatha, M., Arora, V., Sinha, A., & Hayitova, M. (2026b). Multi-omic biomarker detection in ovarian cancer. *Clinica Chimica Acta, 581*, 120758. Advance online publication. DOI: 10.1016/j.cca.2025.120758 PMID: 41349936

Abuhassan, Q., Atoom, A. M., Roopashree, R., Kanwar, J. B., Sudhakar, T., Sharma, V., Chauhan, A. S., & Ruziyev, O. (2026a). Aptasensors in colorectal cancer: Emerging tools for precision diagnostics. *Clinica Chimica Acta, 581*, 120751. Advance online publication. DOI: 10.1016/j.cca.2025.120751 PMID: 41352752

Abuhassan, Q., Saleh, K., Roopashree, R., Kanwar, J. B., Sudhakar, T., Sharma, V., Chauhan, A. S., & Khaitova, S. (2026c). Next-generation nano-biosensors for hepatocellular carcinoma. *Clinica Chimica Acta, 555*, 120805. DOI: 10.1016/j.cca.2025.120805 PMID: 41461225

Agliata, A. K., & Stewart-Spencer, S. (2026). *Mastering resilience: Strategies for high-demand professionals*. C3: Connect. Communicate. Collaborate. https://a.co/d/03xpmiAU

Alang, S., McAlpine, D., McCreedy, E., & Hardeman, R. (2017). Police brutality and Black health: Setting the agenda for public health scholars. *American Journal of Public Health, 107*(5), 662–665. DOI: 10.2105/AJPH.2017.303691 PMID: 28323470

Al-khreisat, M. J., Abdulsahib, W. K., Jasim, I. K., Malathi, H., Nayak, P. P., Anand, D. A., Mukherjee, G., Sinha, A., & Ruziyev, O. (2026). Targeting cancer stem cell plasticity and tumor microenvironment crosstalk: A comprehensive review. *Discover. Oncology, 17*(1), 145. DOI: 10.1007/s12672-025-04297-y PMID: 41422192

Allen, E. S., Atkins, D. C., Baucom, D. H., Snyder, D. K., Gordon, K. C., & Glass, S. P. (2005). Intrapersonal, interpersonal, and contextual factors in engaging in and responding to extramarital involvement. *Clinical Psychology : a Publication of the Division of Clinical Psychology of the American Psychological Association*, *12*(2), 101–130. DOI: 10.1093/clipsy.bpi014

AlRamadneh, T. N., Abdulsahib, W. K., Ismael, S. H., Roopashree, R., Nayak, P. P., Nandhini, S. U., Arora, V., Chauhan, A. S., & Ruziyev, O. (2025). Crossroads of cell fate: miR-34-mediated regulation of apoptosis and autophagy in glioblastoma. *Discover. Oncology*, *16*(1), 2177. Advance online publication. DOI: 10.1007/s12672-025-04021-w PMID: 41313571

American Counseling Association. (2014). *ACA code of ethics*. Author. https://www.counseling.org/resources/aca-code-of-ethics.pdf

American Psychiatric Association. (2022). *Diagnostic and statistical manual of mental disorders* (5th ed., text rev.)., DOI: 10.1176/appi.books.9780890425787

American Psychological Association. (2017). *Ethical principles of psychologists and code of conduct*. https://www.apa.org/ethics/code

American School Counselor Association (ASCA). (2018). *The School Counselor and Equity for All Students*. Author.

American School Counselor Association. (2022). *ASCA ethical standards for school counselors*. Author. https://www.schoolcounselor.org/Standards-Positions/Ethical-Standards

Americans with Disabilities Act of 1990, Pub. L. No. 101-336, 104 Stat. 327 (1990). congress.gov.

Americans with Disabilities Amendments Act of 2008, Pub. L. No. 110-325. (2008). ADA Amendments Act of 2008, Pub. L. No. 325, Stat. 122 (2008), 3553-3559. congress.gov.

Anderson, S., & James, R. (2025). *4 charts on Immigrant Worker Exploitation in America*. Inequality.org. https://inequality.org/article/charts-immigrant-worker-exploitation/

Anderson, K. P. (2023). Biased Opportunities: The Role of Implicit and Explicit Bias in Advanced Placement and Dual Enrollment. *Educational Evaluation and Policy Analysis*, *46*(4), 735–763. DOI: 10.3102/01623737231192487

Andrews, E. E., Forber-Pratt, A. J., Mona, L. R., Lund, E. M., Pilarski, C. R., & Balter, R. (2019). # SaytheWord: A disability culture commentary on the erasure of "disability". *Rehabilitation Psychology, 64*(2), 111–118. DOI: 10.1037/rep0000258 PMID: 30762412

APA Office on Disability Issues in Psychology. (n.d.) *APA Resource guide for psychology graduate students with disabilities* (2nd ed.). American Psychological Association. https://www.apa.org/pi/disability/resources/publications/resource-guide?shem=rimspwouoe,

APA. (1997). *Policy statement of the full participation for psychologists with disabilities.* American Psychological Association. https://www.apa.org/about/policy/participation.pdf

APA. (2008). *Resolution on the Americans with Disabilities Act.* American Psychological Association. https://www.apa.org/about/policy/disabilities-act?shem=rimspwouoe,

APA. (2014). *Resolution in support of the U.N. Convention on the Rights of Persons with Disabilities.* American Psychological Association. https://www.apa.org/about/policy/support-un-convention?shem=rimspwouoe,

APA. (2017). *Ethical principles of psychologists and code of conduct.* American Psychological Association.

APA. (2022). *Guidelines for Assessment and Intervention with Persons with Disabilities.* American Psychological Association. https://www.apa.org/pi/disability/resources/assessment-disabilities

APA. (2026a). *Standards of Accreditation for Health Service Psychology.* APA's Commission on Accreditation Standards of Accreditation. American Psychological Association. https://www.apa.org/ed/accreditation/standards-of-accreditation.pdf

APA. (2026b). *APA Guidelines for clinical supervision in Health Service Psychology.* APA Task Force on Clinical Supervision in Health Service Psychology, American Psychological Association. https://www.apa.org/about/policy/guidelines-supervision.pdf

APPIC (2020). *APPIC member policy for legal and ethical conduct.* Association of Psychology Post-doctoral and Internship Centers. https://www.appic.org/About-APPIC/APPIC-Policies/Member-Policy?shem=rimspwouoe,

Arnsten, A. F. T. (2015). Stress weakens prefrontal networks: Molecular insults to higher cognition. *Nature Neuroscience, 18*(10), 1376–1385. DOI: 10.1038/nn.4087 PMID: 26404712

Asakura, K., Miller, J., Nakash, O., & O'Neill, P. (2023). Toward "Decolonizing" Clinical Social Work Practice and Education. *Smith College Studies in Social Work*, *93*(2–4), 73–82. DOI: 10.1080/00377317.2023.2279389

ASPPB. (n.d.). *Current examination for professional practice in psychology (EPPP)®content areas*. https://asppb.net/exams/asppb-examination-for-professional-psychology-eppp/eppp-exam-topics/

Association for Spiritual, Ethical, and Religious Value in Counseling (2024). *Competencies for Addressing Spiritual and Religious Issues in Counseling*. Alexandria: Association for Spiritual, Ethical, and Religious Value in Counseling https://aservic.org/

Atkins, D. C., Baucom, D. H., & Jacobson, N. S. (2001). Understanding infidelity: Correlates in a national random sample. *Journal of Family Psychology*, *15*(4), 735–749. DOI: 10.1037/0893-3200.15.4.735 PMID: 11770478

Avery, J. C., Morris, H., Galvin, E., Misso, M., Savaglio, M., & Skouteris, H. (2021). Systematic review of school-wide trauma-informed approaches. *Journal of Child & Adolescent Trauma*, *14*(3), 381–397. DOI: 10.1007/s40653-020-00321-1 PMID: 34471456

Avon and Somerset Police Federation. (2021, September 15). *Capture data on traumatic incidents*. Police Federation of England and Wales. https://www.polfed.org/avonsom/news/news-articles/capture-data-on-traumatic-incidents/

Babanataj, R., Mazdarani, S., Hesamzadeh, A., Gorji, M. H., & Cherati, J. Y. (2019). Resilience training: Effects on occupational stress and resilience of critical care nurses. *International Journal of Nursing Practice*, *25*(1), e12697. Advance online publication. DOI: 10.1111/ijn.12697 PMID: 30338603

Bailey, Z. D., Feldman, J. M., & Bassett, M. T. (2021). How structural racism works—Racist policies as a root cause of U.S. racial health inequities. *The New England Journal of Medicine*, *384*(8), 768–773. DOI: 10.1056/NEJMms2025396 PMID: 33326717

Baker, J. (2025). *The overlapping roots of Mental Health Disparities: Poverty, racism, and trauma as Social Determinants - Behavioral Health News*. Behavioral Health News. https://behavioralhealthnews.org/the-overlapping-roots-of-mental-health-disparities-poverty-racism-and-trauma-as-social-determinants/

Ballo, E., & Tribe, R. (2023). Therapeutic work with clients living in poverty. *The International Journal of Social Psychiatry*, *69*(4), 1043–1050. DOI: 10.1177/00207640221139798 PMID: 36609182

Banaji, M. R., & Greenwald, A. G. (2013). *Blind spot: Hidden biases of good people*. Delacorte Press.

Bargeman, M., Abelson, J., Mulvale, G., Niec, A., Theuer, A., & Moll, S. (2022). Understanding the Conceptualization and Operationalization of Trauma-Informed Care Within and Across Systems: A Critical Interpretive Synthesis. *The Milbank Quarterly*, *100*(3), 785–853. DOI: 10.1111/1468-0009.12579

Bargeman, M., Smith, S., & Wekerle, C. (2021). Trauma-informed care as a rights-based "standard of care": A critical review. *Child Abuse & Neglect*, *119*, 104762. DOI: 10.1016/j.chiabu.2020.104762

Bargiela, S., Steward, R., & Mandy, W. (2016). The experiences of late-diagnosed women with autism spectrum conditions: An investigation of the female autism phenotype. *Journal of Autism and Developmental Disorders*, *46*(10), 3281–3294. DOI: 10.1007/s10803-016-2872-8 PMID: 27457364

Barnett, J. E. (2011). Utilizing technology to provide clinical supervision: Opportunities and challenges. *The Clinical Supervisor*, *30*(1), 59–77.

Bauer, K. L., Eskew, S., Tung, G., Leiferman, J. A., Fort, M. P., McManus, B. M., & Johnson-Koenke, R. A. (2025). Marginalization and Intersectionality in Adults' Relationship to Society Explain Increasing Loneliness: A Critical Realist Lens on Thematic Narrative Inquiry. *International Journal of Qualitative Methods*, *24*, 16094069251346264. Advance online publication. DOI: 10.1177/16094069251346264

Baughman, K., Leventhal, L., Black, S., & Friedheim, R. E. (2005). The missing link: Disability inclusion in psychology education, training, and employment. [Poster]. *APA Annual Conference*, Los Angeles.

Bergeman, C. S., & Nelson, N. A. (2024). Building a dynamic adaptational process theory of resilience (ADAPTOR): Stress exposure, reserve capacity, adaptation, and consequence. *The American Psychologist*, *79*(8), 1063–1075. DOI: 10.1037/amp0001280 PMID: 39531707

Berliner, L., & Kolko, D. J. (2016). Trauma Informed Care: A Commentary and Critique. *Child Maltreatment*, *21*(2), 168–172. DOI: 10.1177/1077559516643785

Berring, L. L., Holm, T., Hansen, J. P., Delcomyn, C. L., Søndergaard, R., & Hvidhjelm, J. (2024). Implementing Trauma-Informed Care—Settings, Definitions, Interventions, Measures, and Implementation across Settings: A Scoping Review. *Healthcare (Basel)*, *12*(9), 908. DOI: 10.3390/healthcare12090908

Bhambhani, Y., & Gallo, L. (2021). Developing and adapting a mindfulness-based group intervention for racially and economically marginalized patients in the Bronx. *Cognitive and Behavioral Practice*, *28*(2), 265–277. DOI: 10.1016/j.cbpra.2021.04.010

Billings, J., & Nicholls, H. (2025). PTSD and complex PTSD, current treatments and debates: A review of reviews. *British Medical Bulletin*, *156*(1), ldaf015. Advance online publication. DOI: 10.1093/bmb/ldaf015 PMID: 41004137

Bills, L. J., Hutchison, S. L., Snider, M. D. H., Skrzypek, B. E., Minnich, C. L., Korney, J. M., Taylor, R. M., & Herschell, A. D. (2023). Implementing a trauma-informed system of care: An analysis of learning collaborative outcomes. *Journal of Traumatic Stress*, *36*(2), 433–443. DOI: 10.1002/jts.22931 PMID: 36995179

Blanden, J., Doepke, M., & Stuhler, J. (2023). Educational inequality. In E. A. Hanushek, S. Machin, & L. Woessmann (Eds.), *Handbook of the Economics of Education* (pp. 405-497). (Handbook of the Economics of Education; Vol. 6). Elsevier B.V. https://doi.org/DOI: 10.1016/bs.hesedu.2022.11.003

Bloom, S. L. (2013). *Creating sanctuary: Toward the evolution of sane societies* (2nd ed.). Routledge.

Bogart, K. R., Heydarian, N. M., Hughes, A. S., Lund, E. M., & Rosa, N. M. (2026). Special issue introduction: Creating an anti-ableist psychology curriculum and teaching environment. *Teaching of Psychology*, *1-4*(2), 115–118. Advance online publication. DOI: 10.1177/00986283251412268

Bogart, K. R., Lund, E. M., Rottenstein, A., & Bouchard, L. (2017). Who self-identifies as disabled? An examination of impairment and contextual predictors. *Rehabilitation Psychology*, *62*(4), 553–562. DOI: 10.1037/rep0000132 PMID: 28581320

Bogart, L. R. (2014). The role of disability self-concept in adaptation to congenital or acquired disability. *Rehabilitation Psychology*, *59*(1), 107–115. DOI: 10.1037/a0035800 PMID: 24611927

Bokek-Cohen, Y., & Gabay, G. (2025). Medical gaslighting as a threat to beneficence and patient autonomy: A qualitative study. *BMC Medical Ethics*, *27*(1), 5. Advance online publication. DOI: 10.1186/s12910-025-01324-z PMID: 41272715

Bolton, M. J. (2023). De-centering neuronormativity is an imperative in humanistic psychotherapy: Towards a neurodiversity-informed, person-centered approach. *The Person-Centered Journal*, 1-39. DOI: 10.31234/osf.io/q2t8h

Bor, J., Venkataramani, A. S., Williams, D. R., & Tsai, A. C. (2018). Police killings and their spillover effects on the mental health of Black Americans: A population-based, quasi-experimental study. *Lancet, 392*(10144), 302–310. DOI: 10.1016/S0140-6736(18)31130-9 PMID: 29937193

Bowen, E. A., & Murshid, N. S. (2016). Trauma-informed social policy: A conceptual framework for policy analysis and advocacy. *American Journal of Public Health, 106*(2), 223–229. DOI: 10.2105/AJPH.2015.302970 PMID: 26691122

Bowlby, J. (1982). Attachment and loss: Vol. 1. *Attachment* (2nd ed.). Basic Books. (Original work published 1969)

Bowlby, J. (1988). *A secure base: Parent-child attachment and healthy human development*. Basic Books.

Bride, B. E. (2007). Prevalence of secondary traumatic stress among social workers. *Social Work, 52*(1), 63–70. DOI: 10.1093/sw/52.1.63 PMID: 17388084

Brison, S. J. (1999). Trauma narratives and the remaking of the self. In Bal, M., Crewe, J., & Spitzer, L. (Eds.), *Acts of Memory: Cultural Recall in the Present* (pp. 39–54). University Press of New England.

Bryant-Davis, T., & Ocampo, C. (2005). The trauma of racism: Implications for counseling, research, and education. *The Counseling Psychologist, 33*(4), 574–578. DOI: 10.1177/0011000005276581

Bumgardner, K. (2023). Ableism in education: Professor perpetuation of disability discrimination through accommodation non-compliance. *Scripps Senior Theses*.2184. https://scholarship.claremont.eduScripps_theses/2184

Bunch, L., & Ketema, H. (2025). *Health insurance coverage in the United States: 2024*. Census.gov. https://www.census.gov/library/publications/2025/demo/p60-288.html

Burstow, B. (2003). Toward a radical understanding of trauma and trauma work. *Violence Against Women, 9*(11), 1293–1317. DOI: 10.1177/1077801203255555

California Southern University. (2026). *Statement on suitability and fitness for the profession.* https://calsouthern.smartcatalogiq.com/en/2025-2026/general-catalog/school-of-behavioral-sciences/doctor-of-psychology-clinical-specialization)

Carter, R. T. (2007). Racism and psychological and emotional injury: Recognizing and assessing race-based traumatic stress. *The Counseling Psychologist, 35*(1), 13–105. DOI: 10.1177/0011000006292033

Castillo, L. G., Perez, F. V., Castillo, R., & Ghosheh, M. R. (2010). Construction and initial validation of the Marianismo Beliefs Scale. *Counselling Psychology Quarterly*, *23*(2), 163–175. DOI: 10.1080/09515071003776036

Chafouleas, S. M., Johnson, A. H., Overstreet, S., & Santos, N. M. (2016). Toward a Blueprint for Trauma-Informed Service Delivery in Schools. *School Mental Health*, *8*(1), 144–162. DOI: 10.1007/s12310-015-9166-8

Champine, R. B., Lang, J. M., Nelson, A. M., Hanson, R. F., & Tebes, J. K. (2019). Systems Measures of a Trauma-Informed Approach: A Systematic Review. *American Journal of Community Psychology*, *64*(3–4), 418–437. DOI: 10.1002/ajcp.12388

Chatters, L. M., Taylor, R. J., Bullard, K. M., & Jackson, J. S. (2008). Spirituality and subjective religiosity among African Americans, Caribbean Blacks, and Non-Hispanic Whites. *Journal for the Scientific Study of Religion*, *47*(4), 725–737. DOI: 10.1111/j.1468-5906.2008.00437.x PMID: 21052481

Childers, C. (2023). *Rooted in racism and economic exploitation: The failed Southern Economic Development Model*. Economic Policy Institute. https://www.epi.org/publication/rooted-in-racism/

Chittom, L., & Walter, A. (2024). *Zero-tolerance policies in schools: Overview*. EBSCO. https://www.ebsco.com/research-starters/education/zero-tolerance-policies-schools-overview#about-the-author

Choi, J., Gabay, E. K., Rachel, A., Brown, A., Cruz, R., Yan, Q., & Cuccaro, P. M. (2024). Evaluation of a trauma-informed care (TIC) training program across community health centers in Texas: A qualitative study. *BMC Health Services Research*, *24*(1), 1360. Advance online publication. DOI: 10.1186/s12913-024-11813-3 PMID: 39511566

Chun, Y., Roll, S., Miller, S., Lee, H., Larimore, S., & Grinstein-Weiss, M. (2023). Racial and Ethnic Disparities in Housing Instability During the COVID-19 Pandemic: The Role of Assets and Income Shocks. *Journal of Economics, Race, and Policy*, *6*(2), 63–81. DOI: 10.1007/s41996-022-00109-5 PMID: 36474600

Clandinin, D. J., & Connelly, F. M. (2000). *Narrative inquiry: Experience and story in qualitative research*. Jossey-Bass.

Clark, M., Ausloos, C., Delaney, C., Waters, L., Salpietro, L., & Tippett, H. (2020). Best Practices for Counseling Clients Experiencing Poverty: A Grounded Theory. *Journal of Counseling and Development*, *98*(3), 283–294. DOI: 10.1002/jcad.12323

Clements, A. D., Haas, B., Cyphers, N. A., Hoots, V., & Barnet, J. (2020). Creating a communitywide system of trauma-informed care. *Progress in Community Health Partnerships, 14*(4), 499–507. DOI: 10.1353/cpr.2020.0055 PMID: 33416770

Cloitre, M., Hyland, P., Prins, A., & Shevlin, M. (2021). The International Trauma Questionnaire (ITQ) measures reliable and clinically significant treatment-related change in PTSD and complex PTSD. *European Journal of Psychotraumatology, 12*(1), 1930961. DOI: 10.1080/20008198.2021.1930961 PMID: 34211640

Cochran, C. B. (2019). Infusing the Principles of Trauma-Informed Care Into Emergency Nursing: A Comprehensive Approach to Change Practice. *Journal of Forensic Nursing, 15*(4), 206–213. DOI: 10.1097/JFN.0000000000000267

Collins, P. H. (2000). *Black feminist thought: Knowledge, consciousness, and the politics of empowerment* (2nd ed.). Routledge.

Collins, P. H. (2019). *Intersectionality as Critical Social Theory*. Duke University Press.

Conching, A. K. S., & Thayer, Z. (2021). Biological pathways for historical trauma to affect health: A conceptual model focusing on epigenetic modifications. *Social Science & Medicine, 230*, 74–82. DOI: 10.1016/j.socscimed.2019.04.001 PMID: 30986608

Condon, M., Bloomfield, M. A. P., Nicholls, H., & Billings, J. (2023). Expert international trauma clinicians' views on the definition, composition and delivery of reintegration interventions for complex PTSD. *European Journal of Psychotraumatology, 14*(1), 2165024. Advance online publication. DOI: 10.1080/20008066.2023.2165024 PMID: 37052098

Connor, K. M., & Davidson, J. R. T. (2003). Development of a new resilience scale: The Connor-Davidson Resilience Scale (CD-RISC). *Depression and Anxiety, 18*(2), 76–82. DOI: 10.1002/da.10113 PMID: 12964174

Conover, K. J., Israel, T., & Nylund-Gibson, K. (2017). Development and validation of the Ableist Microaggressions Scale. *The Counseling Psychologist, 45*(4), 570–599. DOI: 10.1177/0011000017715317

Cook, J. M., Simiola, V., Ellis, A. E., & Thompson, R. (2017). Training in trauma psychology: A national survey of doctoral graduate programs. *Training and Education in Professional Psychology, 11*(2), 108–114. DOI: 10.1037/tep0000150

Council for Accreditation of Counseling and Related Educational Programs. (2024). *2024 CACREP standards*. https://www.cacrep.org/for-programs/2024-cacrep-standards/

Covington-Ward, Y., & Jouili, J. S. (2021). *Embodying Black Religions in Africa and Its Diasporas*. Duke University Press.

Crenshaw, K. (1989). Demarginalizing the intersection of race and sex: A Black feminist critique of antidiscrimination doctrine, feminist theory and antiracist politics. *University of Chicago Legal Forum, 1989*(1), 139–167. https://chicagounbound.uchicago.edu/uclf/vol1989/iss1/8

Crenshaw, K. (1989). Demarginalizing the intersection of race and sex: A Black feminist critique of antidiscrimination doctrine, feminist theory, and antiracist politics. *University of Chicago Legal Forum, 1989*(1), 139–167.

Crenshaw, K. (1991). Mapping the margins: Intersectionality, identity politics, and violence against women of color. *Stanford Law Review, 43*(6), 1241–1299. DOI: 10.2307/1229039

Cronholm, P. F., & Dichter, M. E. (2018). The need for systems of care and a trauma-informed approach to intimate partner violence. *American Family Physician, 97*(11). https://www.aafp.org/pubs/afp/issues/2018/0601/p717.html PMID: 30215942

Cronholm, P. F., Forke, C. M., Wade, R., Bair-Merritt, M. H., Davis, M., Harkins-Schwarz, M., Pachter, L. M., & Fein, J. A. (2021). Adverse childhood experiences: Expanding the concept of adversity. *American Journal of Preventive Medicine, 49*(3), 354–361. DOI: 10.1016/j.amepre.2015.02.001 PMID: 26296440

Daoud, E., Abdulsahib, W. K., Ismael, S. H., Roopashree, R., Ray, S., Nellore, J., Mukherjee, G., Chauhan, A. S., & Kholiyeva, M. (2025). Nanomedicine and nutraceutical-based nanocarriers for specific delivery to cancer stem cells: Targeted drug delivery at the STEM frontier. *Discover. Oncology, 16*(1), 4057. DOI: 10.1007/s12672-025-04057-y PMID: 41286210

Dautovich, N. D., Katjijova, M., Cyrus, J. W., & Kliewer, W. (2023). Duty-related stressors, adjustment, and the role of coping processes in first responders: A systematic review. *Psychological Trauma: Theory, Research, Practice, and Policy, 15*(Suppl. 2), S286–S296. DOI: 10.1037/tra0001258 PMID: 35653742

De Vynck, E., Boynton, H. M., & Burns, V. F. (2023). Pulled from the shorelines in search of spacious spirituality: Journeys of spiritual distress, resilience and post-traumatic growth for women for evangelical Christian backgrounds in a Canadian context. *Religions, 14*(9), 1193. DOI: 10.3390/rel14091193

Delgado, R., & Stefancic, J. (2017). *Critical race theory: An introduction* (3rd ed.). NYU Press.

DePrince, A. P., Combs, M. D., & Shanahan, M. E. (2016). Victim advocacy, social support, and trauma recovery: Practice, research, and policy. *Journal of Interpersonal Violence, 31*(1), 110–118.

Downey, J., & Greco, J. (2023). Trauma sensitive schools: A comprehensive guide for the assessment planning and implementation of trauma informed frameworks. *Children and Youth Services Review, 149*, 106930. DOI: 10.1016/j.childyouth.2023.106930

Draper-Clarke, L., & Green, C. (2024). Cultivating well-being, community cohesion, and a sense of purpose through African contemplative practices. *Creative Arts in Education and Therapy, 10*(2), 235–252. DOI: 10.15212/CAET/2024/10/19

Drew, D., Banks, B., & Joseph, R. (2022). Religion and spirituality in clinical practice: An exploration of comfort and discomfort among practitioners. *Social Thought, 41*(1), 104–120. https://psycnet.apa.org/doi/10.1080/15426432.2021.1994099

Dubi, M., Powell, P. W., & Gentry, E. (2017). *Trauma, PTSD, grief & loss: The 10 core competencies for evidence-based treatment*. PESI Publishing & Media.

Duffey, T., & Haberstroh, S. (2020). *Introduction to crisis and trauma counseling*. American Counseling Association.

Du, L. J. (2024). The associations between religiosity and resilience when individuals are challenged by risk factors of suicide and mental illness. *Frontiers in Public Health, 12*, 1442248. DOI: 10.3389/fpubh.2024.1442248 PMID: 39145184

Dunn, D. S., & Burkaw, S. (2013). Disability identity: Exploring narrative accounts of disability. *Rehabilitation Psychology, 58*(2), 148–157. DOI: 10.1037/a0031691 PMID: 23437994

Edgar, N. E., MacLean, S. E., Jormand, M., Paranjkhoo, P., & Hatcher, S. (2025). Designing a trauma informed service to deliver trauma therapy with people experiencing homelessness: A qualitative study. *BMC Health Services Research, 25*(1), 1350. DOI: 10.1186/s12913-025-13428-8 PMID: 41074101

Ekbäck, E., Granåsen, G., Svärling, R., Blomqvist, I., & Henje, E. (2021). Clinical effectiveness of training for awareness resilience and action online compared to standard treatment for adolescents and young adults with depression: Study protocol and analysis plan for a pragmatic, multi-center randomized controlled superiority trial. *Frontiers in Psychiatry, 12*, 674583. Advance online publication. DOI: 10.3389/fpsyt.2021.674583 PMID: 34707516

Elisseou, S., Shamaskin-Garroway, A., Kopstick, A. J., Potter, J., Weil, A., Gundacker, C., & Moreland-Capuia, A. (2024). Leading organizations from burnout to trauma-informed resilience: A vital paradigm shift. *The Permanente Journal, 28*(1), 198–205. DOI: 10.7812/TPP/23.110 PMID: 38332699

El-Khalil, C., Tudor, D. C., & Nedelcea, C. (2025). Impact of intergenerational trauma on second-generation descendants: A systematic review. *BMC Psychology, 13*(1), 668. DOI: 10.1186/s40359-025-03012-4 PMID: 40597246

Elliott, D. E., Bjelajac, P., Fallot, R. D., Markoff, L. S., & Reed, B. G. (2005). Trauma-informed or trauma-denied: Principles and implementation of trauma-informed services for women. *Journal of Community Psychology, 33*(4), 461–477. DOI: 10.1002/jcop.20063

Ellis, B. H., Abdi, S. M., Lazarevic, V., White, M. T., Lincoln, A. K., Stern, J. E., & Horgan, J. G. (2021). Relation of psychosocial factors to diverse behaviors and attitudes among Somali refugee youth in the United States. *The American Journal of Orthopsychiatry, 86*(4), 393–403. DOI: 10.1037/ort0000121 PMID: 26618939

Ellis, H. M., Hook, J. N., Zuniga, S., Hodge, A. S., Ford, K. M., Davis, D. E., & Van Tongeren, D. R. (2022). Religious/spiritual abuse and trauma: A systematic review of the empirical literature. *Spirituality in Clinical Practice, 9*(4), 213–231. DOI: 10.1037/scp0000301

Emerson, L. (2026, January 15). *Servicemembers, veterans are quitting psychotherapy treatment for post-traumatic stress disorder*. U.S. Medicine. https://www.usmedicine.com/clinical-topics/ptsd/servicemembers-veterans-are-quitting-psychotherapy-treatment-for-post-traumatic-stress-disorder/

Erickson, M., & Harvey, T. (2023). A Framework for a Structured Approach for Formulating a Trauma-Informed Environment. *Journal of Education, 203*(3), 666–677. DOI: 10.1177/00220574211046811

Erikson, E. H. (1964). Inner and outer space: Reflections on womanhood. *Daedalus*, •••, 582–606.

Ernstmeyer, K., & Christman, E. (2022). *Nursing: Mental Health and Community Concepts*. Open Resources for Nursing (Open RN). Chippewa Valley Technical College.

Espiritu Gandhi, E. L., & Nguyen, V. (2023). *The Routledge Handbook of Refugee Narratives*. Routledge. DOI: 10.4324/9781003131458

Family Educational Rights and Privacy Act of 1974, 20 U.S.C. §232g. govinfo.gov

Farah, H., Abdulsahib, W. K., Ismael, S. H., Roopashree, R., Ray, S., Nandhini, S. U., Arora, V., Chauhan, A. S., & Buriyeva, D. (2026). Emerging small molecule strategies target cancer stem cells through ferroptosis and metabostemness. *Discover. Oncology*, *17*(1), 111. DOI: 10.1007/s12672-025-04259-4 PMID: 41390898

Farmer, P. (2004). An anthropology of structural violence. *Current Anthropology*, *45*(3), 305–325. DOI: 10.1086/382250

Figley, C. R. (2002). Compassion fatigue: Psychotherapists' chronic lack of self-care. *Journal of Clinical Psychology*, *58*(11), 1433–1441. DOI: 10.1002/jclp.10090 PMID: 12412153

Fishman, D. B. (1999). *The case for pragmatic psychology*. New York University Press.

Flores, N. (2020). From academic language to language architecture: Challenging raciolinguistic ideologies in research and practice. *Theory into Practice*, *59*(1), 22–31. DOI: 10.1080/00405841.2019.1665411

Forester-Miller, H., & Davis, T. (1996). *A practitioner's guide to ethical decision making*. American Counseling Association.

Forkey, H., Szilagyi, M., Kelly, E. T., Duffee, J., Springer, S. H., Fortin, K., Jones, V. F., Vaden Greiner, M. B., Ochs, T. J., Partap, A. N., Davidson Sagor, L., Allen Staat, M., Thackeray, J. D., Waite, D., & Weber Zetley, L. (2021). Trauma-informed care. *Pediatrics*, *148*(2), e2021052580. DOI: 10.1542/peds.2021-052580 PMID: 34312292

Foss-Kelly, L. L., Generali, M. M., & Kress, V. E. (2017). Counseling Strategies for Empowering People Living in Poverty: The I-CARE Model. *Journal of Multicultural Counseling and Development*, *45*(3), 201–213. DOI: 10.1002/jmcd.12074

Foucault, M. (1977). *Discipline and punish: The birth of the prison*. Pantheon.

Foucault, M. (1980). *Power/knowledge: Selected interviews and other writings*. Pantheon.

Fowler, J. W. (1981). *Stages of faith*. Harper & Row.

Frankl, V. E. (1984). *Man's search for meaning* (Rev. ed.). Washington Square Press. (Original work published 1959)

Freed, D., Palmer, J., Minchala, D., Levy, K., Ristenpart, T., & Dell, N. (2017). "A stalker's paradise": How intimate partner abusers exploit technology. *Proceedings of the ACM on Human-Computer Interaction, 1*(CSCW), 1–27.

Freyd, J. J. (1996). *Betrayal trauma: The logic of forgetting childhood abuse*. Harvard University Press.

Freyd, J. J. (2013). Preventing betrayal. *Journal of Trauma & Dissociation, 14*(2), 119–124. PMID: 24060032

Freyd, J. J., Kles, B., & Allard, C. B. (2005). Betrayal trauma: Relationship to physical health, psychological distress, and a written intervention. *Journal of Trauma & Dissociation*, *6*(3), 83–104. DOI: 10.1300/J229v06n03_04 PMID: 16172083

Fricker, M. (2007). *Epistemic Injustice: Power and the Ethics of Knowing*. Oxford University Press., DOI: 10.1093/acprof:oso/9780198237907.001.0001

Fung, L. K. (2021). *Neurodiversity: From phenomenology to neurobiology and enhancing technologies*. American Psychiatric Association. DOI: 10.1176/appi.books.9781615379514

Furnham, A., Richards, S. C., & Palhus, D. L. (2013). The dark triad of personality: A 10-year review. *Social and Personality Psychology Compass*, *7*(3), 199–216. DOI: 10.1111/spc3.12018

Galiana-Simal, A., Vela-Romero, M., Romero-Vela, V. M., Oliver-Tercero, N., García-Olmo, V., Benito-Castellanos, P. J., Muñoz-Martinez, V., & Beato-Fernandez, L. (2020). Sensory processing disorder: Key points of a frequent alteration in neurodevelopmental disorders. *Cogent Medicine*, *7*(1), 1736829. DOI: 10.1080/2331205X.2020.1736829

Gil-Goméz, E. N. (2017). (In)visibilities: A woman faculty of color search for a disabled identity that fits. In Massé, M. A., & Bauer-Maglin, N. (Eds.), *Staging women's lives in academia: Gendered life stages in language and literature workplaces*. SUNY Press.

Glass, S. P., & Wright, T. L. (1985). Sex differences in type of extramarital involvement and marital dissatisfaction. *Journal of Sex Research*, *21*(4), 361–387.

Goldstein, E., Chokshi, B., Melendez-Torres, G., Rios, A., Jelley, M., & Lewis-O'Connor, A. (2024). Effectiveness of Trauma-Informed Care Implementation in Health Care Settings: Systematic Review of Reviews and Realist Synthesis. *The Permanente Journal*, *28*(1), 135–150. DOI: 10.7812/TPP/23.127

Goodkind, J. R., LaNoue, M., Lee, C., Freeland, L., & Freund, R. (2021). Feasibility, acceptability, and initial findings from a community-based cultural mental health intervention for American Indian youth and their families. *Journal of Community Psychology*, *40*(4), 381–405. DOI: 10.1002/jcop.20517 PMID: 25414529

Gottfried, A. W., Gottfried, A. E., Bathurst, K., Guerin, D. W., & Parramore, M. M. (2014). Socioeconomic status in children's development and family environment: Infancy through adolescence. In *Socioeconomic status, parenting, and child development* (pp. 189–207). Routledge.

Gottman, J. M., & Driver, J. L. (2005). Dysfunctional marital conflict and everyday marital interaction. *Journal of Divorce & Remarriage*, *43*(3–4), 63–77. DOI: 10.1300/J087v43n03_04

Gradus, J. L., & Galea, S. (2023). Moving From Traumatic Events to Traumatic Experiences in the Study of Traumatic Psychopathology. *American Journal of Epidemiology*, *192*(10), 1609–1612. DOI: 10.1093/aje/kwad126 PMID: 37218615

Gross, J. J. (1998). The emerging field of emotion regulation: An integrative review. *Review of General Psychology*, *2*(3), 271–299. DOI: 10.1037/1089-2680.2.3.271

Gross, J. J., & John, O. P. (2003). Individual differences in two emotion regulation processes: Implications for affect, relationships, and well-being. *Journal of Personality and Social Psychology*, *85*(2), 348–362. DOI: 10.1037/0022-3514.85.2.348 PMID: 12916575

Guevara, A. M. M., Johnson, S. L., Elam, K., Rivas, T., Berendzen, H., & Gal-Szabo, D. E. (2021). What Does it Mean to be Trauma-Informed? A Multi-System Perspective from Practitioners Serving the Community. *Journal of Child and Family Studies*, *30*(11), 2860–2876. DOI: 10.1007/s10826-021-02094-z

Gupta, D., Azizbek, I., Suxrob, P., & Abdullaeva, I. Ravshan kizi, B. M., Abdukabilovna, T. D., & Jumayev, U. (2026a). Digital hoboism. In E. Kaygisiz (Ed.), *Digital ideologies in the age of algorithmic culture* (pp. 307-338). IGI Global Scientific Publishing. https://doi.org/DOI: 10.4018/979-8-3373-4531-4.ch010

Gupta, D., Nigora, A., Gulkhayo, G., Nuriddin, E., Karimov, S., Otabek, M., & Kuanishbay, S. (2026b). Explainable and transparent AI architectures. In Pakshad, P., & Omar, M. (Eds.), *Examining vulnerabilities and adversarial exploitation of AI and LLMs* (pp. 297–324). IGI Global Scientific Publishing., DOI: 10.4018/979-8-3373-8252-4.ch011

Hagion-Rzepka, C. (2023). The invisible minority: Addressing disability in graduate psychology training programs. In Jesus, Â. (Ed.), *Instructional Approaches for Health Professions Education*. IGI Global Scientific.

Hansen, D. T. (2024). *Trauma-informed spiritual care: Interventions for safety, meaning, reconnection, and justice*. Fortress Press. DOI: 10.2307/jj.12949092

Hanson, R. F., & Lang, J. (2021). A critical look at trauma-informed care among agencies and systems serving maltreated youth and their families. *Child Maltreatment, 21*(2), 95–100. DOI: 10.1177/1077559516635274 PMID: 26951344

Hargons, C. N. (2022). Mindfulness and matter. In Purser, R. E., Forbes, D., & Burke, A. (Eds.), *Beyond white mindfulness: Critical perspectives on race, power, and meditation* (pp. 133–150). North Atlantic Books. DOI: 10.4324/9781003090922-8

Hargrave, A. S., Garcia, C. M., Lightfoot, M., Handley, M. A., Weeks, J., Olsen, P., Knight, K. R., & Kushel, M. B. (2024). "We Remember the Pain": A qualitative study of intergenerational trauma among older adults experiencing homelessness in the HOPE HOME study. *Journal of Social Distress and the Homeless, 33*(1), 103–111. DOI: 10.1080/10530789.2022.2080793 PMID: 38948456

Harrell, S. P., & Malebranche, D. A. (2025). Reclamation and emancipation in mindfulness and nature-based contemplative practice: A Sankofa-oriented collaborative autoethnography. *The American Journal of Orthopsychiatry, 95*(1), 1–15. DOI: 10.1037/ort0000860 PMID: 41166194

Harsey, S., & Freyd, J. J. (2020). Deny, attack, reverse victim and offender (DARVO): What is the influence on perceived perpetrator and victim credibility? *Journal of Aggression, Maltreatment & Trauma, 29*(8), 897–916. DOI: 10.1080/10926771.2020.1774695

Hartinger-Saunders, R. M., Jones, A. S., & Rittner, B. (2019). Improving Access to Trauma-Informed Adoption Services: Applying a Developmental Trauma Framework. *Journal of Child & Adolescent Trauma, 12*(1), 119–130. DOI: 10.1007/s40653-016-0104-1

Hatcher, S. S., Bride, B. E., Oh, H., King, D. M., & Catrett, J. F. (2021). An assessment of secondary traumatic stress in juvenile justice education workers. *Journal of Correctional Health Care, 17*(3), 208–217. DOI: 10.1177/1078345811401509 PMID: 21571748

Henshall, C., Davey, Z., & Jackson, D. (2020). The implementation and evaluation of a resilience enhancement programme for nurses working in the forensic setting. *International Journal of Mental Health Nursing, 29*(3), 508–520. DOI: 10.1111/inm.12689 PMID: 31930654

Herman, J. (1992). Complex PTSD: A Syndrome in survivors of prolonged and repeated trauma. *Journal of Traumatic Stress, 5*(3), 377–391. DOI: 10.1002/jts.2490050305

Herman, J. L. (1992). *Trauma and Recovery: The Aftermath of Violence, from Domestic Abuse To Political Terror*. Basic Books.

Herman, J. L. (1992). *Trauma and recovery: The aftermath of violence—from domestic abuse to political terror*. Basic Books.

Herman, J. L. (1992). *Trauma and recovery: The aftermath of violence—From domestic abuse to political terror*. Basic Books.

Herman, J. L. (2015). Justice from the victim's perspective. *Violence Against Women, 21*(6), 638–658. DOI: 10.1177/1077801205274450 PMID: 16043563

Higginbotham, E. B. (1993). *Righteous discontent: The women's movement in the Black Baptist church, 1880–1920*. Harvard University Press.

Hochschild, A. R. (2003). The managed heart: Commercialization of human feeling (20th anniversary ed.). University of California Press. (Original work published 1983)

Holmes, M. R., King, J. A., Miller, E. K., King-White, D. L., Korsch-Williams, A. E., Johnson, E. M., Oliver, T. S., & Conard, I. T. (2023). Innovations in Trauma-Informed Care: Building the Nation's First System of Trauma-Informed Recreation Centers. *Behavioral Sciences (Basel, Switzerland), 13*(5), 394. DOI: 10.3390/bs13050394

Hook, J. N., Davis, D. E., Owen, J., Worthington, E. L., & Utsey, S. O. (2013). Cultural humility: Measuring openness to culturally diverse clients. *Journal of Counseling Psychology, 60*(3), 353–366. DOI: 10.1037/a0032595 PMID: 23647387

Hopper, E. K., Bassuk, E. L., & Olivet, J. (2010). Shelter from the storm: Trauma-informed care in homelessness services. *The Open Health Services and Policy Journal, 3*, 80–100. htttps://DOI: 10.2174/1874924001003020080

HRC. (2022). *The wage gap among LGBTQ+ workers in the United States*. https://www.hrc.org/resources/the-wage-gap-among-lgbtq-workers-in-the-united-states#:~:text=Economic%20Disparities%20Faced%20by%20the,its%20basic%20necessities%20and%20resources

Huo, Y., Couzner, L., Windsor, T., Laver, K., Dissanayaka, N. N., & Cations, M. (2023). Barriers and enablers for the implementation of trauma-informed care in healthcare settings: A systematic review. *Implementation Science Communications, 4*(1), 49. Advance online publication. DOI: 10.1186/s43058-023-00428-0 PMID: 37147695

Hurtado, A. (1996). *The color of privilege: Three blasphemies on race and feminism*. University of Michigan Press. DOI: 10.3998/mpub.9839

Imel, Z. E., Laska, K., Jakupcak, M., & Simpson, T. L. (2013). Meta-analysis of dropout in treatments for posttraumatic stress disorder. *Journal of Consulting and Clinical Psychology*, *81*(3), 394–404. DOI: 10.1037/a0031474 PMID: 23339535

Jones, T. W., Power, J., & Jones, T. M. (2022). Religious trauma and moral injury from LGBTQA+ conversion practices. *Social science & medicine (1982)*, *305*, 115040. https://doi.org/Top of FormDOI: 10.1016/j.socscimed.2022.115040

Jones, M. N., Elliott, K., Sherman, S. N., Falade, E., Clark, R. L., Lipps, L., Hill-Williams, L., Williams, C., Copeland, K. A., Beck, A. F., Unaka, N., Burkhardt, M. C., & Corley, A. M. S. (2025). "Racism Happens Every Day, All the Time": Black Families' Outpatient Experiences of Racism Across a Large Pediatric System. *Academic Pediatrics*, *25*(1), 102566. Advance online publication. DOI: 10.1016/j.acap.2024.08.011 PMID: 39191371

Jordan, J. V. (2019). Relational-cultural theory: the power of connection to transform our lives. *Journal of Humanistic Counseling, October 2017, 56,* 228-243

Jordan, J. V. (2024). Relational–cultural therapy. *(3rd Ed).* American Psychological Association. Bottom of FormJohnson, D. W. and VanVonderen, J. (1991) *The subtle power of spiritual abuse*. Bethany House Publishers DOI: 10.1037/0000411-000

Jordan, J. V. (2024). *The development of relational-cultural theory*. Jean Baker Miller Training Institute. https://www.wcwonline.org/JBMTI-Site/the-development-of-relational-cultural-theory

Kalisch, R., Müller, M. B., & Tüscher, O. (2015). A conceptual framework for the neurobiological study of resilience. *Behavioral and Brain Sciences*, *38*, e92. Advance online publication. DOI: 10.1017/S0140525X1400082X PMID: 25158686

Karatzias, T., McGlanaghy, E., & Cloitre, M. (2023). Enhanced Skills Training in Affective and Interpersonal Regulation (ESTAIR): A new modular treatment for International Classification of Diseases, 11th revision, complex posttraumatic stress disorder (CPTSD). *Brain Sciences*, *13*(9), 1300. Advance online publication. DOI: 10.3390/brainsci13091300 PMID: 37759901

Kassam-Adams, N., Marsac, M. L., Kohser, K. L., Kenardy, J., March, S., & Winston, F. K. (2021). A new method for assessing content validity in model-based creation and iteration of eHealth interventions. *Journal of Medical Internet Research*, *17*(4), e95. DOI: 10.2196/jmir.3811 PMID: 25881584

Katyal, S., Lumma, A. L., Goldin, P., & Roy, S. K. (2023). Editorial: The varieties of contemplative experiences and practices. *Frontiers in Psychology*, *14*, 1156937. Advance online publication. DOI: 10.3389/fpsyg.2023.1232999 PMID: 37408976

Kauffman, J. M., Hallahan, D. P., & Pullen, P. C. (Eds.). (2017). *Handbook of Special Education* (2nd ed.). Routledge., DOI: 10.4324/9781315517698

Kearns, J., Davidson, G., Shannon, C., & Mulholland, C. (2026). How trauma-informed are we? A comparative framework analysis of early intervention service guidelines for psychosis and trauma-informed principles. *Psychosis*, •••, 1–19. DOI: 10.1080/17522439.2025.2603435

Keast, R., Lengyell, M., Finnigan, C., Brown, J., & Jay, M. (2025). Barriers to Mental Health Care for Low-Income Clients As Perceived By Counsellors. *Journal for Social Action in Counseling and Psychology*, *17*(1), 2–21. DOI: 10.33043/r23873x5

Kenjayev, Y., Khalikova, N., Eshqobilov, O., Axmedov, U., Babamuratov, A., & Xursanov, A. (2026). Utilizing pH-sensitive nanoparticles in cancer radiotherapy: Mechanisms and therapeutic potential. *Journal of Nanoparticle Research*, *28*(2), 36. DOI: 10.1007/s11051-026-06553-w

Kessler, R. C., Aguilar-Gaxiola, S., Alonso, J., Benjet, C., Bromet, E. J., Cardoso, G., Degenhardt, L., de Girolamo, G., Dinolova, R. V., Ferry, F., Florescu, S., Gureje, O., Haro, J. M., Huang, Y., Karam, E. G., Kawakami, N., Lee, S., Lepine, J. P., Levinson, D., & Koenen, K. C. (2017). Trauma and PTSD in the WHO World Mental Health Surveys. *European Journal of Psychotraumatology*, *8*(sup5, Suppl. 5), 1353383. Advance online publication. DOI: 10.1080/20008198.2017.1353383 PMID: 29075426

Kgatle, M. S., & Qiki, V. (2023). The commercialisation of anointed water in two ministries: An African theological perspective. *In die Skriflig*, *57*(1), a2937. DOI: 10.4102/ids.v57i1.2937

Khan, A. U., Jasim, Y. H., Shahid, K., Saidov, J., Atamuratova, Z., & Urazbaeva, D. (2025). Circulating tumor DNA as a predictive biomarker for colorectal cancer postsurgical recurrence: A systematic review and meta-analysis. *Clinical & Translational Oncology*, *28*(4), 1348–1362. Advance online publication. DOI: 10.1007/s12094-025-04073-y PMID: 41107654

Kim, J., Aggarwal, A., Maloney, S., & Tibbits, M. (2021). Organizational assessment to implement trauma-informed care for first responders, child welfare providers, and healthcare professionals. *Professional Psychology, Research and Practice*, *52*(6), 569–578. DOI: 10.1037/pro0000408

Kirkbride, J. B., Anglin, D. M., Colman, I., Dykxhoorn, J., Jones, P. B., Patalay, P., Pitman, A., Soneson, E., Steare, T., Wright, T., & Griffiths, S. L. (2024). The social determinants of mental health and disorder: Evidence, prevention and recommendations. *World Psychiatry; Official Journal of the World Psychiatric Association (WPA)*, *23*(1), 58–90. DOI: 10.1002/wps.21160 PMID: 38214615

Knight, C. (2015). Trauma-informed social work practice: Practice considerations and challenges. *Clinical Social Work Journal*, *43*(1), 25–37. DOI: 10.1007/s10615-014-0481-6

Kohlberg, L. (1981). *The psychology of moral development*. Essays on moral development. Harper & Row.

Kolmes, K. (2012). Social media in the future of professional psychology. *Professional Psychology, Research and Practice*, *43*(6), 606–612. DOI: 10.1037/a0028678

Kress, V. E., Haiyasoso, M., Zolden, C. A., Headley, J. A., & Trepal, H. (2018). The use of relational-cultural theory in counseling clients who have traumatic stress disorder. *Journal of Counseling and Development*, *96*(1), 106–114. https://psycnet.apa.org/doi/10.1002/jcad.12182. DOI: 10.1002/jcad.12182

Kroger, J. (2007). *Identity development: Adolescence through adulthood* (2nd ed.). Sage.

Kuemmel, A., & Wilbur, R. (2020). Thirty-one years after the ADA: The perplexity of disability. *APPIC 2020 Conference*.

Kurz, H. D., & Salvadori, N. (2023). Marx's concept of "exploitation" and the problem of measurement. *Journal of Economic Behavior & Organization*, *212*, 887–896. DOI: 10.1016/j.jebo.2023.06.016

Kvarfordt, C. L., & Herba, K. (2018). Religion and spirituality in social work practice with children and adolescents: A survey of Canadian practitioners. *Child & Adolescent Social Work Journal*, *35*(2), 153–167. DOI: 10.1007/s10560-017-0513-5

Kwah, H., & Fellner, G. L. (2020). Contemplative, visual arts–based research methods for self-care and transformation. *Qualitative Research in Psychology*, *17*(4), 533–550. DOI: 10.1163/9789004446885_009

La Scala, S., Mullins, J. L., Firat, R. B., & Michalska, K. J. (2023). Equity, diversity, and inclusion in developmental neuroscience: Practical lessons from community-based participatory research. *Frontiers in Integrative Neuroscience*, *16*, 1007249. Advance online publication. DOI: 10.3389/fnint.2022.1007249 PMID: 37007188

Langer, K., Wolf, O. T., Merz, C. J., & Jentsch, V. L. (2025). The effects of stress hormones on cognitive emotion regulation: A systematic review and integrative model. *Neuroscience and Biobehavioral Reviews, 170*, 106040. Advance online publication. DOI: 10.1016/j.neubiorev.2025.106040 PMID: 39909150

Lanza, A., Roysircar, G., & Rodgers, S. (2018). First responder mental healthcare: Evidence-based prevention, postvention, and treatment. *Professional Psychology, Research and Practice*, *49*(3), 193–204. DOI: 10.1037/pro0000192

Leedham, A., Thompson, A. R., Smith, R., & Freeth, M. (2020). 'I was exhausted trying to figure it out': The experiences of females receiving an autism diagnosis in middle to late adulthood. *Autism*, *24*(1), 135–146. DOI: 10.1177/1362361319853442 PMID: 31144507

Lee, H., Fawsett, J., & Demarco, R. (2016). Stroytelling/ narrative theory to address health communication with minority populations. *Applied Nursing Research, 30*, 558–560. DOI: 10.1016/j.apnr.2015.09.004 PMID: 27091254

Leitch, L., & McCaw, B. (2024). Time to move forward: Resilience and trauma-informed care. *The Permanente Journal*, *28*(1), 188–192. DOI: 10.7812/TPP/23.076 PMID: 37862407

Lett, K. (2018). *Impact of ableist microaggressions on university students with self-identified disabilities*. University of Regina.

Levenson, J. (2021). Trauma-informed social work practice. *Social Work*, *62*(2), 105–113. DOI: 10.1093/sw/swx001 PMID: 28339563

Lewis, R. K., Martin, P. P., & Guzman, B. L. (2022). COVID-19 and vulnerable populations. *Journal of Community Psychology*, *50*(6), 2537–2541. DOI: 10.1002/jcop.22880 PMID: 35567541

Liasidou, A., & Gregoriou, A. (2024). A systematic literature review of intersectionality and disability in education. *British Journal of Sociology of Education*, *45*(4), 584–608. DOI: 10.1080/01425692.2024.2340562

Lindsay, S., & Fuentes, K. (2022, April 07). It is time to address ableism in academia: A systematic review of the experiences and impact of ableism among faculty and staff. *Disabilities*, *2*(2), 178–203. DOI: 10.3390/disabilities2020014

Liu, S. R., Kia-Keating, M., & Nylund-Gibson, K. (2021). Patterns of adversities and pathways to health among White, Black, and Latinx youth. *Child Abuse & Neglect*, *86*, 89–99. DOI: 10.1016/j.chiabu.2018.09.007 PMID: 30273815

Lodi-Smith, J. (Sep 4, 2025). From the Board: APA council approves major policy changes—Master's-level practice, disability inclusion, and traditional wisdom integration. Society for Personality and Social Psychology. *SPSP News Blog.* https://spsp.org/news/spsp-news/board-apa-council-approves-6-major-policy-changes?shem=rimspwouoe,

Louw, B. (2024). *Neonatal Opioid Withdrawal Syndrome: Speech-Language Pathologists and Interprofessional Care* (1st ed.). Routledge., DOI: 10.4324/9781003397267

Lucchetti, G., Koenig, H. G., & Granero Lucchetti, A. L. (2021). Spirituality, religiousness, and mental health: A review of the current scientific evidence. *World Journal of Clinical Cases, 9*(16), 7620–7631. DOI: 10.12998/wjcc.v9.i26.7620 PMID: 34621814

Lund, E. M. (2023). Addressing the leaking pipeline: Supporting disabled graduate student teachers in psychology. *Teaching of Psychology, 50*(2), 99-104. DOI: 10.1177/0098628321103642

Lund, E. M. (2018). Disability as diversity in professional psychology: A continued call for research and action. *Training and Education in Professional Psychology, 12*(4), 295–296. DOI: 10.1037/tep0000218

Lund, E. M., Khazeem, L. R., & DeJesus, C. R. (2023). Addressing intersectional identities and experiences professional psychology trainees with disabilities. A call for action. *Training and Education in Professional Psychology, 17*(2), 185–190. DOI: 10.1037/tep0000403

Lynch, J. M., Stange, K. C., Dowrick, C., Getz, L., Meredith, P. J., Van Driel, M. L., Harris, M. G., Tillack, K., & Tapp, C. (2025). The sense of safety theoretical framework: A trauma-informed and healing-oriented approach for whole person care. *Frontiers in Psychology, 15*, 1441493. DOI: 10.3389/fpsyg.2024.1441493

MacIntosh, H. B. (2024). Developmental couple therapy for complex trauma: A pilot study of treatment outcomes. *Journal of Marital and Family Therapy, 50*(2), 411–432.

Mahood, E., Shahid, M., Gavin, N., Rahmann, A., Tadakamadla, S. K., & Kroon, J. (2024). Theories, Models, Frameworks, Guidelines, and Recommendations for Trauma-Informed Oral Healthcare Services: A Scoping Review. *Trauma, Violence & Abuse, 25*(2), 869–884. DOI: 10.1177/15248380231165699

Mao, L., Huang, L., & Chen, Q. (2021). Promoting resilience and lower stress in nurses and improving inpatient experience through emotional intelligence training in China: A randomized controlled trial. *Nurse Education Today*, *107*, 105130. Advance online publication. DOI: 10.1016/j.nedt.2021.105130 PMID: 34543939

Mark, K. P., Janssen, E., & Milhausen, R. R. (2011). Infidelity in heterosexual couples: Demographic, interpersonal, and personality-related predictors of extradyadic sex. *Archives of Sexual Behavior*, *40*(5), 971–982. DOI: 10.1007/s10508-011-9771-z PMID: 21667234

Marsac, M. L., Kassam-Adams, N., Hildenbrand, A. K., Nicholls, E., Winston, F. K., Leff, S. S., & Fein, J. (2021). Implementing a trauma-informed approach in pediatric health care networks. *JAMA Pediatrics*, *170*(1), 70–77. DOI: 10.1001/jamapediatrics.2015.2206 PMID: 26571032

Maslow, A. H. (1943). A theory of human motivation. *Psychological Review*, *50*(4), 370–396. DOI: 10.1037/h0054346

Maslow, A. H. (1954). *Motivation and personality*. Harper & Row.

Matthews, C., Leary, K., & Ricks, E. (2022). Intersectionality and trauma-informed care: A framework for culturally responsive practice. *Journal of Counseling Psychology*, *69*(3), 215–229. DOI: 10.1080/10926771.2019.1572403

Mattingly, C. (1998). *Healing Dramas and Clinical Plots: The Narrative Structure of Experience*. Cambridge University Press. DOI: 10.1017/CBO9781139167017

Mboweni, T. J., & De Crom, E. P. (2016). A narrative interpretation of the cultural impressions on water of the communities along the Vaal River, Parys, Free State. *The Journal for Transdisciplinary Research in Southern Africa*, *12*(1), a345. DOI: 10.4102/td.v12i1.345

McDonald, K. E., Keys, C. B., & Balcazar, F. E. (2007). Disability, race/ethnicity and gender: Themes of cultural oppression, acts of individual resistance. *American Journal of Community Psychology*, *39*(1-2), 145–161. DOI: 10.1007/s10464-007-9094-3 PMID: 17294120

McEwen, B. S., & Akil, H. (2020). Revisiting the stress concept: Implications for affective disorders. *The Journal of Neuroscience : The Official Journal of the Society for Neuroscience*, *40*(1), 12–21. DOI: 10.1523/JNEUROSCI.0733-19.2019 PMID: 31896560

McKenzie-Mohr, S., & Lafrance, M. (Eds.). (2014). *Women Voicing Resistance: Discursive and Narrative Explorations*. Routledge. DOI: 10.4324/9780203094365

Mehrotra, S., & Swami, N. (2018). Looking Beyond Distress: A Call for Spanning the Continuum of Mental Health Care. *Cureus, 10*(6), e2815. DOI: 10.7759/cureus.2815 PMID: 30128219

Menjívar, C., & Abrego, L. J. (2012). Legal violence: Immigration law and the lives of Central American immigrants. *American Journal of Sociology, 117*(5), 1380–1421. DOI: 10.1086/663575

Meuris, J., & Gladstone, J. (2023). Contextual Inequality in the Performance Costs of Financial Precarity. *Journal of Management, 50*(3), 014920632311531. DOI: 10.1177/01492063231153136

Meuris, J., & Leana, C. (2018). The Price of Financial Precarity: Organizational Costs of Employees' Financial Concerns. *Organization Science, 29*(3), 398–417. DOI: 10.1287/orsc.2017.1187

Meyer, I. H. (2003). Prejudice, social stress, and mental health in lesbian, gay, and bisexual populations: Conceptual issues and research evidence. *Psychological Bulletin, 129*(5), 674–697. DOI: 10.1037/0033-2909.129.5.674 PMID: 12956539

Middleton, J. S., Bloom, S. L., Strolin-Goltzman, J., & Caringi, J. (2019). Trauma-informed care and the public child welfare system: The challenges of shifting paradigms. *Journal of Public Child Welfare, 13*(3), 235–244. DOI: 10.1080/15548732.2019.1603602

Mikulincer, M., & Shaver, P. R. (2016). *Attachment in adulthood: Structure, dynamics, and change* (2nd ed.). Guilford Press.

Miller, J. B. (2012). *Toward a new psychology of women.* Beacon Press.

Miller, K. K., Brown, C. R., Shramko, M., & Svetaz, M. V. (2021). Applying trauma-informed practices to the care of refugee and immigrant youth: 10 clinical pearls. *Children (Basel, Switzerland), 6*(8), 94. DOI: 10.3390/children6080094 PMID: 31434278

Mirza, S. A., & Rooney, C. (2018). *Discrimination prevents LGBTQ people from accessing health care - center for american progress.* Center for American Progresss. https://www.americanprogress.org/article/discrimination-prevents-lgbtq-people-accessing-health-care/

Mkandawire-Valhmu, L. (2018). *Cultural Safety, Healthcare and Vulnerable Populations: A Critical Theoretical Perspective* (1st ed.). Routledge., DOI: 10.4324/9781315708706

Mohatt, N. V., Thompson, A. B., Thai, N. D., & Tebes, J. K. (2014). Historical trauma as public Narrative: A conceptual review. *Social Science & Medicine*, *106*, 128–136. DOI: 10.1016/j.socscimed.2014.01.043 PMID: 24561774

Morales, A., & Burnett-Zeigler, I. E. (2024). A scoping review of culturally adapted mindfulness-based interventions for communities of color. *Journal of Integrative and Complementary Medicine*, *30*(3), 214–226. DOI: 10.1089/jicm.2023.0457 PMID: 39093941

Najavits, L. M. (2015). The problem of dropout from "gold standard" PTSD therapies. *F1000prime Reports*, *7*, 43. Advance online publication. DOI: 10.12703/P7-43 PMID: 26097716

Nario-Redmond, M. (2024). Ableism: The many manifestations of disability prejudice. In Bennett, G., & Goodall, E. (Eds.), *The Palgrave Encyclopedia of Disability*., DOI: 10.1007/978-3-031-40858-8_8-1

Negi, N. J., Cepeda, A., & Valdez, A. (2021). Crime victimization among immigrant Latino day laborers in post-Katrina New Orleans. *Hispanic Journal of Behavioral Sciences*, *35*(3), 354–369. DOI: 10.1177/0739986313488089 PMID: 39371044

Nerenberg, J. (2020). *Divergent mind: Thriving in a world that wasn't designed for you*. Harper One.

Niles, S., & Harris-Bowlsbey, J. (2016). *Career development interventions in the 21st century* (5th ed.). Pearson.

O'Dwyer, C., Tarzia, L., Fernbacher, S., & Hegarty, K. (2019). Health professionals' experiences of providing care for women survivors of sexual violence in psychiatric inpatient units. *BMC Health Services Research*, *19*(1), 839. Advance online publication. DOI: 10.1186/s12913-019-4683-z PMID: 31727056

O'Hara, C., Chang, C. Y., & Giordano, A. L. (2021). Multicultural Competence in Counseling Research: The Cornerstone of Scholarship. *Journal of Counseling and Development*, *99*(2), 200–209. DOI: 10.1002/jcad.12367

Oakley, L., Kinmond, K., & Humphreys, J. (2018). Spiritual abuse in Christian faith settings: Definition, policy and practice guidance. *Journal of Adult Protection*, *20*(3-4), 144–154. DOI: 10.1108/JAP-03-2018-0005

Office of Disease Prevention and Health Promotion. (2023). *Poverty*. Poverty - Healthy People 2030. https://odphp.health.gov/healthypeople/priority-areas/social-determinants-health/literature-summaries/poverty

Olkin, R. (1999). *What psychotherapists should know about disability*. Guilford Press.

Olkin, R., Hayward, H., Abbene, M. S., & VanHeel, G. (2019). The experiences of microaggressions against women with visible and invisible disabilities. *The Journal of Social Issues*, *75*(3), 757–785. https://doi.org/. DOI: 10.1111/josi.12342

Oral, R., Ramirez, M., Coohey, C., Nakada, S., Walz, A., Kuntz, A., Benoit, J., & Peek-Asa, C. (2021). Adverse childhood experiences and trauma informed care: The future of health care. *Pediatric Research*, *79*(1), 227–233. DOI: 10.1038/pr.2015.197 PMID: 26460523

Osman, J. (2019). *Navigating intersectionality: how race, class, and gender overlap*. Enslow Publishing. https://ebookcentral.proquest.com/lib/jmu/detail.action?docID=5733748

Ott, T. (2025). Purity cultures and the ideology of 'bodies as property'as form of sexual violence. *Theology and Sexuality*, *31*(1-3), 54–73. DOI: 10.1080/13558358.2025.2525613

Oxlander, H. K., & Parrish, D. E. (2018). Integrating clients' religion/ spirituality in clinical practice: A comparison among social workers, psychologists, counselors, and nurses. *Journal of Clinical Psychology*, *74*, 680–694. DOI: 10.1002/jclp.22539 PMID: 29023713

Padilla, A. M. (1994). Ethnic minority scholars: Research, and mentoring. *Educational Researcher*, *23*(4), 24–27.

Palfrey, N., Reay, R. E., Aplin, V., Cubis, J. C., McAndrew, V., Riordan, D. M., & Raphael, B. (2021). Achieving service change through the implementation of a trauma-informed care training program within a mental health service. *Community Mental Health Journal*, *55*(3), 467–475. DOI: 10.1007/s10597-018-0272-6 PMID: 29705979

Papaleontiou - Louca, E.Papaleontiou - Louca. (2025). Spirituality and religiosity in the developing person. *Journal of Beliefs & Values*, *46*(1), 15–46. DOI: 10.1080/13617672.2023.2267924

Paredes, L. G., Wang, Y., Keene, D. E., Gill, T. M., & Becher, R. D. (2024). Population-based estimates of major forms of housing insecurity among community-living older Americans. *Journal of the American Geriatrics Society*, *72*(12), 3773–3783. DOI: 10.1111/jgs.19167 PMID: 39229863

Peeren, S., Montgomery, E., Sweeney, A., Spaducci, G., Kaul, A., Smeeth, D., & Oram, S. (2025). Trauma-informed healthcare from the perspectives of women who have experienced sexual violence in adulthood: A systematic review and meta-ethnography. *BMC Health Services Research*, *26*(1), 13. Advance online publication. DOI: 10.1186/s12913-025-13584-x PMID: 41310653

Perel, E. (2007). *Mating in captivity: Unlocking erotic intelligence*. HarperCollins.

Perry, B. D., & Szalavitz, M. (2017). *The Boy Who Was Raised as a Dog: And Other Stories From a Child Psychiatrist's Notebook* (3rd ed.). Basic Books.

Perry, B. D., & Winfrey, O. (2021). *What Happened to You? Conversations on Trauma, Resilience and Healing*. Flatiron Books.

Perry, S. L. (2024). *Religion for realists: Why we all need the scientific study of religion*. Oxford University Press. DOI: 10.1093/oso/9780197672549.001.0001

Peternelj-Taylor, C. (2018). Trauma-Informed Care: Responding to the Call for Action. *Journal of Forensic Nursing*, *14*(4), 185–186. DOI: 10.1097/JFN.0000000000000224

Piaget, J. (1929). *The child's conception of the world*. Harcourt, Brace.

Pink-Harper, S. A., Davis, R. S., & Burnside, R. (2017). "Justice for all": An examination of self-identified LGBT job satisfaction in the US federal workforce. *Canadian Journal of Administrative Sciences*, *34*(2), 182–197. DOI: 10.1002/cjas.1420

Polinska, W. (2018). Mindfulness meditation as a remedy to "white ignorance" and its consequences. *Journal of Applied Philosophy*, *35*(4), 683–697. DOI: 10.1111/japp.12308

Porges, S. W. (2022). Polyvagal theory: A science of safety. *Frontiers in Integrative Neuroscience*, *16*, 871227. Advance online publication. DOI: 10.3389/fnint.2022.871227 PMID: 35645742

Powers, A., Langhinrichsen-Rohling, R. A., Sonu, S. C., Haynes, T., & Lathan, E. C. (2024). Brief trauma-informed care training to enhance health care providers' knowledge, comfort, and implementation of trauma-informed care in primary care clinics: A pilot effectiveness study. *Psychological Services*, *21*(4), 792–796. DOI: 10.1037/ser0000823 PMID: 37956055

Ptak, M. K., Smith, D., Pridgen, S., & Held, P. (2025). Pre-treatment resilience as a predictor of veterans' post-traumatic stress disorder symptom outcomes immediately and up to 12-months following intensive cognitive processing therapy. *Journal of Clinical Psychology*, *81*(12), 1213–1220. DOI: 10.1002/jclp.70029 PMID: 41074762

Purtle, J. (2021). Systematic review of evaluations of trauma-informed organizational interventions that include staff trainings. *Trauma, Violence & Abuse, 21*(4), 725–740. DOI: 10.1177/1524838018791304 PMID: 30079827

Rafa, A. (2019). *The Status of School Discipline in State Policy.* Education Commission of the States. www.ecs.org/the-status-of-school-discipline-in-state-policy

Reamer, F. G. (2015). Clinical social work in a digital environment: Ethical and risk-management challenges. *Clinical Social Work Journal, 43*(2), 120–132. DOI: 10.1007/s10615-014-0495-0

Reeves, E. (2021). A synthesis of the literature on trauma-informed care. *Issues in Mental Health Nursing, 36*(9), 698–709. DOI: 10.3109/01612840.2015.1025319 PMID: 26440873

Rehabilitation Act of 1973, 29 U.S.C. § 794. 28 CFR 35.104.

Reid, K., Odusanya, A., Lawrence, W., & Hastings, J. (2022). Commentary: An Equitable Approach to Serving Structurally Marginalized Communities. *Family & Community Health, 45*(4), 215–217. DOI: 10.1097/FCH.0000000000000345 PMID: 35985021

Rimon, A., & Shelef, L. (2025). Moral injury among medical personnel and first responders across different healthcare and emergency response settings: A narrative review. *International Journal of Environmental Research and Public Health, 22*(7), 1055. Advance online publication. DOI: 10.3390/ijerph22071055 PMID: 40724122

Robey, N., Margolies, S., Sutherland, L., Rupp, C., Black, C., Hill, T., & Baker, C. N. (2021). Understanding staff- and system-level contextual factors relevant to trauma-informed care implementation. *Psychological Trauma: Theory, Research, Practice, and Policy, 13*(2), 249–257. DOI: 10.1037/tra0000948 PMID: 32915041

Rosen, L. T. (2021). Mapping out epistemic justice in the clinical space. *Philosophy, Ethics, and Humanities in Medicine; PEHM, 16*(1), 9. Advance online publication. DOI: 10.1186/s13010-021-00110-0 PMID: 34696799

Rosenthal, L., & Lobel, M. (2016). Stereotypes of Black American women related to sexuality and motherhood. *Psychology of Women Quarterly, 40*(3), 414–427. DOI: 10.1177/0361684315627459 PMID: 27821904

Rubinstein, D., Abargil, M., Duek, O., & Harpaz-Rotem, I. (2025). RESET posttraumatic stress disorder: Clinical protocol integrating reconsolidation, exposure, and short-term emotional transformation. *European Journal of Psychotraumatology, 16*(1), 2540141. Advance online publication. DOI: 10.1080/20008066.2025.2540141 PMID: 40815290

Rutledge, M. L., & Smith-Durkin, S. D. (2025). Antiracist School Counseling Advocacy Framework. *Professional School Counseling*, *29*(1), 2156759X251340047. Advance online publication. DOI: 10.1177/2156759X251340047

Rutledge, M., Cameron, E., & Susko, J. (2023). *School Counselors as Antiracist and Social Justice Advocates. Foundations of school counseling: Innovation in professional practice*. Springer Publishing., DOI: 10.1891/9780826187536.0001

Rutter, M. (2006). Implications of resilience concepts for scientific understanding. *Annals of the New York Academy of Sciences*, *1094*(1), 1–12. DOI: 10.1196/annals.1376.002 PMID: 17347337

Sabater Minarim, D., Morgan, K. M., Buckley, K., Riviere, P., Ochoa, C., Deshler, L. N., Duran, E. A., Mehtsun, W. T., Rose, B. S., & Banegas, M. P. (2025). Racial and Ethnic Disparities in Perceived Healthcare Discrimination and Health Outcomes: Racial and Ethnic Disparities in Perceived Healthcare Discrimination. *Journal of General Internal Medicine*, *40*(11), 2548–2557. DOI: 10.1007/s11606-025-09627-y PMID: 40447985

Sadusky, A., Berger, E. P., & Toporkova, L. (2021). Examination of trauma training for postgraduate psychology students. *Clinical Psychologist*, *25*(3), 306–315. DOI: 10.1080/13284207.2021.1913047

Schank, J. A., & Skovholt, T. M. (2006). Multiple relationships and boundary challenges for therapists in rural practice. *Journal of Clinical Psychology*, *62*(4), 505–512.

Schön, D. A. (1983). *The reflective practitioner: How professionals think in action*. Basic Books.

Sebton, S. A., Bridger, C. M., Arias, P. A., Okeibunor, C. K., Spencer, S. R., Willis, R. E., Taylor, S. E., & Alsip, B. J. (2025). Comprehensive trauma-informed organizational change at an academic medical center in South Texas. *BMC Health Services Research*, *25*(1), 1433. Advance online publication. DOI: 10.1186/s12913-025-13381-6 PMID: 41185002

Seshadri, A., Fuller-Tyszkiewicz, M., Harper, L., Clark, M. M., Singh, B., Chesak, S., Kung, S., Bobo, W. V., & Wieneke, K. (2025). Randomized controlled trial of stress management and resiliency training for depression (SMART-D)—Pilot study. *PLoS One*, *20*(8), e0328539. Advance online publication. DOI: 10.1371/journal.pone.0328539 PMID: 40828809

Shin, R. Q., Smith, L. C., Welch, J. C., & Ezeofor, I. (2017). Is Allison more likely than Lakisha to receive a callback from counseling professionals? A racism audit study. *Journal of Counseling Psychology*, *64*(1), 41–52. DOI: 10.1037/cou0000179 PMID: 28068130

Siegel, D. J. (2012). *The developing mind: How relationships and the brain interact to shape who we are* (2nd ed.). Guilford Press.

Simon, R. W. (1995). Gender, multiple roles, role meaning, and mental health. *Journal of Health and Social Behavior*, *36*(2), 182–194. DOI: 10.2307/2137224 PMID: 9113142

Singh, R. P. (2025). Promoting Social and Economic Justice in Black Communities in the Current Anti-DEI Climate. *Societies (Basel, Switzerland)*, *15*(10), 280. DOI: 10.3390/soc15100280

Sinkler, M. A., Alejo, A., Agel, J., Hendrickson, S., Breslin, M. A., & Vallier, H. A. (2023). The development of a Trauma Resiliency Scale (tRS-18). *Journal of Orthopaedic Research*, *41*(9), 2040–2045. DOI: 10.1002/jor.25550 PMID: 36919222

Siotia, S. (2024, June 25). AP-LS Student Committee Preparing for the EPPP: Essential Tips and Tricks. [blog post]. American-Psychology Law Society. http://www.apls-students.org/the-intersection-a-blog/preparing-for-the-eppp-essential-tips-and-tricks

Smith, C. P., & Freyd, J. J. (2014). Institutional betrayal. *The American Psychologist*, *69*(6), 575–587. DOI: 10.1037/a0037564 PMID: 25197837

Smith, L. T. (2021). *Decolonizing Methodologies: Research and Indigenous Peoples* (3rd ed.). Zed Books., DOI: 10.5040/9781350225282

Sonu, S., Mann, K., Potter, J., Rush, P., & Stillerman, A. (2024). Toward integration of trauma, resilience, and equity theory and practice: A narrative review and call for consilience. *The Permanente Journal*, *28*(1), 151–168. DOI: 10.7812/TPP/23.105 PMID: 38206776

Sparks, G., Lopes, L., Montero, A., Presiado, M., & Hamel, L. (2026). *Americans' challenges with health care costs*. KFF. https://www.kff.org/health-costs/americans-challenges-with-health-care-costs/

Spivak, G. C. (1988). Can the subaltern speak? In C. Nelson & L. Grossberg (Eds.), *Marxism And the Interpretation of Culture* (pp. 271–313). Macmillan.

Stake, R. E. (2005). Qualitative case studies. In Denzin, N. K., & Lincoln, Y. S. (Eds.), *The Sage handbook of qualitative research* (3rd ed., pp. 443–466). Sage.

Stanton, M. C., Ali, S., McCormick, K. A., Stanley, M., Traylor, M., Johnson, V., & Scruggs, L. (2025). Implementation outcomes of trauma-informed organizational change among HIV service organizations in the Southern United States. *SSM. Mental Health, 8*, 100500. Advance online publication. DOI: 10.1016/j.ssmmh.2025.100500

Stepney, S. (2022). Multicultural and diversity perspectives in art therapy: Transforming image into substance. .DOI: 10.1016/B978-0-12-824308-4.00010-7

Stopforth, S., Kapadia, D., Nazroo, J., & Bécares, L. (2022). The enduring effects of racism on health: Understanding direct and indirect effects over time. *SSM - Population Health, 19*, 101217. DOI: 10.1016/j.ssmph.2022.101217 PMID: 36091297

Stout, M. (2005). *The sociopath next door*. Broadway Books.

Substance Abuse and Mental Health Services Administration. (2014). *SAMHSA's concept of trauma and guidance for a trauma-informed approach* (HHS Publication No. SMA 14-4884). https://ncsacw.acf.hhs.gov/userfiles/files/SAMHSA_Trauma.pdf

Substance Abuse and Mental Health Services Administration. (2014). *SAMHSA's concept of trauma and guidance for a trauma-informed approach* (HHS Publication No. SMA 14-4884). https://ncsacw.samhsa.gov/userfiles/files/SAMHSA_Trauma.pdf

Substance Abuse and Mental Health Services Administration. (2014). *SAMHSA's concept of trauma and guidance for a trauma-informed approach (HHS Publication No. SMA 14-4884).* U.S. Department of Health and Human Services.

Swidler, E. (2018). Invisible Exploitation: How Capital Extracts Value Beyond Wage Labor. *Monthly Review (New York. 1949), 69*(10), 29–36. https://doi.org/ DOI: 10.14452/MR-069-10-2018-03_2

Tebes, J. K., Champine, R. B., Matlin, S. L., & Strambler, M. J. (2019). Population Health and Trauma-Informed Practice: Implications for Programs, Systems, and Policies. *American Journal of Community Psychology, 64*(3–4), 494–508. DOI: 10.1002/ajcp.12382

Templeman, K., & Robinson, A. (2011). Integrative medicine models in contemporary primary health care. *Complementary Therapies in Medicine, 19*(2), 84–92. DOI: 10.1016/j.ctim.2011.02.003

Thoits, P. A. (1991). On merging identity theory and stress research. *Social Psychology Quarterly, 54*(2), 101–112. DOI: 10.2307/2786929

Tolstoy, A. (2023). Culture and Economic Justice in America. *Sustainability and Climate Change, 16*(1), 83–94. DOI: 10.1089/scc.2022.0066

Torshizi, S. S., Aboqader, R. F., Muhammadov, N., Khujaniyozova, O., Ruzmetova, Z., Hayitova, M., Shahreza, M. S., Girish, M. S., Dehkordi, F. S., & Vahed, S. (2026). Curcumin in redox and inflammatory signaling: Mechanistic insights into NF-κB and Nrf2 pathway regulation. *Journal of Chemical Health Risks*, *16*(1), 1–13. DOI: 10.60829/jchr.2025.1205763

Tran, S., Krauter, M., & Bogart, K. R. (2025). Ableism: The time has come to understand bias against people with disabilities. In Nelson, T. D. (Ed.), *Handbook of prejudice, stereotyping, and discrimination* (3rd ed., pp. 276–299). Routledge.

Treleaven, D. A. (2018). *Trauma-sensitive mindfulness: Practices for safe and transformative healing*. WW Norton & Company.

Tsomo, K. L. (2024). Being Black and Buddhist. *Religious Studies Review*, *50*(1), 12–15. DOI: 10.1111/rsr.17079

Umberson, D., Thomeer, M. B., & Lodge, A. C. (2006). Intimacy and emotion work in lesbian, gay, and heterosexual relationships. *Journal of Marriage and Family*, *77*(2), 542–556. DOI: 10.1111/jomf.12178 PMID: 25814771

Unjai, S., Forster, E. M., Mitchell, A. E., & Creedy, D. K. (2024). Interventions to promote resilience and passion for work in health settings: A mixed-methods systematic review. *International Journal of Nursing Studies Advances*, *7*, 100242. Advance online publication. DOI: 10.1016/j.ijnsa.2024.100242 PMID: 39380624

van der Kolk, B. A. (2014). *The body keeps the score: Brain, mind, and body in the healing of trauma*. Viking.

Varghese, L., & Emerson, A. (2022). Trauma-informed care in the primary care setting: An evolutionary analysis. *Journal of the American Association of Nurse Practitioners*, *34*(3), 465–473. DOI: 10.1097/JXX.0000000000000663

Vella, S. C., & Pai, N. B. (2019). A theoretical review of psychological resilience: Defining resilience and resilience research over the decades. *Archives of Medicine and Health Sciences*, *7*(2), 233–239. DOI: 10.4103/amhs.amhs_119_19

Verissimo, A. D., Henley, N., Gee, G. C., Davis, C., & Grella, C. (2021). Homelessness and discrimination among US adults: The role of intersectionality. *Journal of Social Distress and the Homeless*, *32*(1), 1–15. DOI: 10.1080/10530789.2021.1935650

Verlenden, J. V., Fodeman, A., Wilkins, N., Jones, S. E., Moore, S., Cornett, K., Sims, V., Saelee, R., & Brener, N. D. (2024). Mental health and suicide risk among high school students and protective factors—Youth Risk Behavior Survey, United States, 2023. *MMWR Supplements*, *73*(4), 73. DOI: 10.15585/mmwr.su7304a9 PMID: 39378246

Wang, Y., Ashokan, A., & Mitra, R. (2023). Physical exercise as a resilience factor in depression and anxiety: A systematic review and meta-analysis. *Neuroscience and Biobehavioral Reviews, 146*, 105071. Advance online publication. DOI: 10.1016/j.neubiorev.2023.105071

Ward, K. (2011). *Is religion dangerous?* Lion Books.

Watson, N. (2002). Well, I know this is going to sound very strange to you, but I don't see myself as a disabled person: Identity and disability. *Disability & Society, 17*(5), 509–527. DOI: 10.1080/09687590220148496

Watson-Singleton, N. N., Black, A. R., & Spivey, B. N. (2019). Recommendations for a culturally-responsive mindfulness-based intervention for African Americans. *Complementary Therapies in Clinical Practice, 34*, 132–138. DOI: 10.1016/j.ctcp.2018.11.013 PMID: 30712717

Weng, H. Y., Ikeda, M. P., Lewis-Peacock, J. A., Chao, M., Fullwiley, D., Goldman, V., Skinner, S., Duncan, L. G., Gazzaley, A., & Hecht, F. M. (2020). Toward a compassionate intersectional neuroscience: Increasing diversity and equity in contemplative neuroscience. *Frontiers in Psychology, 11*, 573594. Advance online publication. DOI: 10.3389/fpsyg.2020.573134

Wepener, C., & Müller, B. (2012). Water rituals as a source of (Christian) life in an African Independent Church: To be healed and (re)connected. *Studia Liturgica, 42*(1–2), 255–269. DOI: 10.1177/0039320712042001-216

Whittle, H. J., Leddy, A. M., Shieh, J., Tien, P. C., Ofotokun, I., Adimora, A. A., Turan, J. M., Frongillo, E. A., Turan, B., & Weiser, S. D. (2020). Precarity and health: Theorizing the intersection of multiple material-need insecurities, stigma, and illness among women in the United States. *Social science & medicine (1982), 245*, 112683. DOI: 10.1016/j.socscimed.2019.112683

Wilbur, R. C., Kuemmel, A., & Lackner, R. J. (2019). Who's on first? Supervising psychology trainees with disabilities and establishing accommodations. *Training and Education in Professional Psychology, 13*(2), 111–118. DOI: 10.1037/tep0000231

Williams, D. R., & Etkins, O. S. (2021). Racism and mental health. *World Psychiatry; Official Journal of the World Psychiatric Association (WPA), 20*(2), 194–195. DOI: 10.1002/wps.20845 PMID: 34002496

Williams, M. T. (2020). Psychology cannot afford to ignore the many harms caused by microaggressions. *Perspectives on Psychological Science, 15*(1), 38–43. DOI: 10.1177/1745691619893362 PMID: 31801042

Williams, M. T., Metzger, I. W., Leins, C., & DeLapp, C. (2021). Assessing racial trauma within a DSM-5 framework: The UConn Racial/Ethnic Stress & Trauma Survey. *Practice Innovations (Washington, D.C.)*, *3*(4), 242–260. DOI: 10.1037/pri0000076

Wilson, C., Pence, D. M., & Conradi, L. (2013). Trauma-Informed Care. In C. Wilson, D. M. Pence, & L. Conradi, *Encyclopedia of Social Work*. NASW Press and Oxford University Press. DOI: 10.1093/acrefore/9780199975839.013.1063

Wilson-Ching, M., & Berger, E. (2024). Relationship building strategies within trauma informed frameworks in educational settings: A systematic literature review. *Current Psychology (New Brunswick, N.J.)*, *43*(4), 3464–3485. DOI: 10.1007/s12144-023-04590-5

Wolbring, G., & Nasir, L. (2024). Intersectionality of disabled people through a Disability Studies, Ability-based studies, and intersectional pedagogy lens: A survey and a scoping review. *Societies (Basel, Switzerland)*, *14*(9), 176. DOI: 10.3390/soc14090176

World Health Organization. (2019). *International statistical classification of diseases and related health problems* (11th ed.). (ICD-11). https://icd.who.int/

Yatchmenoff, D. K., Sundborg, S. A., & Davis, M. A. (2017). Implementing trauma-informed care: Recommendations on the process. *Advances in Social Work*, *18*(1), 167–185. DOI: 10.18060/21311

Young, J., Edosomwan, K., & Young, J. (2024). Advanced Placement and Black High School Students: A Logistical Regression of College Persistence Factors. *Journal of Urban Learning, Teaching, and Research.*

Zaeske, L. M., Dye, A. R., Spadoni, S., Strothkamp, R., Kane, M. L., Ridgway, K., Dugan, A. J., Patterson, T. P., McEathron, S. R., & Cole, B. P. (2024). Addressing harm from adverse religious/ spiritual experiences in psychotherapy: A scoping review. *Practice Innovations (Washington, D.C.)*, *9*(1), 1–18. https://psycnet.apa.org/doi/10.1037/pri0000237. DOI: 10.1037/pri0000237

Zaki, J., & Williams, W. C. (2013). Interpersonal emotion regulation. *Emotion (Washington, D.C.)*, *13*(5), 803–810. DOI: 10.1037/a0033839 PMID: 24098929

Zembylas, T. (Ed.). (2014). *Artistic Practices* (0 ed.). Routledge., DOI: 10.4324/9781315863092

Zieff, G., Kerr, Z. Y., Moore, J. B., & Stoner, L. (2020). Universal Healthcare in the United States of America: A Healthy Debate. *Medicina (Kaunas, Lithuania)*, *56*(11), 580. DOI: 10.3390/medicina56110580 PMID: 33143030

Zur, O. (2007). *Boundaries in psychotherapy: Ethical and clinical explorations.* American Psychological Association. DOI: 10.1037/11563-000

About the Contributors

Sara Pickett is the Director of Counseling and Psychological Services (CaPS) at Spalding University and an adjunct instructor in the Counseling and Student Affairs Department at Western Kentucky University. A licensed professional counselor with more than a decade of clinical experience, Dr. Pickett has worked extensively in counselor education, clinical supervision, and mental health leadership. Prior to assuming the directorship at Spalding, she served as a full-time faculty member at Western Kentucky University and previously held a faculty appointment at Spalding University. Her professional interests include trauma-informed care, intersectionality, disaster mental health, counselor development, resilience, and social justice–oriented approaches to counseling and supervision. Dr. Pickett is an active scholar, presenter, and editor whose research explores topics such as internalized sexism, gendered experiences in counseling, trauma recovery, and mental health equity. She is the recipient of the Kentucky Counseling Association Outstanding Counselor Educator Award and has secured multiple competitive research and teaching grants in support of her scholarly work. In addition to leading CaPS and teaching graduate counseling students, Dr. Pickett maintains a private counseling practice, provides clinical supervision to counselors-in-training, and is committed to expanding access to evidence-based, culturally responsive mental health services for diverse communities.

***

Albrina Burger is a 3rd year doctoral student in the James Madison University's Counselor Education and Supervision program. Her research interests include advocacy for students of marginalized identities, anti-bias and anti-racist policies, and social justice attitudes in schools and school counseling programs. Albrina has 15 years of experience as a certified educator in Georgia, with 5 years of experience as a school counselor in middle and high schools. She is a National Certified School

Counselor and a Licensed Associate Professional Counselor in the State of Georgia. In her leisure time, Albrina spends time with her husband, Terence, and three children: Tristan (9), Torrian (6), and Teaghan (3).

Yuridia Carrete is a passionate educator with almost twenty years of experience providing students with comprehensive school counseling services and multi-tiered systems of support. Once an undocumented student in the state of California, she was brought to the United States at a very young age and faced adversity and racism in education. Her experience spans all levels and both private and public education. She also served on the state counseling association for almost ten years as the Southern California Area Representative. She has been successful in leading post-secondary courses at the university level and providing mentoring, professional development, and coaching to educators on counseling best practices. Dedicated to enhancing learning environments for diverse student populations through comprehensive counseling strategies that address equity and access barriers through the use of data. She was the 2016 California School Counselor of the Year for the California Association of School Counselors and was named one of the top five counselors of the year by the American School Counselors Association (ASCA) in 2017. She was named the Top Student Advisor by the mayor's office for the city of Riverside in 2018 and awarded the Champion for Justice Award in 2017 by the Fair Housing Council for her support of at-risk youth. She serves as a reviewer for the American School Counseling Association *ASCA) Recognized ASCA Model Program and serves on the College Board's Counselor Community Advisory Board.

Maritza Cha graduated from Garfield High School in East Los Angeles and became the first in her family to attend and graduate from college, the University of California, Los Angeles. She graduated in 2005 with two Bachelor's Degrees in Political Science and History, with a minor in Education. UCLA was so nice she went there twice, earning a Master's Degree in Education, as well as a teaching credential, from UCLA's Teacher Education Program in 2007. She taught social studies at her alma mater, Garfield High School for 4 years. In 2010, Mrs. Cha and several colleagues designed and launched a pilot school within Los Angeles Unified School District – Social Justice Leadership Academy at Esteban Torres High School. Mrs. Cha then decided to work towards her lifelong dream of becoming a college counselor. Mrs. Cha earned her second Master's Degree, a counseling credential and child welfare and attendance credential, from Cal State Dominguez Hills in 2015. Mrs. Cha currently works for Alhambra Unified School District as a school counselor and completed her PhD at Claremont Graduate University in Education/ Urban Leadership.

Mukhayya Djumaniyazova is working at Pedagogy and Psychology Department, Urganch State University, Uzbekistan.

Deepak Gupta is a distinguished academician with over 20 years of teaching experience and expertise in Computer Science and Engineering. He holds a Ph.D. in Computer Engineering and has an extensive research portfolio, including many international journal papers, multiple conference proceedings, and several books. His research interests span machine learning, artificial intelligence, and data mining. Currently, Dr. Gupta serves as an Associate Professor and Head of Department of CSE (Emerging Branches) at ITM Gwalior, MP, India. He has also contributed significantly to the field through patents and copyrights and actively engages as a reviewer, conference chair and editor.

Nasiba Jumaniyazova is a faculty member in the Department of Psychology at Mamun University, Khiva, Uzbekistan. She is engaged in teaching and academic activities related to psychological science, human behavior, and educational psychology. Her academic interests include cognitive and developmental psychology, student mental well-being, and the application of psychological principles in educational settings. She is committed to fostering students' analytical thinking, emotional intelligence, and academic growth through learner-centered instruction. Nasiba Jumaniyazova actively contributes to academic and institutional initiatives aimed at strengthening psychology education and promoting research-informed teaching practices in higher education.

Pardeep Kumar Assistant Professor, Department of Mathematics, Lovely Professional University, Phagwara, Punjab, India Dr. Pardeep Kumar holds a Ph.D. in Mathematics from Lovely Professional University (2021). His research expertise lies in Stochastic Processes, with a specialized focus on Markov Models, Engineering System Reliability, and Reliability Theory. He actively contributes to the modeling and reliability analysis of IoT-enabled and sensor-integrated systems for next-generation engineering applications. Dr. Kumar has a profound command of Stochastic Modelling, Reliability Testing, and advanced analytical methods for complex system behavior under uncertainty. His work emphasises practical implementations in smart technologies and cyber-physical systems. He has an exceptional academic track record, having qualified the prestigious CSIR-UGC NET twice, securing All India Ranks (AIR) of 15 and 32, respectively. To date, Dr. Kumar has published 26 high-quality research papers in reputed national and international journals, reflecting his continued contribution to the advancement of mathematical reliability and its engineering applications.

Sanjeev Kumar Is a Professor in Lovely Professional University Punjab India. He received Undergraduate in Hotel Management from Osmania University, Postgraduate in Tourism Management from Madurai Kamaraj University. He completed Doctor of Philosophy in Hospitality Management in 2019 from Amity University Jaipur India. His research areas lies in food Service Industry, his research focuses on Alcoholic beverages, Event management and Sustainable Management Practices, Metaverse, AI Machine Learning and Artificial Intelligence. He published more than 80 research papers, articles and chapters in Scopus Indexed, UGC Approved and peer reviewed Journals and books. Dr. Sanjeev Kumar participated and acted as resource person in various National and International conferences, seminars, session chair, research workshops and industry talks and his work has been widely cited. Dr. Sanjeev also edited more than 20 books with various International Publishers such as IGI Global, Cambridge Scholars, Emerald, CABI, Bentham Science, Taylor & Francis. Dr Sanjeev is an active researcher and has published numerous research articles in prestigious National and International journals and books.

Eva Yifan Li is an MSW student at the University of Pittsburgh School of Social Work. Her academic and practice interests include trauma-informed social work, attachment, emotional identity, relational systems, occupational stress, and community-based mental health support. Her current work explores the Dual-Track Emotional System as a conceptual framework for understanding emotional selfhood, long-term relational functioning, and extradyadic emotional attachment.

Yolanda Loften Sims, M.Ed., RMHCI, is a doctoral candidate in the Counselor Education and Supervision program at National Louis University, a Registered Mental Health Counseling Intern in Florida, and a devoted school counselor serving diverse adolescent populations. Her professional identity is deeply rooted in multicultural counseling, social justice advocacy, and strength-based clinical practice, with a particular commitment to supporting older adults, adolescents, and women of color. Guided by an ethic of intentionality, cultural humility, and human dignity, Yolanda's work bridges research, teaching, supervision, and clinical practice to expand equitable access to mental health care for marginalized and underrepresented communities. As a military spouse, she brings lived insight into the unique challenges faced by service members, veterans, and their families, enriching her advocacy for women of color navigating military and post-military identities. Yolanda's scholarship centers on Positive Aging, resilience, culturally responsive practice, and the intersectional experiences of marginalized groups across the lifespan. Her research and clinical commitments emphasize empowering older adults through strength-based counseling, promoting visibility and voice among women of color in military spaces, and fostering emotional wellness and identity development in adolescents. Grounded in Multicultural and Social Justice Counseling Competencies–informed and internationally aligned ethical frameworks, her work promotes belonging, purpose, and holistic well-being at every stage of life.

Wednesdae Reim Ifrach is an art therapist and counselor whose work focuses on gender-affirming care, LGBTQ+ issues, trauma-informed care, body image, and eating disorders. They are full-time faculty members in the School of Behavioral and Community Health at Moravian University and co-own and operate Rainbow Recovery, which provides clinical supervision, consultations, training, workshops, clinical counseling, and art therapy to clients across Connecticut and Pennsylvania. They serve on the GLMA board as the Health Professionals in Training Co-Chair, they are also a board member with Prism Counseling and Advocacy as the Secretary and the chair of the Fundraising Committee. Their past art therapy-based work includes participating in the Monument Quilt, which is housed at the Baltimore Museum of Art, as well as being a guest creator for the Museum of Modern Art's Artful Practices of Well-being Program. They have presented workshops and trainings nationally and internationally, include at the Expressive Art Therapy Summit, American Art Therapy Association, GLMA, the CT State Department of Mental Health and Addiction Services, MEDA, Project HEAL, the National Alliance for Eating Disorders, the International Association for Eating Disorder Professionals, Yale University's Summer Spiral program, Smith College, PA NASW, Fenway Health Collective, Drexel University, and the Longmore Institute of Disabilities with SFSU. Their book, Queer Expressions: Expressive Art and Somatic Therapy Practices for Healing Body Trauma, is scheduled for release by North Atlantic Books in June 2026, and they have a forthcoming poetry chapbook, Skeletons, Sequin, and Kin through Finishing Line Press and Hex & Flesh: 35 Incantations of Queer Becoming through Rebel Satori. Their book, Queer Expressions: Expressive Art and Somatic Therapy Practices for Healing Body Trauma, was released in June 2026 by North Atlantic Books and covers how expressive arts and somatics can help heal trauma and body-related issues in the Queer community. Outside of their academic work, they are an artist and poet with two poetry chapbooks out now, Skeletons, Sequin, and Kin through Finishing Line Press, and Hex & Flesh: 35 Incantations of Queer Becoming through Rebel Satori.

Sarah Stewart-Spencer is a clinical provider specializing in trauma and an accomplished leader in higher education and counseling. Dr. Stewart-Spencer is a Licensed Professional Counselor, a Licensed Mental Health Counselor, and Nationally Certified Counselor. She is also certified as a First Responder Provider, Hypnotherapist and a Clinical Trauma Professional. Dr. Stewart-Spencer is the founder of the Integrated Wellness Institute and Stewart-Spencer Consulting, where she trains clinical professionals, educates the public on wellbeing, and provides clinical services to high trauma-exposure populations. She serves as an educator at The Chicago School, University of West Alabama, and is a course developer for the International Trauma Training Institute. Formerly Dean of Behavioral Sciences at Yorkville University, she helped shape Canada's largest online counseling graduate programs. Her books include Mastering Resilience: Strategies for High-Demand Professionals, Metaphors in Therapy, and Metaphors in Counselor Education and Supervision. She is the creator of First Responder Treatment Provider certification, which established a national standard for helping professionals providing services to first responders. With a career spanning emergency services, mental health community agencies, private practice, and academic leadership, Dr. Stewart-Spencer brings a uniquely integrative, trauma-informed lens to every space she serves.

Samantha Swift, MA, LPC, NCC, is a PhD candidate in Counselor Education and Supervision at National Louis University. She is a licensed professional counselor whose clinical and scholarly interests include trauma-informed systems, grief and relational loss, spirituality in counseling, and women's mental health. Her work focuses on bridging research and practice to support trauma-responsive clinical care and organizational change.

Index

A

B

C

D

E

F

G

H

I

L

M

N

O

P

R

S

T

V

W

www.ingramcontent.com/pod-product-compliance
Lightning Source LLC
LaVergne TN
LVHW080903300926
849162LV00003B/531